Oral Inflammations and Systemic Diseases

Oral Inflammations and Systemic Diseases

Special Issue Editors
Udo Seedorf
Ghazal Aarabi

MDPI • Basel • Beijing • Wuhan • Barcelona • Belgrade

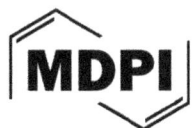

Special Issue Editors
Udo Seedorf
Universitatsklinikum
Hamburg-Eppendorf und
Medizinische Fakultät
Germany

Ghazal Aarabi
Universitatsklinikum
Hamburg-Eppendorf und
Medizinische Fakultät
Germany

Editorial Office
MDPI
St. Alban-Anlage 66
4052 Basel, Switzerland

This is a reprint of articles from the Special Issue published online in the open access journal *International Journal of Molecular Sciences* (ISSN 1422-0067) in 2019 (available at: https://www.mdpi.com/journal/ijms/special_issues/oral_ijms).

For citation purposes, cite each article independently as indicated on the article page online and as indicated below:

LastName, A.A.; LastName, B.B.; LastName, C.C. Article Title. *Journal Name* **Year**, *Article Number*, Page Range.

ISBN 978-3-03936-288-2 (Hbk)
ISBN 978-3-03936-289-9 (PDF)

© 2020 by the authors. Articles in this book are Open Access and distributed under the Creative Commons Attribution (CC BY) license, which allows users to download, copy and build upon published articles, as long as the author and publisher are properly credited, which ensures maximum dissemination and a wider impact of our publications.

The book as a whole is distributed by MDPI under the terms and conditions of the Creative Commons license CC BY-NC-ND.

Contents

About the Special Issue Editors vii

Preface to "Oral Inflammations and Systemic Diseases" ix

Hessam Tabeian, Beatriz F. Betti, Cinthya dos Santos Cirqueira, Teun J. de Vries,
Frank Lobbezoo, Anouk V. ter Linde, Behrouz Zandieh-Doulabi, Marije I. Koenders,
Vincent Everts and Astrid D. Bakker
IL-1β Damages Fibrocartilage and Upregulates MMP-13 Expression in Fibrochondrocytes in
the Condyle of the Temporomandibular Joint
Reprinted from: *Int. J. Mol. Sci.* **2019**, *20*, 2260, doi:10.3390/ijms20092260 1

Dorina Lauritano, Alberta Lucchese, Dario Di Stasio, Fedora Della Vella, Francesca Cura,
Annalisa Palmieri and Francesco Carinci
Molecular Aspects of Drug-Induced Gingival Overgrowth: An In Vitro Study on Amlodipine
and Gingival Fibroblasts
Reprinted from: *Int. J. Mol. Sci.* **2019**, *20*, 2047, doi:10.3390/ijms20082047 16

Hiromichi Yumoto, Katsuhiko Hirota, Kouji Hirao, Masami Ninomiya, Keiji Murakami,
Hideki Fujii and Yoichiro Miyake
The Pathogenic Factors from Oral Streptococci for Systemic Diseases
Reprinted from: *Int. J. Mol. Sci.* **2019**, *20*, 4571, doi:10.3390/ijms20184571 24

C.M. Figueredo, R. Lira-Junior and R.M. Love
T and B Cells in Periodontal Disease: New Functions in A Complex Scenario
Reprinted from: *Int. J. Mol. Sci.* **2019**, *20*, 3949, doi:10.3390/ijms20163949 42

Siddharth Garde, Rahena Akhter, Mai Anh Nguyen, Clara K. Chow and Joerg Eberhard
Periodontal Therapy for Improving Lipid Profiles in Patients with Type 2 Diabetes Mellitus:
A Systematic Review and Meta-Analysis
Reprinted from: *Int. J. Mol. Sci.* **2019**, *20*, 3826, doi:10.3390/ijms20153826 55

Yasuyoshi Miyata, Yoko Obata, Yasushi Mochizuki, Mineaki Kitamura, Kensuke Mitsunari,
Tomohiro Matsuo, Kojiro Ohba, Hiroshi Mukae, Tomoya Nishino, Atsutoshi Yoshimura and
Hideki Sakai
Periodontal Disease in Patients Receiving Dialysis
Reprinted from: *Int. J. Mol. Sci.* **2019**, *20*, 3805, doi:10.3390/ijms20153805 68

Sadayuki Hashioka, Ken Inoue, Tsuyoshi Miyaoka, Maiko Hayashida, Rei Wake,
Arata Oh-Nishi and Masatoshi Inagaki
The Possible Causal Link of Periodontitis to Neuropsychiatric Disorders: More Than
Psychosocial Mechanisms
Reprinted from: *Int. J. Mol. Sci.* **2019**, *20*, 3723, doi:10.3390/ijms20153723 89

Mineaki Kitamura, Yasushi Mochizuki, Yasuyoshi Miyata, Yoko Obata, Kensuke Mitsunari,
Tomohiro Matsuo, Kojiro Ohba, Hiroshi Mukae, Atsutoshi Yoshimura, Tomoya Nishino and
Hideki Sakai
Pathological Characteristics of Periodontal Disease in Patients with Chronic Kidney Disease
and Kidney Transplantation
Reprinted from: *Int. J. Mol. Sci.* **2019**, *20*, 3413, doi:10.3390/ijms20143413 101

Kübra Bunte and Thomas Beikler
Th17 Cells and the IL-23/IL-17 Axis in the Pathogenesis of Periodontitis and Immune-Mediated Inflammatory Diseases
Reprinted from: *Int. J. Mol. Sci.* **2019**, *20*, 3394, doi:10.3390/ijms20143394 . . . . **120**

Mark Kaschwich, Christian-Alexander Behrendt, Guido Heydecke, Andreas Bayer, Eike Sebastian Debus, Udo Seedorf and Ghazal Aarabi
The Association of Periodontitis and Peripheral Arterial Occlusive Disease—A Systematic Review
Reprinted from: *Int. J. Mol. Sci.* **2019**, *20*, 2936, doi:10.3390/ijms20122936 . . . . **144**

About the Special Issue Editors

Udo Seedorf born in Hamburg, Germany, is a Professor for the Department of Prosthetic Dentistry at the University Medical Center Hamburg-Eppendorf, Germany. He received his diploma in Molecular Biology in 1981 and his Ph.D. in 1984 from the University of Constance, Germany. He completed his post-doctoral fellowship in Molecular Cardiology at the Children's Hospital, Harvard Medical School, Boston, USA, in 1987. Subsequently, he served as Senior Scientist at the Institute of Arteriosclerosis Research at the University of Munster, Germany until 2004, as a Professor of Biochemistry and Molecular Biology at the University Medical Center Hamburg-Eppendorf from 2004 to 2006, and as Head of the Department of Epidemiology and Lipid Metabolism at the Leibniz-Institute of Arteriosclerosis Research from 2006 to 2013. In 2014 he joined the Department of Prosthetic Dentistry to conduct research on the impact of chronic oral infections on systemic diseases.

Ghazal Aarabi born in Tehran, Iran, is a Senior Physician and research group leader at the Department of Prosthetic Dentistry of the University Medical Center Hamburg-Eppendorf, Germany. She studied dentistry at the University of Freiburg, Germany, and completed her final examination in dental medicine in 2010. Subsequently, she became a dentist and scientific associate at the Department of Prosthetic Dentistry of the University Medical Center Hamburg-Eppendorf. She received her DDS (Dr. med. dent.) from the University of Freiburg in 2012 and was appointed Qualified Advanced Trained Specialist of Prosthodontics by the German Society of Prosthodontics and Biomaterials (DGPro). She received her MSc in Prosthodontics from the University of Greifswald, Germany in 2015, and in 2019 she was appointed Senior Physician at the Department of Prosthetic Dentistry of the University Medical Center Hamburg-Eppendorf. She is a member of the board of the Center for Health Care Research of the University Hospital Hamburg-Eppendorf, a member of the Expert Group for Dental Health and the Expert Group for Infectiology of the NAKO Health Study, as well as deputy spokeswoman for the Working Group for Dental Public Health of the German Society for Social Medicine and Prevention.

Preface to "Oral Inflammations and Systemic Diseases"

Oral infections occur frequently in humans and often lead to chronic inflammations affecting the teeth (i.e., as caries), the gingival tissues surrounding the teeth (i.e., as gingivitis and endodontic lesions), and the tooth-supporting structures (i.e., as periodontitis). It has been proposed that these inflammations are not restricted to specific sites in the oral cavity and may have a negative impact on the general health of the affected patients by increasing their risk of several widespread diseases, such as diabetes, coronary heart disease, peripheral arterial disease, ischemic stroke, and small vessel disease in the brain. At least four basic pathogenic mechanisms involving oral inflammation in the pathogenesis of widespread diseases have been proposed: (1) low level bacteremia by which oral bacteria enter the blood stream and invade the body; (2) systemic inflammation induced by inflammatory mediators released from the sites of the oral inflammation into the blood stream; (3) autoimmunity to host proteins caused by the host immune response to specific components of oral pathogens; and (4) pathogenic effects resulting from specific bacterial toxins produced by oral pathogenic bacteria.

This Special Issue focuses on several aspects of the interaction between oral infections and widespread systemic diseases. We collected contributions in the form of reviews and original papers written by highly reputed experts in this field.

Udo Seedorf, Ghazal Aarabi
Special Issue Editors

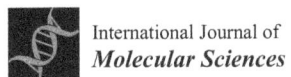

Article

IL-1β Damages Fibrocartilage and Upregulates MMP-13 Expression in Fibrochondrocytes in the Condyle of the Temporomandibular Joint

Hessam Tabeian [1,†], Beatriz F. Betti [1,2,3,†], Cinthya dos Santos Cirqueira [4], Teun J. de Vries [5], Frank Lobbezoo [2], Anouk V. ter Linde [1], Behrouz Zandieh-Doulabi [1], Marije I. Koenders [6], Vincent Everts [1] and Astrid D. Bakker [1,*]

[1] Oral Cell Biology, Academic Centre for Dentistry Amsterdam, University of Amsterdam and Vrije Universiteit Amsterdam, 1081 LA Amsterdam, The Netherlands; h.tabeian@acta.nl (H.T.); b.f.betti@acta.nl (B.F.B.); anouk.terlinde@student.auc.nl (A.V.t.L.); b.zandiehdoulabi@acta.nl (B.Z.-D.); v.everts@acta.nl (V.E.)
[2] Oral Kinesiology, Academic Centre for Dentistry Amsterdam, University of Amsterdam and Vrije Universiteit Amsterdam, 1081 LA Amsterdam, The Netherlands; f.lobbezoo@acta.nl
[3] Orthodontics, Academic Centre for Dentistry Amsterdam, University of Amsterdam and Vrije Universiteit Amsterdam, 1081 LA Amsterdam, The Netherlands
[4] Núcleo de Anatomia Patológica, Instituto Adolfo Lutz, São Paulo 01246-000, Brazil; cinthyaquiron@gmail.com
[5] Periodontology, Academic Centre for Dentistry Amsterdam, University of Amsterdam and Vrije Universiteit Amsterdam, 1081 LA Amsterdam, The Netherlands; teun.devries@acta.nl
[6] Rheumatology, Radboud University Medical Center, 6525 GA Nijmegen, The Netherlands; marije.koenders@radboudumc.nl
* Correspondence: a.bakker@acta.nl; Tel.: +31-(0)20-5980224
† These authors contributed equally to this work.

Received: 14 April 2019; Accepted: 1 May 2019; Published: 7 May 2019

Abstract: The temporomandibular joint (TMJ), which differs anatomically and biochemically from hyaline cartilage-covered joints, is an under-recognized joint in arthritic disease, even though TMJ damage can have deleterious effects on physical appearance, pain and function. Here, we analyzed the effect of IL-1β, a cytokine highly expressed in arthritic joints, on TMJ fibrocartilage-derived cells, and we investigated the modulatory effect of mechanical loading on IL-1β-induced expression of catabolic enzymes. TMJ cartilage degradation was analyzed in 8–11-week-old mice deficient for IL-1 receptor antagonist (IL-1RA$^{-/-}$) and wild-type controls. Cells were isolated from the juvenile porcine condyle, fossa, and disc, grown in agarose gels, and subjected to IL-1β (0.1–10 ng/mL) for 6 or 24 h. Expression of catabolic enzymes (ADAMTS and MMPs) was quantified by RT-qPCR and immunohistochemistry. Porcine condylar cells were stimulated with IL-1β for 12 h with IL-1β, followed by 8 h of 6% dynamic mechanical (tensile) strain, and gene expression of MMPs was quantified. Early signs of condylar cartilage damage were apparent in IL-1RA$^{-/-}$ mice. In porcine cells, IL-1β strongly increased expression of the aggrecanases ADAMTS4 and ADAMTS5 by fibrochondrocytes from the fossa (13-fold and 7-fold) and enhanced the number of MMP-13 protein-expressing condylar cells (8-fold). Mechanical loading significantly lowered (3-fold) IL-1β-induced MMP-13 gene expression by condylar fibrochondrocytes. IL-1β induces TMJ condylar cartilage damage, possibly by enhancing MMP-13 production. Mechanical loading reduces IL-1β-induced MMP-13 gene expression, suggesting that mechanical stimuli may prevent cartilage damage of the TMJ in arthritic patients.

Keywords: ADAMTS4; ADAMTS5; fossa; cartilage degradation; arthritis; mechanical loading; MMP-13; IL1β; temporomandibular joint; juvenile idiopathic arthritis

1. Introduction

The temporomandibular joint (TMJ) is a unique joint, consisting of a fossa, disc, and condyle that is essential for mastication, speech, and deglutition [1]. The major difference between the TMJ and other synovial joints is that the TMJ contains fibrocartilage rather than hyaline cartilage, i.e., it contains collagen type I in addition to collagen type II and proteoglycans [2]. More precisely, the matrix of all three anatomical structures of the TMJ contained collagen type I. The condyle and the fossa stained positive for collagen type II and proteoglycans, but the condyle contained considerably more collagen type II and proteoglycans than the fossa. The disc did not contain collagen type II, and the disc did not stain positive for proteoglycans [2]. The TMJ is an under-recognized joint in arthritic disease, while it is one of the most commonly affected joints in patients with juvenile idiopathic arthritis (JIA) [3]. It has been suggested that at the time of diagnosis, approximately 75% of JIA patients have problems with the TMJ [3]. JIA, the most prevalent type of arthritis of unknown cause in young children, is initiated before the age of 16 years old and is characterized by chronic inflammation of the joints, which can result in joint degradation. Affected children suffer from jaw pain but also jaw dysfunction, which can manifest in malocclusion [4] and a reduced maximum mouth opening [5]. How the cartilage of the TMJ is affected by inflammation in JIA and in other arthritic diseases with involvement of the TMJ remains elusive.

One of the most potent inflammatory factors involved in hyaline cartilage degradation in many forms of arthritis is interleukin (IL)-1β [6]. This cytokine is responsible for hyaline cartilage matrix degradation by inducing expression of matrix metalloproteinases (MMPs) and disintegrin and metalloproteinase with thrombospondin motifs (ADAMTS) by chondrocytes [7,8]. The importance of IL-1β in the pathogenesis of systemic arthritic diseases is demonstrated by the success of treatment with IL-1 receptor antagonist (IL-1RA) [9]. However, it is unknown whether IL-1β also affects the integrity of the cartilaginous structures of the TMJ.

Since the TMJ is a secondary growth center, damage induced by catabolic factors during JIA can introduce growth abnormalities, resulting in asymmetric growth of the mandible [10] undersized jaw, and abnormal positioning of the maxilla [11]. Therefore, strategies to prevent TMJ joint damage, particularly in JIA patients, are highly desirable. Preferably, a non-invasive treatment should be deployed that inhibits the catabolic effect of inflammatory factors on TMJ cartilage. Mechanical loading of inflamed joints can be a promising approach towards achieving this. Moderate exercise has been shown to have a systematic anti-inflammatory effect by reducing the disease activity in rheumatoid arthritis (RA) patients [12]. Furthermore, mechanical loading reduced the expression of MMP-13 in synovial cells from RA patients [13]. However, it is not known whether mechanical loading will also reduce IL-1β-induced expression of catabolic factors in cells derived from the TMJ condyle, which is especially susceptible to damage in JIA [14].

We hypothesize that IL-1β plays an important role in inducing degradation of the TMJ cartilage, that it enhances expression of catabolic factors such as MMPs and ADAMTSs, and that mechanical stimuli can revert IL-1β-induced expression of catabolic factors. We have used different model systems to investigate this hypothesis. First of all, an IL1RA knock-out mouse model was used to investigate whether overactive IL-1β signaling induces histological signs of damage in the fibrocartilage tissue of the temporomandibular joint. The second and third part of the hypothesis was challenged using pig TMJ-derived cells. Pigs were chosen to isolate cells because they will yield more cells than mice and because the TMJ of this species is comparable with that of humans in cellular composition [15–19].

2. Results

2.1. IL-1βRA$^{-/-}$ Mice Showed Early Signs of Condylar Cartilage Damage

To investigate the role of IL-1β in TMJ damage, we assessed whether young mice that lack IL1-RA develop arthritis in the TMJ. Discs were barely visible in sections of mouse TMJ. Because of the similar histological appearance of fossa and disc tissue in both wild-type (WT) and IL-1RA$^{-/-}$ mice, only the condyles were quantified. Safranin O staining was more intense in IL-1RA$^{-/-}$ condyles compared to WT condyles (Figure 1A,B). In addition, the most superficial layer of the cartilage in IL-1RA$^{-/-}$ condyles was positive for Safranin O staining (Figure 1B), which was not the case in WT mice (Figure 1A). The IL-1RA$^{-/-}$ TMJ samples had a significantly higher Mankin score compared to the joints of the WT mice ($p < 0.01$) (Figure 1C). The IL-1RA$^{-/-}$ condyles contained 11-fold more empty lacunae than the WT mice ($p < 0.001$) (Figure 1D).

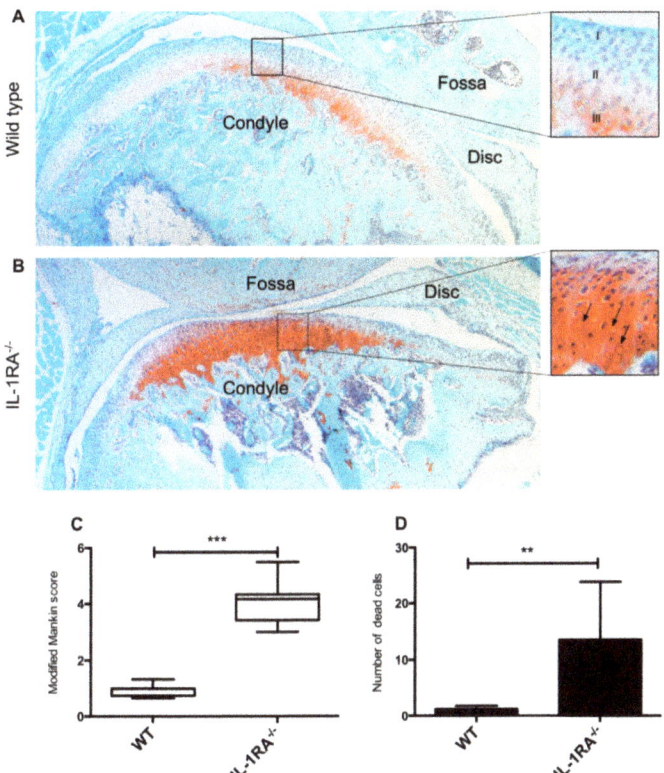

Figure 1. Histologic assessment of the temporomandibular joint (TMJ) of IL-1 receptor antagonist (IL-1RA$^{-/-}$) and wild-type (WT) mice. Sagittal section of the condyles of IL-1RA$^{-/-}$ and WT mice stained with Safranin O. (**A**) WT TMJ, original magnification 10×. The condyle cartilage can be divided into the fibrous, proliferative, and hypertrophic zones, indicated in the figure as I, II, III, respectively. In the WT sample the modest red staining is limited to zone III. (**B**) The IL-1R$^{-/-}$ mice condyle showed a higher level of Safranin O staining in comparison to WT. In the IL-1R$^{-/-}$ mice, Safranin O staining was not limited to the hypertrophic and the proliferative zone of the condyle but extended to the fibrous layer. Empty lacunae were frequently seen (arrows). (**C**) The Mankin score of the IL-1RA$^{-/-}$ mice was higher than the WT. (**D**) The number of empty lacunae in the condyles of the IL-1RA$^{-/-}$ mice was higher than in the WT. ** Significant difference between IL-1RA$^{-/-}$ and WT mice, $p < 0.01$; *** significant difference between IL-1R$^{-/-}$ and WT mice, $p < 0.001$, a t-test is used.

2.2. Cells from the Fossa, Disc, and Condyle Expressed IL-1 Receptors

The ability of the cells isolated from porcine fossa, disc, and condyle cartilaginous structures to react to IL-1β was assessed by measuring gene expression of receptors for IL-1β. All cells from the three types of TMJ cartilage displayed similar gene expression levels for IL-1RI as well as of the mock receptor of IL-1β, IL-1RII (Figure 2A,B). The ratio of IL-1RI to IL-1RII gives a rough indication of the effectiveness of IL-1β to elicit downstream signaling. The three cartilaginous structures displayed similar IL-1RI/IL-1RII ratios (Figure 2C). Expression of IL-1RA and IL-1β was in most cases undetectable, and therefore no statistical analysis could be performed.

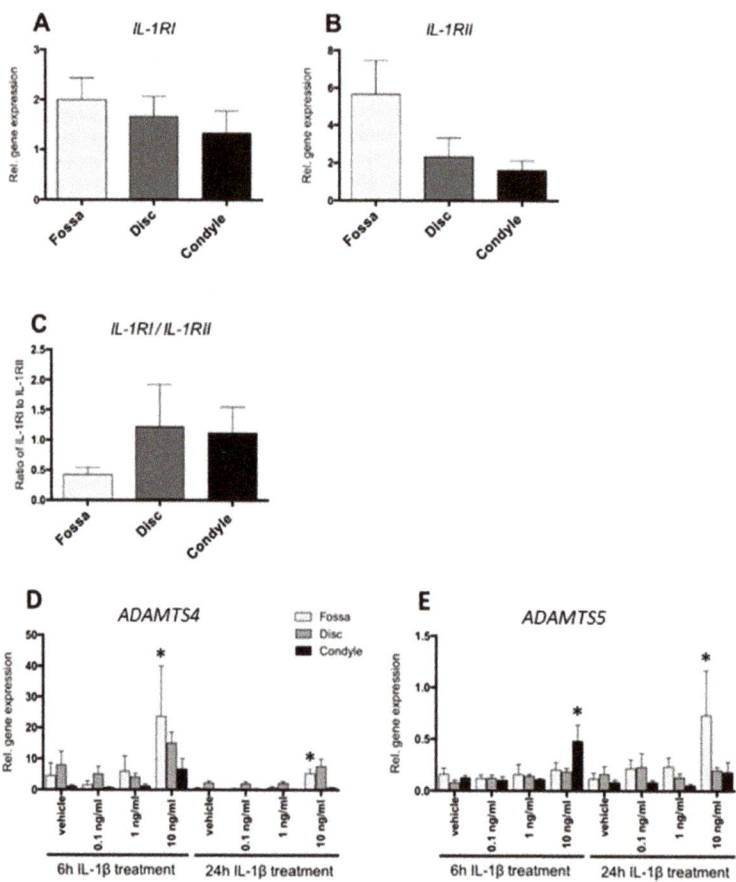

Figure 2. Relative gene expression of IL-1 receptor (IL-1R)I, IL-1RII, disintegrin and metalloproteinase with thrombospondin motifs (ADAMTS)4 and ADAMTS5 by porcine fossa, condyle and disc cells. (**A**) IL-1RI and (**B**) IL-1RII expression of the cells from fossa, disc, and condyle. All cells expressed IL-1RI and RII gene at similar levels. (**C**) The ratio between *IL-1RI* and *IL-1RII*. The ratio IL-1RI/IL-1RII was comparable for all cells. (**D**) *ADAMTS4* expression in the cells from the fossa, disc, and condyle. IL-1β incubation for 6 h enhanced ADAMTS4 expression in condyle cells. After 24 h of incubation with 10 ng/mL IL-1β, both fossa and discs showed an increase in ADAMTS4 expression in comparison to the vehicle-treated cells. (**E**) *ADAMTS5* expression in the cells from the fossa, disc, and condyle. Six hours of 10 ng/ml IL-1β treatment enhanced ADAMTS5 gene expression in condyle cells. After 24 h of 10 ng/mL IL-1β, the fossa cells showed an increased *ADAMTS5* expression. * Significant effect of treatment with IL-1β relative to vehicle, $p < 0.05$.

2.3. IL-1β Increased ADAMTS4 and ADAMTS5 Gene Expression

IL-1β at 10 ng/mL enhanced ADAMTS4 gene expression by 5-fold after 6 h in cells from the fossa ($p < 0.01$) (Figure 2D). After 24 h incubation, fossa cells showed a 13-fold increased expression of ADAMTS4 in response to 10 ng/mL IL1β ($p < 0.01$) (Figure 2D).

Six hours of IL-1β stimulation (10 ng/mL) also enhanced ADAMTS5 by 4-fold, but only in condylar cells ($p < 0.01$) (Figure 2E). After 24 h incubation with 10 ng/mL IL-1β, only fossa cells demonstrated enhanced ADAMTS5 gene expression (7-fold) in comparison to vehicle-treated cells ($p < 0.017$) (Figure 2E).

2.4. MMP-2 Activity Was Higher in Condyle Than Disc and Fossa Cells; MMP9 mRNA Upregulated in Condyle by IL-1β

Six hours of IL-1β treatment did not affect MMP-9 gene expression in any of the TMJ-derived cell types (Figure 3B). After 24 h of stimulation with 10 ng/mL IL-1β, there was a 3-fold increase of MMP-9 gene expression by condyle cells ($p < 0.01$, Figure 3B). MMP-9 enzyme activity was undetectable by zymographic analysis of the conditioned medium of fossa, disc, and condyle cells, regardless of the IL-1β treatment (Figure 3C), suggesting that the mRNA for MMP-9 was not sufficiently converted into active protein. Though not statistically significant at the mRNA level (Figure 3A), MMP-2 enzyme activity appeared higher in condyle cells than in the disc and fossa (Figure 3C). IL-1β did not visibly affect the level of MMP-2 activity in any of the cells (Figure 3C).

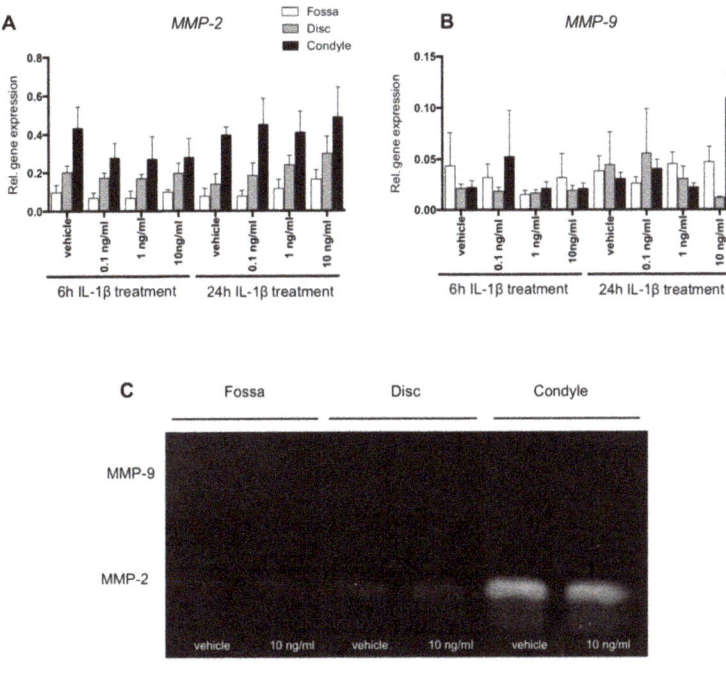

Figure 3. Matrix metalloproteinase (MMP)-2 and MMP-9 gene expression and activity. (**A**) IL-1β did not affect *MMP-2* expression by the cells from the fossa, disc, and condyle at any time point tested. (**B**) After 24 h of 10 ng/mL IL-1β incubation, the *MMP-9* gene expression of the disc and condyle cells were higher than that of the vehicle-treated samples. (**C**) Zymogram of the conditioned medium from fossa, disc, and condyle cells after 24 h of incubation with IL-1β. There was no MMP-9 activity detected. The condyle showed strong MMP-2 activity, but no effect of IL-1β was apparent. * Significant effect of treatment with IL-1β, relative to vehicle, $p < 0.05$. Results are shown from one out of three identical experimental replicates.

2.5. IL-1β Induced MMP-13 Expression by Condylar Cells Only

After 6 and 24 h of 10 ng/mL IL-1β stimulation, MMP-13 gene expression by cells of the condyle was up-regulated by 3.4- and 9-fold, respectively ($p < 0.001$ and $p < 0.0001$, respectively) (Figure 4A). MMP-13 gene expression was almost undetectable in the cells from the disc and fossa and remained low after IL-1β incubation (Figure 4A).

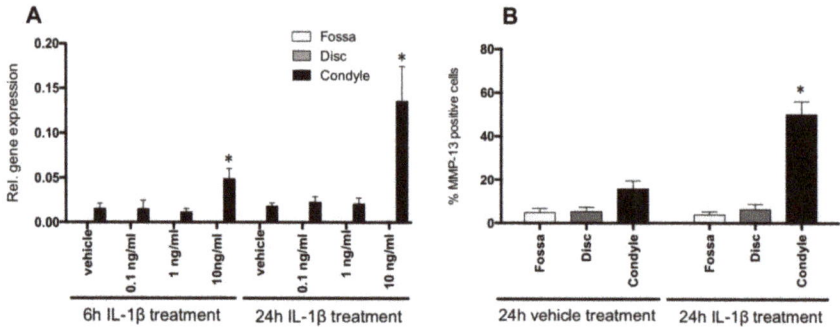

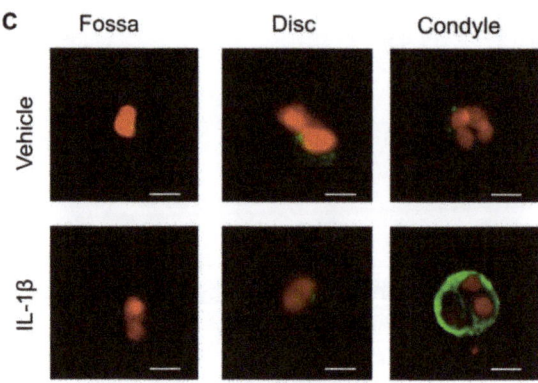

Figure 4. MMP-13 gene and protein expression. (**A**) MMP-13 gene expression by the cells from the fossa, disc, and condyle. IL-1β for 6 h and 24 h at 10 ng/mL increased MMP-13 expression in condyle cells in comparison to vehicle. (**B**) Number of MMP-13-positive cells. Condylar cells incubated with 10 ng/mL IL-1β for 24 h showed the highest number of MMP-13-positive cells. (**C**) Image of MMP-13-positive cells after 24 h of 10 ng/mL IL-1β treatment. The green label indicates the presence of MMP-13, and the nuclei are red. * Significant effect of treatment with IL-1β relative to vehicle treatment, $p < 0.05$. Scale bar represents 5 μm.

Next, we analyzed the number of cells expressing MMP-13 by immunostaining. Twenty-four hours of 10 ng/mL IL-1β incubation increased the percentage of MMP-13-positive condylar cells (3.5-fold increase, $p < 0.001$) (Figure 4B). The number of MMP-13-positive cells derived from the condyle compared to the fossa and disc was remarkably higher (Figure 4C).

2.6. Cyclic Tensile Strain Reduced IL-1β-Induced MMP-13 Expression

Six percent cyclic tensile strain (CTS) reduced IL-1β-induced MMP-13 gene expression by 3-fold ($p < 0.05$) (Figure 5B). CTS neither affected expression of MMP-2, IL-12RI, IL-1RII nor the ratio of IL-1RI and IL-1RII in control condylar cells or in those incubated with IL-1β (Figure 5A,C,D).

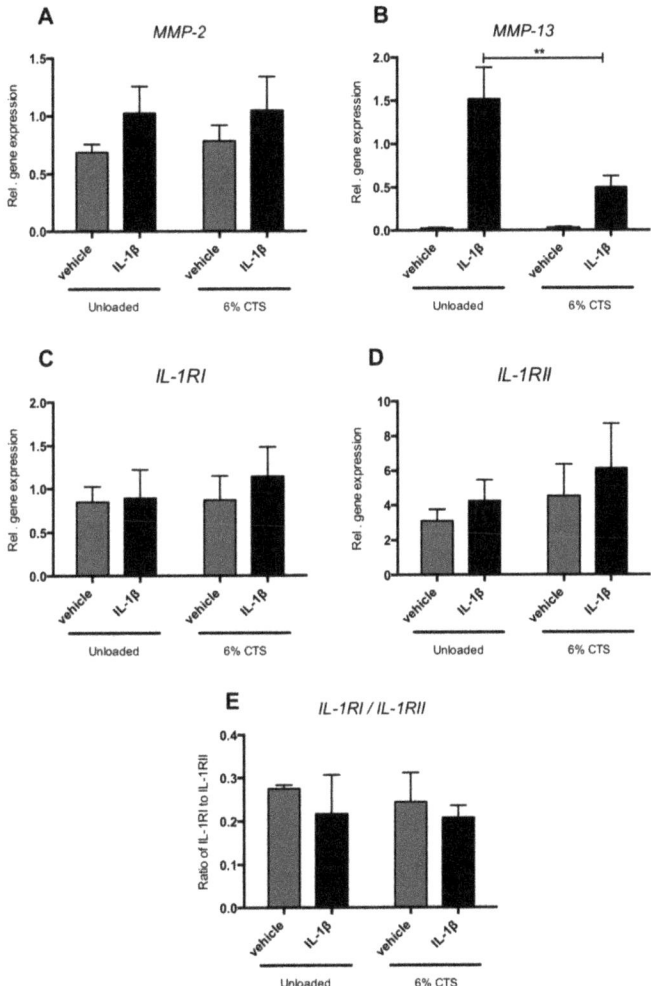

Figure 5. Mechanical strain reduces MMP-13 expression of condylar cells incubated with IL1-β. Gene expression of (**A**) MMP-13, (**B**) MMP-2, (**C**) IL1-RI, and (**D**) IL1-RII. (**E**) Ratio between IL-1RI and IL-1RII by condylar cells. Mechanical loading reduced IL-1β-induced gene expression of MMP-13. ** Significant effect of mechanical loading, $p < 0.01$.

3. Discussion

The TMJ is frequently affected in patients with chronic inflammation, which can result in permanent damage to the joint, especially in young patients. Since biological sampling of the TMJ of children for research purposes is unethical, the role of specific inflammatory factors in the degradation of the TMJ of young individuals remains elusive. In the present study, we made use of relatively young mice and juvenile porcine TMJs to investigate the effect of the inflammatory cytokine IL-1β on its three cartilaginous structures. Our findings strongly suggest that excess IL-1β induces degradation of TMJ cartilage. Young mice deficient for IL-1RA showed early histological signs of TMJ degradation, an effect preferentially found in the condyle. In culture, porcine cells isolated from the three cartilaginous structures expressed different catabolic enzymes in response to IL-1β, e.g., IL-1β at 10 ng/mL induced the expression of ADAMTS4 and ADAMTS5 by cells from the fossa, while cells isolated from the condyle responded to IL-1β with an increased expression of MMP-9, and MMP-13. Mechanical loading reduced MMP-13 expression in IL-1β-treated condylar fibrochondrocytes.

Horai et al. previously demonstrated that IL-RA$^{-/-}$ mice developed spontaneous arthritis due to unopposed excess of IL-1 signaling. In this systemic arthritis model, between 5–20% of the front paws developed arthritis, which depended on, for instance, the microbiological status of the animal facility [20]. We used these mice to investigate whether an excess of IL-1 signaling could result in TMJ damage. We did indeed find some remarkable changes in the condyle. A high level of staining for proteoglycans was seen around the condyles and also in the fibrous areas of the condyle. This area normally does not contain proteoglycans. Condyles of the IL-RA$^{-/-}$ mice showed, overall, more clustering of cells, more intense proteoglycan staining, and higher Mankin score in comparison to WT mice. Over-production of proteoglycans and cluster formation of chondrocytes may represent signs of local repair of articular cartilage, an indication of the onset of the cartilage degradation process. Proteoglycans are unlike collagen in a continuous turnover [20], therefore overshoot in matrix synthesis might occur more easily with proteoglycans. Other studies have also found an increased level of proteoglycans in the early phases of condyle cartilage degradation [21–23]. In these studies, at later stages, a gradual loss of proteoglycans occurred together with cleaving of collagen fibrils. This pattern of degeneration implies that there may be a common chain of molecular events underlying degeneration [21]. Further studies in older IL-1RA$^{-/-}$ mice should indicate whether these mice will undergo loss of proteoglycans together with cleaving of the collagen fibrils in their TMJ by, for instance, MMP-13, which was upregulated in the porcine model. Taken together, our results with IL-1RA$^{-/-}$ mice suggest that overactive IL-1β signaling induces damage in the fibrocartilage tissue of the condyle of the TMJ.

We assumed initially that the fossa and disc cells would not express the genes of the receptors related to IL-1β signaling, since these cartilage parts seemed to be unaffected in the inflamed joint of JIA patients [14]. However, we found that the cells from the fossa and disc expressed mRNA for these receptors, and cells from the fossa responded to IL-1β with an enhanced expression of ADAMTS4 and ADAMTS5. This shows that the receptors are present and functional in the fossa and disc, even though these structures are damaged to a lesser extent than the condyle in JIA patients. Increased ADAMTS5 expression in response to IL-1β in combination with lack of tissue damage was also observed in articular cartilage from knees of Sox9 knockout animals [24]. In addition, very limited numbers of proteoglycans are present in the fossa and disc. Therefore, with ADAMTS4 and ADAMTS5 being the catalytic enzymes that degrade proteoglycans, damage by these aggrecanases would be limited in comparison to the condyle.

Condylar cells responded to IL-1β by increasing the expression of the catabolic enzymes ADAMTS5, MMP-9 and MMP-13. These cells also expressed constitutively active MMP-2. These enzymes are able to cleave the matrix proteins of the condylar cartilage. The aggrecanases ADSMTS5, MMP-13 and MMP-2 are capable of cleaving proteoglycans [25,26], and both MMP-13 and MMP-2 are able to unwind and cleave collagen fibrils [27]. The resulting fragments will form an excellent substrate for the gelatinase MMP-2. This enzyme is also able to cleave the pro-MMP-13, thereby activating this collagenase [28]. We found that IL-1β enhanced MMP-13 expression in cells isolated from the porcine condyle. The isolated cells constitute a mix of more fibroblast-like cells from the upper layer of the condyle and chondrocyte-like cells from the deeper layers. It is possible that only one of these subtypes of cells responds to IL-1β with increased MMP-13 expression. We found in a limited set of histological slides that MMP-13 protein was mostly expressed by chondrocyte-like cells of the deeper layers of mouse condyles (data not shown). It is thus possible that the response to IL-1β was most pronounced in the chondrocyte-like cells within our mix of isolated condyle cells. The importance of MMP-13 in cartilage degradation in arthritis was demonstrated in transgenic mice overexpressing MMP-13 [29] and elevated levels of MMP-13 were found in synovial fluid of arthritic patients [30]. Therefore, MMP-13 can be considered as one of the prime suspects in the degradation of condylar cartilage in JIA. Taken together, we found that IL-1β enhances the expression of catabolic enzymes by TMJ-derived cells, thereby possibly explaining cartilage damage as observed after overactive IL-1 signaling.

One limitation of this study is that we cannot be certain that histological changes indicative of degeneration in the condylar fibrocartilage of the TMJ of IL-1R$^{-/-}$ mice can be attributed to MMP-13 over-expression. Studies using IL-1R$^{-/-}$ mice treated with MMP-13 inhibitors could provide clarity, but such experiments were beyond the scope of the current study. In addition, our in vitro studies showing the effect of IL-1β on MMP-13 expression in condyle-derived fibrochondrocytes were performed with cells from pig TMJs but not mice, and species differences can occur. We have performed immunohistochemistry for MMP-13 on sections of mouse TMJs, but the resulting quality prevented accurate quantitative assessment, though roughly 60% of the condylar cells seemed positive in wildtype animals and nearly 100% in IL-RA knock-out mice (data not shown), which indicates that the effects of overactive IL-1β with regards to MMP-13 expression is similar between pig and mouse. Another limitation is the selection of only one mechanical loading regime of tensile forces, whereas compressive forces are also occurring in the moving jaw.

Since MMP-13 plays an important role in many biological processes, including growth and development [31], inhibition of activity of this enzyme could have severe, undesirable side-effects in the children with JIA that are still growing. This important role of MMP-13 in many biological processes [31] requires a *direct* inhibition. Pharmaceutical intervention should therefore be based on tempering IL-1β's destructive effects [32,33]. A potential non-invasive, non-pharmaceutical approach to inhibit inflammation-induced MMP-13 expression is exercise or physical therapy of inflamed joints. We found that 6% cyclic tensile strain exerted on the condylar cells significantly reduced the IL-1β-induced MMP-13 gene expression, similar to our previous finding that tensile strain exerted on condylar cells significantly reduced TNFα-induced MMP-13 gene expression [34]. These findings are in line with several other studies, in which the anti-catabolic capacity of cyclic strain was analyzed [34–36]. In our study, the cells maintained their pericellular matrix when they were embedded in an agarose gel, thereby allowing proper transmission of mechanical forces to the cells. The condylar cartilage undergoes considerable tensile forces due to compression and shear [37]. For this reason, we used 6% cyclic tensile strain. This percentage was calculated by using the following literature data. Deschner et al. used 20% of strain to stimulate rat disc cells [35], but Chain et al. calculated that the maximal tensile strain that the condyle cartilage would experience would be 3.7-fold lower than the disc [38]. Further in vivo studies are needed to assess whether 6% tensile strain is effective in downregulating catabolic enzymes induced by inflammation.

In conclusion, overactive IL-1 signaling can induce changes in condyle cartilage metabolism indicative of degeneration, and cells from the three cartilaginous structures of the TMJ react to exposure to the inflammatory cytokine IL-1β, whereby the condyle seems particularly sensitive in terms of catabolic enzyme expression. This might explain why only the condyle is disproportionately degraded in children with JIA. MMP-13 induced by IL-1β might be a prime suspect in causing degradation of the condyle in JIA patients, and mechanical loading could inhibit expression. Future studies should confirm whether a direct link exists between JIA, IL-1β and MMP-13 over-expression, and whether controlled exercise can reduce MMP-13 expression in the condyle of the TMJ in vivo. These are important future steps with high clinical relevance because controlled physical exercise could provide a therapeutic intervention in children with JIA, potentially preventing serious effects of TMJ inflammation such as pain, dysfunction, and even malformations. Non-invasive studies, for instance using MRI, could be useful to monitor the effect of motion on the progression of JIA.

4. Materials and Methods

4.1. Mice

IL-1RA-deficient (IL-1RA$^{-/-}$) mice on a BALB/c background were kindly supplied by Martin Nicklin (Sheffield, UK). Wild-type control mice were 8–10 weeks old and were purchased from Charles River (Sulzfeld, Germany). Before the age of 12 weeks, mice were sacrificed, heads were dissected and fixed in 4% formaldehyde for 6–12 weeks. Ethical permission was obtained in July 2013 at the Radboud University Nijmegen, RU-DEC 2013-096.

4.2. Histological Analysis of Murine TMJ

Mouse heads (four mice per strain) were decalcified for 6 days in 10% formic acid and 10% sodium citrate solution. The heads were then dehydrated, embedded in paraffin, and 5 μm-thick sagittal sections were cut. Safranin O-fast green and hematoxylin and eosin staining were performed. Mouse TMJ cartilage was evaluated by a blinded observer based on pericellular staining, chondrocyte arrangement, and structural appearance of the articular cartilage, using a modified Mankin score [21] (Table 1).

Table 1. Modified Mankin score.

1) Pericellular Safranin O staining	
a. Normal	0
b. Slightly enhanced	1
c. Intensely enhanced	2
2) Background Safranin O staining	
a. Normal	0
b. Slight decrease/increase	1
c. Severe decrease/increase	2
d. No staining	3
3) Arrangement of Chondrocytes	
a. Normal	0
b. Appearance of clustering	1
b. Hypocellularity	2
4) Cartilage Structure	
a. Normal	0
b. Fibrillation in superficial layer	1
c. Fibrillation beyond superficial layer	2
d. Missing articular cartilages	3

4.3. Cell Isolation and Culture

Because mouse TMJs only contain few cells, all in vitro studies were performed with cells isolated from pig TMJs. Heads of Dutch Landrace pigs (*Sus scrofa*), with a body weight in the range of 70–80 kg and aged 6–8 months old, were obtained from a local abattoir (Westford, Gorinchem, The Netherlands). Approval by the Animal Ethics Committee of the VU University was not required as the animals were not sacrificed for the purpose of the experiment. Within 4 h after sacrifice, the entire articular cartilage of the fossa and condyle and the whole disc were dissected. The cells were isolated as previously described [39,40]. The medium containing the cells was mixed 1:1 with 6% ultrapure low melting point agarose (Invitrogen, Carlsbad, CA, USA) to a final concentration of 1×10^6 cells/mL, 3% agarose, 1× DMEM supplemented with 50 μg/mL ascorbic acid (Merck, Darmstadt, Germany), 10% fetal bovine serum (FBS) (Thermo Fisher Scientific, Waltham, MA, USA), and 1% penicillin/streptomycin/fungizone (Invitrogen). The non-solidified gel was poured in a 2 mL syringe with a diameter of 8 mm of which the needle end was cut off, leaving a cylinder with an open needle-end. After gelation, the cell-gel construct was gently pressed out using the plunger and was cut into slices with a 2 mm thickness and transferred into a 24-wells plate. The 3D constructs were cultured for 6 days (Table 2) using a previously described protocol that is suitable for culturing chondrocytes [41]. On day 6, the cells were incubated with vehicle (PBS) or with 0.1, 1, or 10 ng/mL (7) recombinant porcine IL-1β (R&D Systems, Minneapolis, MN, USA) for 6 or 24 h.

Table 2. Timetable of progressive substitution of serum for ITS in the cell-agarose construct.

	Fetal Bovine Serum (%)	ITS (%)	Ascorbic Acid (µg mL^{-1})	PSF (%)
Day 0	10	-	50	2
Day 1	5	-	50	2
Day 2	1	1	50	1
Day 4	-	1	50	1
Day 6	-	1	50	1

For mechanical loading experiments, the cell-gel solution was poured on the silicone membrane of a Flexcell tissue train plate (Dunn Labortechnik, Asbach, Germany) on which two Velcro strips were glued. The Velcro strips ensured that the agarose cell-gel constructs would stick to the membrane of the tissue train plate. The rectangular shape of the cell-gel construct was confined by a 3D-printed mold to match the standard dimensions of gels on a tissue train plate. The cell-gel constructs were cultured as described in Table 2 for 6 days before performing tensile strain experiments. In the cyclic tensile strain experiments, the cells were incubated first for 12 h with IL-1β (10 ng/mL, R&D Systems), followed by 6% of sinusoidal mechanical strain at 0.5 Hz for 8 h, which was applied using the Flexcell system. Cells were post-incubated without strain for 24 h with IL-1β.

4.4. RNA Extraction and Real-Time Quantitative PCR

After 6 and 24 h of incubation with IL-1β, the cell-gel constructs were snap-frozen, and the RNA was extracted according to the protocol developed by Bougault and co-workers [41], cDNA was made using SuperScript® VILO™ cDNA Synthesis Kit according to the manufacturer's instructions (Life Technologies, Carlsbad, CA, USA). Real-time PCR reactions were performed according to the manufacturer's instructions in a LightCycler480® (Roche Diagnostics, Switzerland). The sequences of the primer pairs are presented in Table 3.

Table 3. Primers used for real-time PCR.

Genes	Primers	Primer Sequences [a]
YWHAZ (reference gene)	Forward:	GATGAAGCCATTGCTGAAACTTG
	Reverse:	CTATTTGTGGGACAGCATGGA
HPRT (reference gene)	Forward:	GCTGACCTGCTGGATTACAT
	Reverse:	CTTGCGACCTTGACCATCT
IL-1RI	Forward:	CATGACTGCCCATTGTTGAG
	Reverse:	AGGGCAGAAGCCTAGGAAG
IL-1RII	Forward:	GTGCCTGTTGAGCCTCATT
	Reverse:	GGCCTTCATGGGCAAATGTCA
ADAMTS4	Forward:	CATCCTACGCCGGAAGAGTC
	Reverse:	GGATCACTAGCCGAGTCACCA
ADAMTS5	Forward:	GTGGAGGAGGAGTCAGTTTG
	Reverse:	TTCAGTGCCATCGGTCACCTT
MMP-2	Forward:	CCGTGGTGAGATCTTCTTCTTC
	Reverse:	GCGGTCAGTGGCTGGGGTA

Table 3. *Cont.*

Genes	Primers	Primer Sequences [a]
MMP-9	Forward:	ACAGGCAGCTGGCAGAGGA
	Reverse:	GCCGGCAAGTCTTCCGAGTA
MMP-13	Forward:	GGAGCATGGCGACTTCTAC
	Reverse:	GAGTGCTCCAGGGTCCTT

[a] Only primers with equal efficacy were used.

4.5. Zymography

MMP-2 and MMP-9 activities in the conditioned medium of IL-1β-treaded cells (10 ng/mL for 24 h) were analyzed by zymography. The medium was lyophilized and concentrated three times. Novex® 10% Zymogram (Gelatin) Protein Gels, 1.0 mm, 15-wells (Life Technologies) were used for electrophoresis. After 1.5 h of electrophoresis, the gel was incubated for 30 min at room temperature in renaturing buffer (Life Technologies) with gentle agitation. The buffer was replaced with developing buffer (Life Technologies) for 30 min at room temperature and subsequently replaced for fresh buffer. After overnight incubation, the gels were washed with demi water and stained for 1 h with SimplyBlue SafeStain (Life Technologies). MMP-2 and MMP-9 activity was displayed as unstained bands.

4.6. Immunohistochemistry

Cell-gel constructs were fixed with formaldehyde and incubated for 2 h at room temperature with blocking buffer. Immunolocalization of MMP-13 was performed by using rabbit polyclonal anti-human MMP-13 (1:1000) (ab84594; Abcam, Cambridge, MA, USA) overnight at 4 °C. The secondary antibody alexa-555 goat anti-rabbit (1:2000 dilution) (A31630; Invitrogen) was incubated for 2 h at room temperature. Negative control staining was performed with Dako rabbit negative control (Dako, Glostrup, Denmark). Nuclei were stained with 4′,6-diamidino-2-phenylindole (DAPI).

Six µm optical sections were made of the gels with an Axio ZoomV16 microscope (Zeiss, Munich, Germany). The micrographs were then superimposed, and the number of positive cells was counted. With this technique, we were able to scan through 200 µm gel and count the MMP-13-positive cells in these areas.

4.7. Statistical Analysis

Prism (GraphPad Software Inc., San Diego, CA, USA) was used for statistical analyses. Mean values and standard errors of the mean (SEM) were calculated and depicted in the figures throughout the manuscript. Differences in pericellular staining of extracellular matrix (proteoglycans), chondrocyte arrangement, and structural appearance of the articular cartilage between four wild-type and four IL-1RA$^{-/-}$ mice were tested using the Mann–Whitney U test ($n = 4$). For each parameter measured, the null hypothesis was that cartilage damage-related changes scored equally in TMJs from WT and IL-1RA$^{-/-}$ mice. Experiments with pig cells were performed at three separate occasions. Data obtained at one separate occasion were considered $n = 1$ (thus, total $n = 3$). At each separate occasion, a *new* cell pool (derived from three pig heads) per anatomical region was created. Cell pools derived from the condyle, fossa, and disc were kept separate, and all were treated with or without IL-1β. To determine whether IL-1β (0.1, 1, or 10 ng/mL) significantly affected gene expression of ADAMTS4, ADAMTS5, MMP-2, MMP-9 and MMP-13, as well as protein expression for MMP-13, and activity of MMP-2 and MMP-9, compared to vehicle, in TMJ-derived cell populations, Dunnett's multiple comparison test was performed. Bonferoni correction was applied, as three tests were performed per parameter (one for fossa, one for disc and one for condyle) at the 6 h and at the 24 h time point, separately. At a $p < 0.017$, the null hypothesis, i.e., IL-1β (at either 0.1, 1, or 10 ng/mL) did not affect gene or protein expression of the catabolic factor of interest in pig TMJ cells, was rejected. To test the effect of mechanical strain on

IL-1β-induced gene expression by pig condylar fibrochondrocytes, one-way ANOVA was performed. Differences were regarded significant at values of $p < 0.05$.

Author Contributions: H.T. performed most of the practical work, and supervised A.V.t.L. B.F.B. was involved in experiments concerning mechanical loading, B.Z.-D. was involved in the protein analysis and zymography, C.d.S.C. performed immunohistochemistry. M.I.K. contributed on the IL1-RA$^{-/-}$ part, T.J.d.V. and A.D.B. were the daily PhD supervisors of H.T., F.L. and V.E. the formal PhD supervisors. All work was discussed on a weekly basis between H.T., T.J.d.V., A.D.B., F.L. and V.E. H.T. initiated writing, all authors have contributed to the writing of the submitted version.

Funding: This research was funded by research institute MOVE.

Acknowledgments: We thank Jolanda Hogervorst for her assistance with the qPCR; Rebecca Rogier and Debbie Roeleveld for collecting the mouse heads; Regina Maria Catarino for help with MMP-13 immunostaining; and Ben Nelemans and Manual Schmitz for their assistance with the Axio-zoom.

Conflicts of Interest: The authors declare no conflict of interest. Hessam Tabeian received funding from the MOVE Research Institute Amsterdam, Amsterdam, The Netherlands. The funding source had no other role in this study.

References

1. Mercuri, L.G. Temporomandibular joint reconstruction. *Alpha Omegan* **2009**, *102*, 51–54. [CrossRef] [PubMed]
2. Tabeian, H.; Bakker, A.D.; De Vries, T.J.; Zandieh-Doulabi, B.; Lobbezoo, F.; Everts, V. Juvenile porcine temporomandibular joint: Three different cartilaginous structures? *Arch. Oral Biol.* **2016**, *72*, 211–218. [CrossRef]
3. Weiss, P.F.; Arabshahi, B.; Johnson, A.; Bilaniuk, L.T.; Zarnow, D.; Cahill, A.M.; Feudtner, C.; Cron, R.Q. High prevalence of temporomandibular joint arthritis at disease onset in children with juvenile idiopathic arthritis, as detected by magnetic resonance imaging but not by ultrasound. *Arthritis Rheum.* **2008**, *58*, 1189–1196.
4. Hu, Y.; Billiau, A.D.; Verdonck, A.; Wouters, C.; Carels, C. Variation in dentofacial morphology and occlusion in juvenile idiopathic arthritis subjects: A case-control study. *Eur. J. Orthod.* **2009**, *31*, 51–58. [CrossRef] [PubMed]
5. Ringold, S.; Torgerson, T.R.; Egbert, M.A.; Wallace, C.A. Intraarticular corticosteroid injections of the temporomandibular joint in juvenile idiopathic arthritis. *J. Rheumatol.* **2008**, *35*, 1157–1164.
6. McInnes, I.B.; Schett, G. Cytokines in the pathogenesis of rheumatoid arthritis. *Nat. Rev. Immunol.* **2007**, *7*, 429–442. [CrossRef]
7. Ge, X.; Ma, X.; Meng, J.; Zhang, C.; Ma, K.; Zhou, C. Role of Wnt-5A in interleukin-1β-induced matrix metalloproteinase expression in rabbit temporomandibular joint condylar chondrocytes. *Arthritis Rheum.* **2009**, *60*, 2714–2722.
8. Su, S.-C.; Tanimoto, K.; Tanne, Y.; Kunimatsu, R.; Hirose, N.; Mitsuyoshi, T.; Okamoto, Y.; Tanne, K. Celecoxib exerts protective effects on extracellular matrix metabolism of mandibular condylar chondrocytes under excessive mechanical stress. *Osteoarthr. Cartil.* **2014**, *22*, 845–851. [CrossRef]
9. Pascual, V.; Allantaz, F.; Arce, E.; Punaro, M.; Banchereau, J. Role of interleukin-1 (IL-1) in the pathogenesis of systemic onset juvenile idiopathic arthritis and clinical response to IL-1 blockade. *J. Exp. Med.* **2005**, *201*, 1479–1486. [CrossRef] [PubMed]
10. Kjellberg, H. Craniofacial growth in juvenile chronic arthritis. *Acta Odontol. Scand.* **1998**, *56*, 360–365. [CrossRef] [PubMed]
11. Twilt, M.; Schulten, A.J.; Nicolaas, P.; Dulger, A.; van Suijlekom-Smit, L.W. Facioskeletal changes in children with juvenile idiopathic arthritis. *Ann. Rheum. Dis.* **2006**, *65*, 823–825. [CrossRef] [PubMed]
12. Sun, H.B. Mechanical loading, cartilage degradation, and arthritis. *Ann. N. Y. Acad. Sci.* **2010**, *1211*, 37–50. [CrossRef]
13. Tani-Ishii, N.; Tsunoda, A.; Teranaka, T.; Umemoto, T. Autocrine regulation of osteoclast formation and bone resorption by IL-1 alpha and TNF alpha. *J. Dent.* **1999**, *78*, 1617–1623.
14. Svensson, B.; Larsson, A.; Adell, R. The mandibular condyle in juvenile chronic arthritis patients with mandibular hypoplasia: A clinical and histological study. *Int. J. Oral Surg.* **2001**, *30*, 300–305. [CrossRef]
15. Herring, S.W. The dynamics of mastication in pigs. *Arch. Oral Biol.* **1976**, *21*, 473–480. [CrossRef]

16. Bermejo, A.; González, O.; Gonzalez, J. The pig as an animal model for experimentation on the temporomandibular articular complex. *Oral Surg. Oral Med. Oral Pathol.* **1993**, *75*, 18–23. [CrossRef]
17. Wang, L.; Detamore, M.S. Effects of growth factors and glucosamine on porcine mandibular condylar cartilage cells and hyaline cartilage cells for tissue engineering applications. *Arch. Oral Biol.* **2009**, *54*, 1–5. [CrossRef] [PubMed]
18. Springer, I.N.; Fleiner, B.; Jepsen, S.; Acil, Y. Culture of cells gained from temporomandibular joint cartilage on non-absorbable scaffolds. *Biomaterials* **2001**, *22*, 2569–2577. [CrossRef]
19. Vapniarsky, N.; Aryaei, A.; Arzi, B.; Hatcher, D.C.; Hu, J.C.; Athanasiou, K.A. The Yucatan Minipig Temporomandibular Joint Disc Structure–Function Relationships Support Its Suitability for Human Comparative Studies. *Tissue Eng. Part. C Methods* **2017**, *23*, 700–709. [CrossRef] [PubMed]
20. Horai, R.; Tanioka, H.; Nakae, S.; Okahara, A.; Ikuse, T.; Iwakura, Y.; Saijo, S.; Sudo, K.; Asano, M. Development of Chronic Inflammatory Arthropathy Resembling Rheumatoid Arthritis in Interleukin 1 Receptor Antagonist-Deficient Mice. *J. Exp. Med.* **2000**, *191*, 313–320. [CrossRef]
21. Xu, L.; Polur, I.; Lim, C.; Servais, J.M.; Dobeck, J.; Li, Y.; Olsen, B.R. Early-onset osteoarthritis of mouse temporomandibular joint induced by partial discectomy. *Osteoarthr. Cartil.* **2009**, *17*, 917–922. [CrossRef]
22. Hu, K.; Xu, L.; Cao, L.; Flahiff, C.M.; Brussiau, J.; Ho, K.; Setton, L.A.; Youn, I.; Guilak, F.; Olsen, B.R.; et al. Pathogenesis of osteoarthritis-like changes in the joints of mice deficient in type IX collagen. *Arthritis Rheum.* **2006**, *54*, 2891–2900.
23. Lam, N.P.; Li, Y.; Waldman, A.B.; Brussiau, J.; Lee, P.L.; Olsen, B.R.; Xu, L. Age-dependent increase of discoidin domain receptor 2 and matrix metalloproteinase 13 expression in temporomandibular joint cartilage of type IX and type XI collagen-deficient mice. *Arch. Oral Biol.* **2007**, *52*, 579–584. [CrossRef] [PubMed]
24. Henry, S.P.; Liang, S.; Akdemir, K.C.; De Crombrugghe, B. The Postnatal Role of Sox9 in Cartilage. *J. Bone* **2012**, *27*, 2511–2525. [CrossRef]
25. Fosang, A.J.; Last, K.; Neame, P.J.; Murphy, G.; Knäuper, V.; Tschesche, H.; Hughes, C.E.; Caterson, B.; Hardingham, T.E. Neutrophil collagenase (MMP-8) cleaves at the aggrecanase site E373–A374 in the interglobular domain of cartilage aggrecan. *Biochem. J.* **1994**, *304*, 347–351. [CrossRef] [PubMed]
26. Takaishi, H.; Kimura, T.; Dalal, S.; Okada, Y.; D'Armiento, J. Joint Diseases and Matrix Metalloproteinases: A Role for MMP-13. *Pharm. Biotechnol.* **2008**, *9*, 47–54. [CrossRef]
27. Aimes, R.T.; Quigley, J.P. Matrix metalloproteinase-2 is an interstitial collagenase. Inhibitor-free enzyme catalyzes the cleavage of collagen fibrils and soluble native type I collagen generating the specific 3/4- and 1/4-length fragments. *J. Biol. Chem.* **1995**, *270*, 5872–5876. [CrossRef]
28. Mort, J.S.; Billington, C. Articular cartilage and changes in arthritis: Matrix degradation. *Arthritis Res.* **2001**, *3*, 337–341. [CrossRef]
29. Neuhold, L.A.; Killar, L.; Zhao, W.; Sung, M.-L.A.; Warner, L.; Kulik, J.; Turner, J.; Wu, W.; Billinghurst, C.; Meijers, T.; et al. Postnatal expression in hyaline cartilage of constitutively active human collagenase-3 (MMP-13) induces osteoarthritis in mice. *J. Clin. Investig.* **2001**, *107*, 35–44. [CrossRef]
30. Yoshihara, Y.; Nakamura, H.; Obata, K.; Yamada, H.; Hayakawa, T.; Fujikawa, K.; Okada, Y. Matrix metalloproteinases and tissue inhibitors of metalloproteinases in synovial fluids from patients with rheumatoid arthritis or osteoarthritis. *Ann. Rheum. Dis.* **2000**, *59*, 455–461. [CrossRef]
31. Inada, M.; Wang, Y.; Byrne, M.H.; Rahman, M.U.; Miyaura, C.; López-Otín, C.; Krane, S.M. Critical roles for collagenase-3 (Mmp13) in development of growth plate cartilage and in endochondral ossification. *Proc. Natl. Acad. Sci. USA* **2004**, *101*, 17192–17197. [CrossRef]
32. Cheleschi, S.; Pascarelli, N.A.; Valacchi, G.; Di Capua, A.; Biava, M.; Belmonte, G.; Giordani, A.; Sticozzi, C.; Anzini, M.; Fioravanti, A. Chondroprotective effect of three different classes of anti-inflammatory agents on human osteoarthritic chondrocytes exposed to IL-1β. *Int. Immunopharmacol.* **2015**, *28*, 794–801. [CrossRef]
33. Bai, X.; Guo, A.; Li, Y. Protective effects of calcitonin on IL-1 stimulated chondrocytes by regulating MMPs/TIMP-1 ratio via suppression of p50-NF-κB pathway. *Biosci. Biotechnol. Biochem.* **2019**, *83*, 598–604. [CrossRef]
34. Tabeian, H.; Bakker, A.D.; Betti, B.F.; Lobbezoo, F.; Everts, V.; de Vries, T.J. Cyclic Tensile Strain Reduces TNF-alpha Induced Expression of MMP-13 by Condylar Temporomandibular Joint Cells. *J. Cell. Physiol.* **2017**, *232*, 1287–1294. [CrossRef]
35. Deschner, J.; Rath-Deschner, B.; Agarwal, S. Regulation of matrix metalloproteinase expression by dynamic tensile strain in rat fibrochondrocytes. *Osteoarthr. Cartil.* **2006**, *14*, 264–272. [CrossRef]

36. Agarwal, S.; Long, P.; Gassner, R.; Piesco, N.P.; Buckley, M.J. Cyclic tensile strain suppresses catabolic effects of interleukin-1β in fibrochondrocytes from the temporomandibular joint. *Arthritis. Rheum.* **2001**, *44*, 608–617. [CrossRef]
37. Singh, M.; Detamore, M.S. Tensile properties of the mandibular condylar cartilage. *J. Biomech. Eng.* **2008**, *130*, 011009. [CrossRef] [PubMed]
38. Chen, J.; Akyuz, U.; Xu, L.; Pidaparti, R. Stress analysis of the human temporomandibular joint. *Med. Eng. Phys.* **1998**, *20*, 565–572. [CrossRef]
39. Lee, G.M.; Poole, C.A.; Kelley, S.S.; Chang, J.; Caterson, B. Isolated chondrons: A viable alternative for studies of chondrocyte metabolism in vitro. *Osteoarthr. Cartil.* **1997**, *5*, 261–274. [CrossRef]
40. Vonk, L.A.; Doulabi, B.Z.; Huang, C.; Helder, M.N.; Everts, V.; Bank, R.A. Preservation of the chondrocyte's pericellular matrix improves cell-induced cartilage formation. *J. Cell. Biochem.* **2010**, *110*, 260–271. [CrossRef]
41. Bougault, C.; Paumier, A.; Aubert-Foucher, E.; Mallein-Gerin, F. Investigating conversion of mechanical force into biochemical signaling in three-dimensional chondrocyte cultures. *Nat. Protoc.* **2009**, *4*, 928–938. [CrossRef] [PubMed]

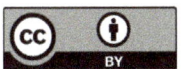

© 2019 by the authors. Licensee MDPI, Basel, Switzerland. This article is an open access article distributed under the terms and conditions of the Creative Commons Attribution (CC BY) license (http://creativecommons.org/licenses/by/4.0/).

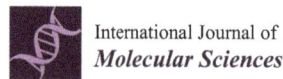

Communication

Molecular Aspects of Drug-Induced Gingival Overgrowth: An In Vitro Study on Amlodipine and Gingival Fibroblasts

Dorina Lauritano [1,*,†], Alberta Lucchese [2,†], Dario Di Stasio [2], Fedora Della Vella [3], Francesca Cura [4], Annalisa Palmieri [4] and Francesco Carinci [5]

1. Department of Medicine and Surgery, Centre of Neuroscience of Milan, University of Milano-Bicocca, 20126 Milan, Italy
2. Multidisciplinary Department of Medical and Dental Specialties, University of Campania- Luigi Vanvitelli, 80138 Naples, Italy; alberta.lucchese@unicampania.it (A.L.); dario.distasio@unicampania.it (D.D.S.)
3. Interdisciplinary Department of Medicine, University of Bari, 70121 Bari, Italy; fedora.dellavella@uniba.it
4. Department of Experimental, Diagnostic and Specialty Medicine, University of Bologna, via Belmoro 8, 40126 Bologna, Italy; cura.francesca@tiscali.it (F.C.); annalisa.palmieri@unife.it (A.P.)
5. Department of Morphology, Surgery and Experimental Medicine, University of Ferrara, 44121 Ferrara, Italy; crc@unife.it
* Correspondence: dorina.lauritano@unimib.it; Tel.: +39-335-679-0163
† Co-first authorship.

Received: 2 April 2019; Accepted: 24 April 2019; Published: 25 April 2019

Abstract: Gingival overgrowth is a serious side effect that accompanies the use of amlodipine. Several conflicting theories have been proposed to explain the fibroblast's function in gingival overgrowth. To determine whether amlodipine alters the fibrotic response, we investigated its effects on treated gingival fibroblast gene expression as compared with untreated cells. Materials and Methods: Fibroblasts from ATCC® Cell Lines were incubated with amlodipine. The gene expression levels of 12 genes belonging to the "Extracellular Matrix and Adhesion Molecules" pathway was investigated in treated fibroblasts cell culture, as compared with untreated cells, by real time PCR. Results: Most of the significant genes were up-regulated. (*CTNND2*, *COL4A1*, *ITGA2*, *ITGA7*, *MMP10*, *MMP11*, *MMP12*, *MMP26*) except for *COL7A1*, *LAMB1*, *MMP8*, and *MMP16*, which were down-regulated. Conclusion: These results seem to demonstrate that amlodipine has an effect on the extracellular matrix of gingival fibroblast. In the future, it would be interesting to understand the possible effect of the drug on fibroblasts of patients with amlodipine-induced gingival hyperplasia.

Keywords: Gingival overgrowth; gene expression; drugs; amlodipine

1. Introduction

Gingival overgrowth may have multiple causes, however drugs assumption is the most common [1,2]. In addiction, drug-induced gingival overgrowth may be associated with a patient's genetic predisposition [3,4].

The three main classes of drugs inducing gingival overgrowth are anticonvulsants, immunosuppressive, and antihypertensive agents [3,5–7]. The first report regarding gingival overgrowth by the administration of amlodipine was published in 1994 [8]. Subsequently, other authors reported the onset of gingival overgrowth as a side effect in patients who received 10 mg per day of amlodipine within two months [9]. Gingival overgrowth manifests as a side effect within one to three months after amlodipine administration [7,10]. Amlodipine shows a pharmacological profile, as follows: long-acting dihydropyridine; coronary and peripheral arterial vasodilatation; headaches, facial flushing, dizziness, and oedema. The main oral side effect that is induced by amlodipine is gingival overgrowth [11,12].

Gingival overgrowth that is induced by amlodipine (GOIA) must be stimulated by a threshold concentration of amlodipine [13]. However the severity of GOIA is supposed to be related to the concentration of amlodipine in oral fluids [13]. The mean dose of amlodipine reported to cause GOIA in most of the subjects is 5 mg/day. Therefore, it may be suggested that the dosage and duration of amlodipine may have an impact on GOIA [13]. Usually, the gingival manifestations of GOIA appear within the first three months of the drug administration [14]. A longer duration of therapy may increase the exposure of cells to amlodipine, and this may modify the apoptosis of cells, resulting in hyperplasia [14]. Genetic susceptibility is one the factors influencing the severity of GOIA; in fact multidrug resistant (*MDR1*) gene polymorphisms is supposed to alter the inflammatory response to the amlodipine [15].

Poor plaque control is another risk factor in developing of GOIA. In fact, GOIA hampered routine oral hygiene measures. Additionally, GOIA can favour the accumulation of bacterial plaque, which in turn determines gingival inflammation, causing gingival overgrowth [14]. Amlodipoine, in presence of proinflammatory cytokines (for example TNF-α), may favour the inhibition of apoptosis of human gingival fibroblasts, thus promoting hyperplasia [16].

1.1. Genetic Factors

Evidence suggests that genetic factors, along with patient susceptibility, may play an important role in the pathogenesis of GOIA [15]. A genetic predisposition can influence a number of factors in the drug interactions, cells, and plaque-induced inflammation. These include the functional heterogeneity of gingival fibroblasts, the collagenolytic activity, the drug-receptor binding, the drug metabolism, collagen synthesis, and many other factors.

Since most types of pharmacological agents that are implicated in GOIA can have negative effects on the flow of calcium ions across cell membranes, it has been postulated that these agents can interfere with the synthesis and function of the collagenase [17]. This mechanism of action has been demonstrated for Cyclosporine. In fact, a recent study in vitro have shown that human gingival fibroblasts that were treated with relevant doses of Cyclosporine show significantly reduced levels of secretion of MMP-1 and MMP-3; these reduced levels can contribute to the accumulation of components of the extracellular matrix [18]. An animal study that showed low mRNA levels of collagenase in situ further supported these results, accompanied by a decrease in phagocytosis and degradation of collagen [19]. The genetic predisposition to GOIA has been studied for cyclosporine, while, for what we know, not yet for amlodipine.

1.2. Objective

To determine whether amlodipine can alter the matrix deposition, we investigated its effects on treated gingival fibroblast gene expression as compared with untreated cells.

2. Results

The PrestoBlue™ cell viability test was conducted to determine the optimal concentration of amlodipine to be used for cell treatment that did not significantly affect cell viability. Based on this test, the concentration used for the treatment was 1000 ng/mL.

The gene expression profile of 12 genes belonging to the "Extracellular Matrix and Adhesion Molecules" pathway was analysed using Real time PCR (Figure 1). Table 1 reported the list gene and their fold change.

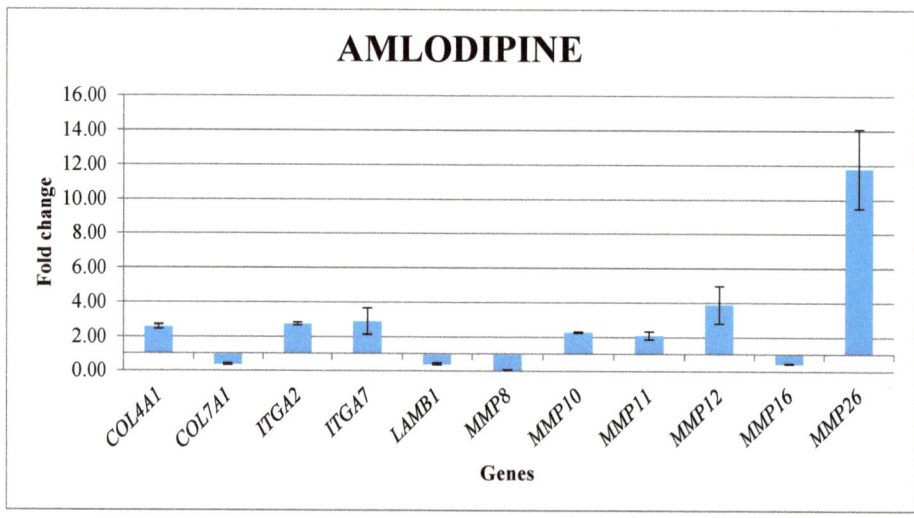

Figure 1. Gene expression profile of fibroblast treated with Amlodipine 1000 ng/mL.

Table 1. Significant gene expression levels after 24 h treatment with Amlodipine, as compared with untreated cells.

Gene	Fold Change	SD (+/−)	Gene Function
CTNND2	**2.29**	0.03	Cell Adhesion Molecule
COL4A1	**2.57**	0.13	Collagens & Extracellular Matrix Structural constituent
COL7A1	**0.38**	0.04	Collagens & Extracellular Matrix Structural constituent
ITGA2	**2.75**	0.08	Transmembrane Receptor
ITGA7	**2.90**	0.77	Transmembrane Receptor
LAMB1	**0.41**	0.05	Basement Membrane Constituent
MMP8	**0.06**	0.01	Extracellular Matrix Protease
MMP10	**2.27**	0.03	Extracellular Matrix Protease
MMP11	**2.09**	0.24	Extracellular Matrix Protease
MMP12	**3.88**	1.09	Extracellular Matrix Protease
MMP16	**0.44**	0.02	Extracellular Matrix Protease
MMP26	**11.78**	2.31	Extracellular Matrix Protease

Bold fonts indicate significant variation of gene expression level: fold change ≥ 2 and p value ≤ 0.05 for up-regulated genes, and fold change ≤ 0.5 and p value ≤ 0.05 for the significantly down-regulated genes.

Among the up-regulated genes, there was *CTNND2*, which code for the cell adhesion protein Catenin Delta 2. Other up-regulated gens were the transmembrane receptor *ITGA2* and *ITGA7* and the basement membrane constituent *LAMB1*. Most of the extracellular matrix proteases were up-regulated (*MMP10*, *MMP11*, *MMP12*, *MMP26*), except for *MMP8* and *MMP16*, which were down-regulated. Other genes that were significantly deregulated genes following the treatment with Amlodipine were *COL7A1*, which was down-regulated and the *COL4A1* that was up-regulated. In Figure 1 the significantly expression levels of the genes up- and down-regulated in fibroblast cells treated with amlodipine were represented.

3. Discussion

The prevalence of GOIA might be as high as 38%, and it is 3.3 times more common in men than in women [20,21]. The pathogenesis may be different for different drugs, even if the oral manifestations of gingival overgrowth are similar. GOIA starts as an enlargement of the interdental papilla of keratinized portions of the gingiva, and it is characterized by an increase in the connective tissue component. Bacteria accumulation appears to be an important uncomfortable effect of GOIA. GOIA may impair oral hygiene and lead to increased oral infections. Oral infection itself is a cause of gingival overgrowth [22]. In addiction, oral infection can potentially impair systemic health and could possibly compromise the general health of patients [22].

The mechanism of action of GOIA is still unknown, however it may be a consequence of the interaction between gingival fibroblasts, cellular and biochemical mediators of inflammation, and drug metabolites [22,23].

Gingival overgrowth is documented more frequently after intake of with phenytoin and rarely with others antihypertensive [24]. Furthermore, poor oral hygiene is indicated as an important risk factor for the expression of GOIA [25,26].

Cross-sectional studies have reported the relationship between bacterial plaque and GOIA. In fact, as previously reported, GOIA can favour the accumulation of bacterial plaque, which in turn determines gingival inflammation, causing gingival overgrowth [26]. The underlying mechanism of GOIA still remains to be fully understood, however two main inflammatory and non-inflammatory pathways have already been suggested [27–29]. One hypothesis may be that amlodipine may induce the alteration of collagenase activity as a consequence of decreased uptake of folic acid, blockage of aldosterone synthesis in adrenal cortex, and consequent feedback increase in the adrenocorticotropic hormone level and the up-regulation of keratinocyte growth factor [30]. Besides, inflammation may be a consequence of the toxic effect of amlodipine in periodontal pocket associated with C pathogens, leading to the up-regulation of several cytokine factors, such as transforming growth factor-beta 1 (TGF-β1) [9]. Another pathogenic mechanism of GOIA is focusing on the effects of amlodipine on gingival fibroblast metabolism and genetic predisposition. In fact, only a subgroup of patients that were treated with this amlodipine will develop GOIA, so it has been hypothesized that these individuals show an abnormal susceptibility to the drug. In fact, elevated levels of protein synthesis, most of which is collagen, characterize the fibroblast of GOIA in these patients. Treatment of GOIA is generally targeted on drug substitution and preventive protocols [12,31]. Surgical intervention is recommended when these measures fail to cause the resolution of GOIA. These treatment modalities, although effective, do not necessarily prevent the recurrence of the lesions [12]. Surgery for treatment of GOIA must be carefully assessed and it is normally performed for cosmetic/aesthetic needs before any functional consequences are present [1,32]. Most reports of GOIA have required surgical intervention [25].

To our knowledge, our study is the first one analysing the effect of amlodipine on genes that belong to the "Extracellular Matrix and Adhesion Molecules" pathway. In this study, gingival fibroblasts were treated for 24 h with 1000 ng/mL of amlodipine. The gene expression profile of 12 genes that belong to the "Extracellular Matrix and Adhesion Molecules" pathway was analysed. Most of the significant genes were up-regulated. (*CTNND2, COL4A1, ITGA2, ITGA7, MMP10, MMP11, MMP12, MMP26*), except for *COL7A1, LAMB1, MMP8*, and *MMP16*, which were down-regulated. These proteins preferentially induce extra cellular matrix deposition. This study demonstrated that, in human gingival fibroblasts that were cultivated in vitro, amlodipine could promote the activities of genes belonging to the "fibroblast matrix and receptors".

It might be part of the underlying reason for the persistent overgrowth of gingiva that was seen when bacterial plaque and local inflammation are present during amlodipine therapy. In fact, GOIA does not allow patient to maintain a good oral hygiene, and this is the reason why GOIA always determines the presence of bacterial plaque and inflammation, which in turn determines gingival overgrowth.

The data presented here suggest that amlodipine may contribute to an extracellular matrix deposition of human gingival fibroblasts inducing gingival overgrowth.

4. Materials and Methods

4.1. Primary Human Fibroblast Cells Culture

We used cells from ATCC® Cell Lines. The cryopreserved cells at the second passage were cultured in 75 cm^2 culture flasks containing DMEM medium (Sigma Aldrich, Inc., St Louis, Mo, USA) supplemented with 20% fetal calf serum, antibiotics (Penicillin 100U/ml and Streptomycin 100 micrograms/ml-Sigma Aldrich, Inc., St Louis, Mo, USA).

Cell cultures were replicated for subsequent experiments and maintained in a water saturated atmosphere at 37 °C and 5% CO_2.

4.2. Cell Viability Test

A stock solution of amlodipine 1 mg/mL was prepared. Further dilutions were made with the culture medium to the desired concentrations just before use. The cell lines were seeded into 96-well plates at a density of 10^4 cells per well containing 100 µL of cell culture medium and incubated for 24 h to allow cell adherence. Serial dilution of amlodipine (5000 ng/mL, 2000 ng/mL, 1000 ng/mL, 500 ng/mL, 100 ng/mL) was added (three wells for each concentration). The cell culture medium alone was used negative control.

After 24 h of incubation, cell viability was measured while using PrestoBlue™ Reagent Protocol (Invitrogen, Carlsbad, CA, USA) according to the manufacturer's instructions. Briefly, the PrestoBlue™ solution (10 µL) was added into each well containing 90 µL of treatment solution. The plates were then placed back into the incubator for 1 h, after which absorbance was measured at wavelengths of 570 nm excitation and 620 nm emission by an automated microplate reader (Sunrise™, Tecan Trading AG, Switzerland). Comparing the average absorbance in drug treated wells with average absorbance in control wells exposed to vehicle alone determined the percentage of viable cells.

4.3. Cell Treatment

Gingival fibroblasts were seeded at a density of 1.0×10^5 cells/ml into 9 cm^2 (3 mL) wells and then subjected to serum starvation for 16 hours at 37 °C. Cells were treated with 1000 ng/mL amlodipine solution for 24 h. This solution was obtained in DMEM that was supplemented with 2% FBS, antibiotics and aminoacids. Cell medium alone was used as control negative. The cells were maintained in a humidified atmosphere of 5% CO_2 at 37 °C. After the end of the exposure time, the cells were trypsinized and processed for RNA extraction.

4.4. RNA Isolation, Reverse Transcription and Quantitative Real-Time RT-PCR

Total RNA was isolated from cultured cells using GenElute mammalian total RNA purification miniprep kit (Sigma-Aldrich, Inc., St Louis, Mo, USA), according to manufacturer's instructions. Pure RNA was quantified at NanoDrop 2000 spectrophotometer (Thermo Scientific, Waltham, Massachusetts, USA).

cDNA synthesis was performed, starting from 500 ng of total RNA, using PrimeScript RT Master Mix (Takara Bio Inc, Kusatsu, Japan). The reaction was incubated at 37 °C for 15 min. and inactivated by heating at 70 °C for 10 s.

cDNA was amplified by Real Time Quantitative PCR using the ViiA™ 7 System (Applied Biosystems, Foster City, CA, USA).

All of the PCR reactions were performed in a 20 µL volume. Each reaction contained 10 µL of 2x qPCRBIO SYGreen Mix Lo-ROX (Pcrbiosystems, London, UK), 400 nM concentration of each primer, and cDNA. Table 2 reported the sequences of the primer that was used in the reaction.

Table 2. Primers sequences of SYBR® Green assay.

Gene Name	Forward Sequence 5' > 3'	Reverse Sequence 5' > 3'
CTNND2	AGAGAATTTGGATGGAGAGAC	TTGTTGTCTCCAAAACAGAG
COL4A1	AAAGGGAGATCAAGGGATAG	TCACCTTTTTCTCCAGGTAG
COL7A1	ATGACCTTGGCATTATCTTG	TGAATATGTCACCTCTCAAGG
ITGA2	GGTGGGGTTAATTCAGTATG	ATATTGGGATGTCTGGGATG
ITGA7	CATGAACAATTTGGGTTCTG	GCCCTTCCAATTATAGGTTC
LAMB1	GTGTGTATAGATACTTCGCC	AAAGCACGAAATATCACCTC
MMP8	AAGTTGATGCAGTTTTCCAG	CTGAACTTCCCTTCAACATTC
MMP10	AGCGGACAAATACTGGAG	GTGATGATCCACTGAAGAAG
MMP11	GATAGACACCAATGAGATTGC	TTTGAAGAAAAAGAGCTCGC
MMP12	AGGTATGATGAAAGGAGACAG	AGGTATGATGAAAGGAGAACAG
MMP16	ACCCTCATGACTTGATAACC	TCTGTCTCCCTTGAAGAAATAG
MMP26	AAGGATCCAGCATTTGTATG	CTTTGATCCTCCAATAAACTCC
RPL13	AAAGCGGATGGTGGTTCCT	GCCCAGATAGGCAAACTTTC

Custom primers belonging to the "Extracellular Matrix and Adhesion Molecules" pathway were purchased from Sigma Aldrich. All of the experiments were performed, including non-template controls to exclude reagents contamination. PCR was performed, including two analytical replicates.

The amplification profile was initiated by 10 min. incubation at 95 °C, followed by two-step amplification of 15 s at 95 °C and 60 s at 60 °C for 40 cycles. As final step, a melt curve dissociation analysis was performed.

4.5. Statistical Analysis

The gene expression levels were normalized to the expression of the reference gene (RPL13) and they were expressed as fold changes relative to the expression of the untreated cells. Quantification was done with the delta/delta Ct calculation method.

5. Conclusions

In this study, most of the significantly genes belonging to the "extracellular matrix proteases" pathway were up-regulated. These results seem to indicate that amlodipine has an effect on the modulation of fibrosis response in gingival fibroblasts, up-regulating extracellular matrix proteases, and favouring the deposition of fibrotic tissue. More explanatory results could probably be obtained by using gingival fibroblasts in which the use of amlodipine seems to aggravate the fibrotic response and the gingival overgrowth.

GOIA is no longer a rare occurrence. From one side, plaque accumulation is an inevitable consequence of GOIA, and from the other, it favours gingival inflammation and overgrowth. The duration of therapy, dosage, and individual genetic susceptibility are considered important risk factors for the development of GOIA. Amlodipine is a widely used drug for the treatment of hypertension and angina, so it is very important that doctors inform patients about side effects, such as GOIA, and about the importance of preventive protocols. Dentists should be able to identify the changes in the oral cavity that are related to the general health of their patients. The patients must be informed of the tendency of certain drugs to cause gingival overgrowth and the associated oral changes and the importance of effective oral hygiene.

Combination therapy consisting of surgical and non-surgical periodontal therapy with drug substitution is the most reliable method in the management of GOIA.

Author Contributions: Conceptualization, D.L.; Data curation, A.L. and F.C. (Francesca Cura); Investigation, D.D.S.; Supervision, F.C. (Francesco Carinci); Visualization, F.D.V.; Writing—review & editing, A.P.

Funding: This research received no external funding.

Conflicts of Interest: All authors declare they have no conflict of interest.

References

1. Amit, B.; Shalu, B.V. Gingival enlargement induced by anticonvulsants, calcium channel blockers and immunosuppressants: A review. *IRJP* **2012**, *3*, 116–119.
2. Ellis, J.S.; Seymour, R.A.; Steele, J.G.; Roberston, P.; Butler, T.J.; Thomason, J.M. Prevalence of gingival overgrowth induced by calcium channel blockers: A community based study. *J. Periodontol.* **1999**, *70*, 63–67.
3. Bharati, T.; Mukesh Tehmina Veenita Jain, V.V.; Jajoo, U.N. Amlodipine induced gum hypertrophy—A rare case report. *J. Mgims* **2012**, *17*, 63–64.
4. Newman, M.G.; Takei, H.H.; Klokkevold, P.R.; Carranza, F.A. *Carranza's Clinical Periodontology*, 10th ed.; Saunders: St Louis, MO, USA, 2006; pp. 373–377.
5. Drug associated gingival enlargement. *J. Periodontol.* **2004**, *75*, 1424–1431. [CrossRef]
6. Jorgensen, M.G. Prevalence of amlodipine-related gingival hyperplasia. *J. Periodontol.* **1997**, *68*, 676–678.
7. Jose, J.; Santhosh, Y.L.; Naveen, M.R.; Kumar, V. Case report of amlodipine induced gingival hyperplasia—Late onset at a low use. *Asian J. Pharm. Clin. Res.* **2011**, *4*, 65–66.
8. Seymour, R.A.; Ellis, J.S.; Thomason, J.M.; Monkman, S.; Idle, J.R. Amlodipine induced gingival overgrowth. *J. Clin. Periodontal* **1994**, *21*, 281–283.
9. Lafzi, A.; Farahani, R.M.; Shoja, M.A. Amlodipine induced gingival hyperplasia. *Med. Oral Patol. Oral Cir. Bucal.* **2006**, *11*, 480–482.
10. Meraw, S.J.; Sheridan, P.J. Medically induced gingival hyperplasia. *Mayo Clin. Proc.* **1996**, *73*, 1196–1199.
11. Ellis, J.S.; Seymour, R.A.; Monkman, S.C.; Idle, J.R. Gingival sequestration of nifedipine induced overgrowth. *Lancet* **1992**, *39*, 1382–1383.
12. Grover, V.; Kapoor, A.; Marya, C.M. Amlodipine induced gingival hyperplasia. *J. Oral Health Comm. Dent.* **2007**, *1*, 19–22.
13. Daley, T.D.; Wysocki, G.P.; Day, C. Clinical and pharmacologic correlations in cyclosporine-induced gingival hyperplasia. *Oral Surg. Oral Med. Oral Pathol.* **1986**, *62*, 417–421.
14. Pasupuleti, M.K.; Musalaiah, S.V.; Nagasree, M.; Kumar, P.A. Combination of inflammatory and amlodipine induced gingival overgrowth in a patient with cardiovascular disease. *Avicenna J. Med.* **2013**, *3*, 68–72.
15. Meisel, P.; Giebel, J.; Kunert-Keil, C.; Dazert, P.; Kroemer, H.K.; Kocher, T. MDR1 gene polymorphisms and risk of gingival hyperplasia induced by calcium antagonists. *Clin. Pharm. Ther.* **2006**, *79*, 62–71.
16. Takeuchi, R.; Matsumoto, H.; Akimoto, Y.; Fujii, A. The inhibitory action of amlodipine for TNF-α-induced apoptosis in cultured human gingival fibroblasts. *Oral Ther. Pharmacol.* **2012**, *31*, 45–52.
17. Hassell, T.M. Evidence for production of an inactive collagenase by fibroblasts from phenytoin-enlarged human gingiva. *J. Oral Pathol.* **1982**, *11*, 310–317.
18. Bolzani, G.; Della Coletta, R.; Martelli Junior, H.; Martelli Junior, H.; Graner, E. Cyclosporin A inhibits production and activity of matrix metalloproteinases by gingival fibroblasts. *J. Periodontal Res.* **2000**, *35*, 51–58.
19. Kataoka, M.; Shimizu, Y.; Kunikiyo, K.; Asahara, Y.; Yamashita, K.; Ninomiya, M.; Morisaki, I.; Ohsaki, Y.; Kido, J.-I.; Nagata, T. Cyclosporin A decreases the degradation of type I collagen in rat gingival overgrowth. *J. Cell Physiol.* **2000**, *182*, 351–358.
20. Sucu, M.; Yuce, M.; Davatoglu, V. Amlodipine induced massive gingival hypertrophy. *Can. Fam. Phys.* **2011**, *57*, 436–437.
21. Prisant, L.M.; Herman, W. Calcium channel blocker induced gingival overgrowth. *J. Clin. Hypertens.* **2002**, *4*, 310–311.
22. Pradhan, S.; Mishra, P.; Joshi, S. Drug induced gingival enlargement—A review. *PGNM* **2009**, *8*.
23. Amgelpoulous, A.P.; Goaz, P.W. Incidence of diphenylhydantoin gingival hyperplasia. *Oral Surg. Oral Med. Oral Pathol.* **1972**, *34*, 898–906.

24. Hegde, R.; Kale, R.; Jain, A.S. Cyclosporine and amlodipine induced severe gingival overgrowth–etiopathogenesis and management of a case with electrocautery and carbon-dioxide (CO_2) laser. *J. Oral Health. Comm. Dent.* **2012**, *6*, 34–42.
25. Taib, H.; Ali, T.B.T.; Kamin, S. Amlodipine induced gingival overgrowth: A case report. *Arch. Orofac. Sci.* **2007**, *2*, 61–64.
26. Srivastava, A.K.; Kundu, D.; Bandyopadhyay, P.; Pal, A.K. Management of amlodipine induced gingival enlargement: A series of three cases. *J. Indian Soc. Perodontol.* **2010**, *14*, 279.
27. Khan, S.; Mittal, A.; Kanteshwari, I.K. Amlodipine induced gingival overgrowth: A case report. *NJDSR* **2012**, *1*, 65–69.
28. Routray, S.N.; Mishra, T.K.; Pattnaik, U.K.; Satapathy, C.; Mishra, C.K.; Behera, M. Amlodipine induced gingival hyperplasia. *J. Assoc. Phys. India* **2003**, *51*, 818–819.
29. Sharma, S.; Sharma, A. Amlodipine induced gingival enlargement—A clinical report. *Compend. Contin. Educ. Dent.* **2012**, *33*, 78–82.
30. Triveni, M.G.; Rudrakshi, C.; Mehta, D.S. Amlodipine induced gingival overgrowth. *J. Indian Soc. Periodontol.* **2009**, *13*, 160–163.
31. Marshall, R.I.; Bartold, P.M. A clinical review of drug induced gingival overgrowth. *Oral Surg. Oral Med. Oral Pathol.* **1993**, *76*, 543–548.
32. Lombardi, T.; Fiore, D.G.; Belser, U.; Di, F.R. Felodipine induced gingival hyperplasia: A clinical and histologic study. *J. Oral Pathol. Med.* **1991**, *20*, 89–92.

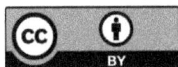

© 2019 by the authors. Licensee MDPI, Basel, Switzerland. This article is an open access article distributed under the terms and conditions of the Creative Commons Attribution (CC BY) license (http://creativecommons.org/licenses/by/4.0/).

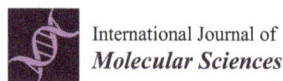

Review

The Pathogenic Factors from Oral Streptococci for Systemic Diseases

Hiromichi Yumoto [1,*], Katsuhiko Hirota [2], Kouji Hirao [3], Masami Ninomiya [1], Keiji Murakami [4], Hideki Fujii [4] and Yoichiro Miyake [5]

1. Department of Periodontology and Endodontology, Institute of Biomedical Sciences, Tokushima University Graduate School, Tokushima 770-8504, Japan; masami.ninomiya@tokushima-u.ac.jp
2. Department of Medical Hygiene, Dental Hygiene Course, Kochi Gakuen College, Kochi 780-0955, Japan; khirota@kochi-gc.ac.jp
3. Department of Conservative Dentistry, Institute of Biomedical Sciences, Tokushima University Graduate School, Tokushima 770-8504, Japan; koujihirao@tokushima-u.ac.jp
4. Department of Oral Microbiology, Institute of Biomedical Sciences, Tokushima University Graduate School, Tokushima 770-8504, Japan; kmurakami@tokushima-u.ac.jp (K.M.); hfujii@tokushima-u.ac.jp (H.F.)
5. Department of Oral Health Sciences, Faculty of Health and Welfare, Tokushima Bunri University, Tokushima, Tokushima 770-8514, Japan; miyake@tks.bunri-u.ac.jp
* Correspondence: yumoto@tokushima-u.ac.jp; Tel.: +81-88-633-7340

Received: 9 August 2019; Accepted: 14 September 2019; Published: 15 September 2019

Abstract: The oral cavity is suggested as the reservoir of bacterial infection, and the oral and pharyngeal biofilms formed by oral bacterial flora, which is comprised of over 700 microbial species, have been found to be associated with systemic conditions. Almost all oral microorganisms are non-pathogenic opportunistic commensals to maintain oral health condition and defend against pathogenic microorganisms. However, oral Streptococci, the first microorganisms to colonize oral surfaces and the dominant microorganisms in the human mouth, has recently gained attention as the pathogens of various systemic diseases, such as infective endocarditis, purulent infections, brain hemorrhage, intestinal inflammation, and autoimmune diseases, as well as bacteremia. As pathogenic factors from oral Streptococci, extracellular polymeric substances, toxins, proteins and nucleic acids as well as vesicles, which secrete these components outside of bacterial cells in biofilm, have been reported. Therefore, it is necessary to consider that the relevance of these pathogenic factors to systemic diseases and also vaccine candidates to protect infectious diseases caused by Streptococci. This review article focuses on the mechanistic links among pathogenic factors from oral Streptococci, inflammation, and systemic diseases to provide the current understanding of oral biofilm infections based on biofilm and widespread systemic diseases.

Keywords: Streptococci; Biofilm; Pathogenic factor; Oral infection; Systemic Diseases

1. Introduction

The human oral microbiome is comprised of over 700 microbial species, as characterized by both cultivation and culture-independent molecular approaches such as the 16S rRNA gene-based method [1]. Almost all oral microorganisms are non-pathogenic opportunistic commensals to maintain oral health condition and defend against pathogenic microorganisms [2]. The most remarkable feature of oral microflora is that numerous oral bacteria form a biofilm, so called dental plaque, which is defined as microbial communities embedded in a self-produced matrix of extracellular polymeric substances and a dynamic metabolically structure, on tooth surface and oral mucosa [3,4]. Within biofilm formed in oral niche, the polymicrobial interactions between interspecies, such as recombination and horizontal gene transfer, are caused and then specialized clones are selected [5]. Several pressures by bacterial communities and the host as well as the change in oral environment caused by the administration of antibiotics also affect the selection of bacterial species and the characterizations of their virulence. Once this homeostasis of oral microflora is disturbed by changing the local environments as well as the metabolic and physiological activities of bacteria in biofilm, oral infectious diseases such as dental caries and periodontitis, which are major two prevalent chronic diseases in oral cavity, are caused. Moreover, in the last two decades, numerous studies regarding the association between oral biofilm infectious diseases and various systemic diseases, such as cardiovascular diseases, atherosclerosis, diabetes mellitus, aspiration pneumonia, and autoimmune diseases, have been reported. To date, it has been considered that there are two major pathways by which oral bacterial infectious diseases affect systemic diseases (Figure 1). Bacteremia as direct pathway, oral bacteria residing in the oral cavity invade blood vessels in dental pulp and periodontal tissues, and then reach not only the heart but also the large blood vessels and various organs to cause systemic diseases. Another direct pathway involving aspiration, which often occurs in elderly people, involves oral bacteria reaching a respiratory organ, such as the lung via a pharynx and airway route, and causing respiratory diseases. Several bacterial products, such as endotoxin (lipopolysaccharide: LPS) and heat shock protein (HSP), as well as antigens, also involved in various systemic diseases due to the indirect causes of triggering immune responses. Therefore, the oral cavity is recognized as a source or reservoir of microbial infection and the establishment of methods to prevent oral infections is one of the most important and urgent issues in dentistry. From the viewpoint of oral biofilm infection, understanding the roles of oral microorganisms and their pathogenic factors and elucidating various systemic diseases and their onset mechanisms related to oral infections would lead to the development of novel preventive measures.

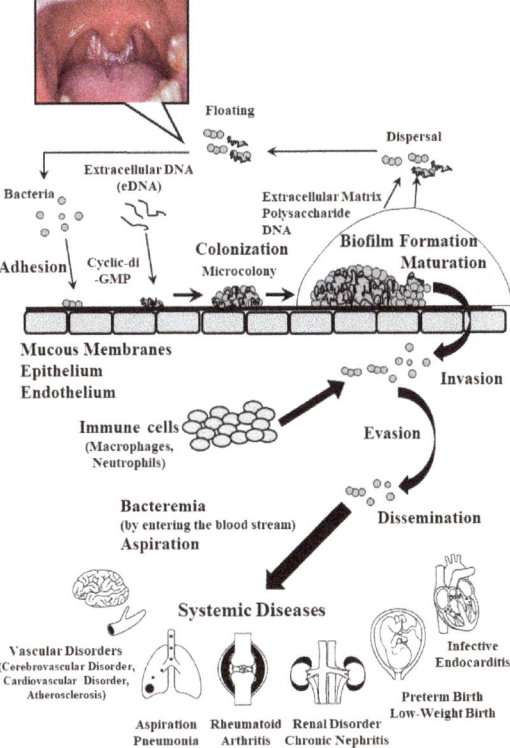

Figure 1. Life style of biofilm and the conceptual pathogenic mechanisms of oral bacterial infection leading to various systemic diseases.

Among oral bacterial species, over 100 identified oral Streptococci, which can colonize shortly after birth and play important roles in the formation of oral physiological microflora, are the predominant commensal and opportunistic inhabitants in the oral cavity and upper respiratory tract in humans, and cause opportunistic infections at sites distant from the oral cavity as well as oral infections, especially in immunocompromised patients and elderly people [6]. Pathogenic Streptococci are identified as sources of invasive infections in humans and their infections are still one of the most serious diseases in modern medical world [7]. Table 1 shows systemic diseases affected and caused by oral Streptococcal infections. Therefore, it has been recently considered that the genus Streptococci severely impacts on human health by carrying a significant number of worldwide human infections, and has been separated into following 8 distinct groups: mitis, sanguinis, anginosus, salivalius, downei, mutans, pyogenic, and bovis using gene clustering, as well as phylogenetic and gene gain/loss analyses (Figure 2) [8]. The distribution of oral Streptococcal species in the oral cavity has been also reported [9,10]. The mitis and sanguinis groups, such as *S. sanguinis*, *S. mitis*, *S. gordonii*, and *S. oralis* are common commensals, primarily involved in initial dental plaque formation as the first colonizers of the tooth surface, but are also associated with an increased risk of systemic diseases and invasive infections, including infective endocarditis, by entering the bloodstream through transient bacteremia after daily activities such as brushing and flossing, as well as invasive dental procedures such as tooth extraction. A recent descriptive epidemiological study has reported the distribution of Streptococci causing infective endocarditis [11]. Figure 3 shows one clinical case of infective endocarditis mainly caused by oral *S. sanguinis*. We encountered the patient with infective endocarditis caused by oral Streptococci, who had severe systemic conditions such as mitral and tricuspid regurgitations and a continuous fever over 37 °C, and who was urgently hospitalized in our university hospital. This case was rigorously diagnosed by the detection of oral *Streptococcus sanguinis*, as well as the examination of chest radiograph and echocardiogram at the time of the onset of infective endocarditis. Therefore, as the presentative case of infective endocarditis, the detailed therapeutic course following the guideline is described below and in Figure 3. The guideline for systemic complications, such as infective endocarditis, shows that bactericidal antibiotics are selected based on the results from microbiological examination, such as blood culture, and long-term antibiotic treatment is performed at high doses in order to kill the causative bacteria and to prevent recurrence. It is also very important to identify the causative bacteria in order to suppress side effects as much as possible. Following this guideline, the patient received viccilin (ampicillin sodium: 6000 mg/day) and gentamicin (a type of aminoglycoside: 60 mg/day) after microbiological examination. Afterwards, the symptoms were improved and no bacteria were detected by blood culture. It has been recognized that *S. mutans* playing important roles in the initiation and progression of dental caries is inversely associated with oral health [12]. The *S. anginosus* group is detected as part of the oropharyngeal microflora and is commonly associated with a variety of purulent infections and abscess formations in the brain, meninx, heart, liver, lung, and spleen. It is caused by bacteremia, as well as periapical odontogenic lesions [13–17]. In particular, *S. intermedius* and *S. constellatus* found in dental plaque has been associated with the development of periodontal diseases [18]. In contrast, *S. salivarius* group, in which *S. salivarius* is predominant in the saliva and on the surface of oral mucosa, is related to oral health rather than disease by producing bacteriocins targeting cariogenic *S. mutans* in addition to some enzymes such as dextranase and urease, which can inhibit the accumulation of dental plaque and acidification, respectively. A previous probiotic study reported that *S. salivarius* provides potential oral benefits to children [19].

Table 1. Systemic diseases affected by oral Streptococcal infections.

Bacteremia and Sepsis
Infective Endocarditis, Pericarditis
Heart Valve Disease
Aortic Aneurysm

Table 1. *Cont.*

Deep-seated purulent Abscess (Brain, Tonsillar, Abdominal, Spleen or Liver Abscess)
Pleural Empyema
Meningitis
Cerebrovascular Disease (Cerebral Hemorrhage etc.)
Gastrointestinal Diseases (Exacerbation and Chronicity of Enteritis)
Kidney Diseases (IgA Nephropathy)
Pneumonia
Pharyngitis, Tonsillitis
Sinusitis
Premature Birth, Neonatal Infections, Puerperal Sepsis
Urinary Tract Infection
Central Nerve System Infections
Arthritis, Necrotizing Fasciitis
Pyarthrosis
Toxic Shock Syndrome
Osteomyelitis
Vulvovaginitis
Peritonitis
Impetigo, Cellulitis, Pyoderma
Otitis Media
Conjunctivitis
Scarlet Fever

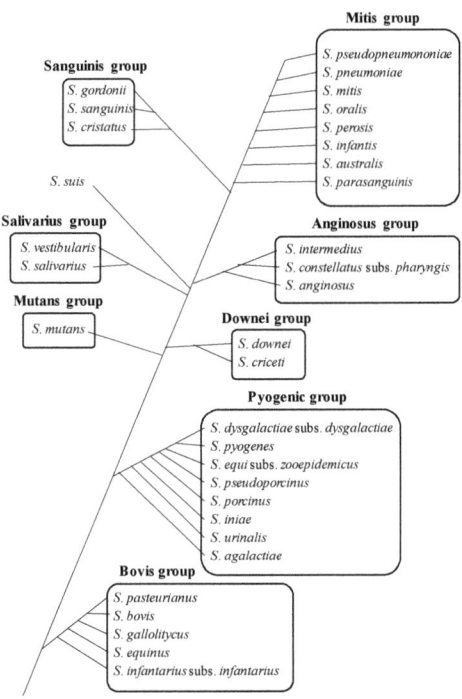

Figure 2. The phylogenetic relationship among 8 major groups of human Streptococcal species.

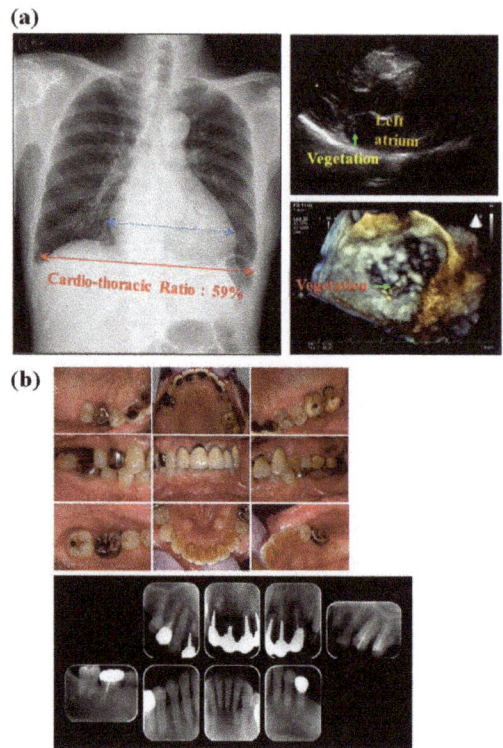

Figure 3. A clinical case of infective endocarditis caused by oral *Streptococcus sanguinis*. A 72 years-old male patient with mitral and tricuspid regurgitations was urgently hospitalized for continuous fever over 37 °C and diagnosed as infective endocarditis by detection of oral Streptococcus, *S. sanguinis*. During the hospitalization for 1 month, patient received viccilin (ampicillin sodium: 6000 mg/day) and gentamicin (a type of aminoglycoside: 60 mg/day). After the improvement of symptoms and no bacterial detection by blood culture, patient underwent artificial valve replacement and tricuspid ring annuloplasty, and then was discharged from hospital due to the stabilization of symptoms. The patient came to our dental department for the prevention of recurrence with a referral from the medical doctor. (**a**) Chest radiograph and echocardiogram at the time of the onset of infective endocarditis. Cardiac hypertrophy (Cardio-thoracic Ratio: CTR: $\geq$ 50%) was observed due to abnormalities in the mitral valve, and the left atrium was enlarged markedly. Vegetation (green arrow) was observed in the mitral valve. (**b**) Oral and X-ray photographs of patient with infective endocarditis. Gingival redness and slight swelling were observed in full mouth, and dental calculus deposition were observed on mandibular anterior teeth and upper left molars. Mobility of upper anterior teeth and left premolars was also observed. From dental X-ray radiographs, root fractures of upper right central and lateral incisors, and a endodontic-periodontal combined lesion of the upper left incisor and canines were found. Severe alveolar bone loss around the upper anterior teeth and left premolars as well as root caries on the upper lateral incisor and 1st premolar was also observed. The number of total Streptococci in 10 µL of saliva was 1.0×10^7 copies and various periodontal pathogens, such as *Porphyromonas gingivalis*, *Aggregatibacter actinomycetemcomitans*, *Tannerella forsythia*, *Treponema denticola* and *Fusobacterium nucleatum*, were also detected at significantly high level.

Streptococci have an array of virulence factors, which include surface proteins for adhesion, invasion/internalization, extracellular enzymatic proteases, and toxins delivered to cell surface as well as extracellular environments, which are associated with their colonization at various sites in the human body, dissemination, evasion from immune system for survival, destruction of host tissues, and modulation of the host immune function [20,21]. Some vaccine candidates are currently being considered to protect against infectious diseases caused by SStreptococci. This review article focuses on the mechanistic links among crucial pathogenic factors from oral Streptococci, inflammation, and systemic diseases to provide the current understanding of oral infections and widespread systemic diseases. In particular, our recent findings regarding the roles of histone-like DNA binding protein and extracellular DNA in biofilm formation and systemic diseases are also summarized.

2. Pathogenic Factors Involved in Adhesion, Colonization, Internalization and Invasion

In general, the first step on bacterial infections is adherence of bacterial cells with host tissues via the interaction between bacterial adhesion factor, adhesin, and its receptor. This step is extremely important for bacterial survival in bacterial multicellular communities and the establishment of infections. Streptococci express a wide range of adhesins that are specific for the surface of host tissues to colonize, grow, and form biofilm (Table 2). These adhesion and colonization factors of oral Streptococci also play pivotal roles in resistant to antimicrobial peptides and protection against host innate immune defense system. Among the numerous adhesion factors, representative molecules are described below.

Table 2. The pathogenic factors expressed in oral Streptococci for colonization, inflammation, infection causing systemic diseases.

Pathogenic Factors	References
Factors for adhesion, colonization, and evasion from host immune defense	
Antigen I/II	[22–24]
Fibronectin-binding proteins	[23,25–27]
Collagen-binding proteins	[20,28]
Laminin-binding proteins	
Fibrinogen-binding proteins	
Platelet-binding proteins	
Serine-rich repeat proteins	[23,29,30]
Pili	[20,23,31–37]
Major surface adhesins (M protein)	[38–41]
Enolase	[23,42,43]
Proteases	
SpeB	[44–47]
C5a peptidase	[26,48–51]
Capsule	
Lipoteichoic acid as pathogen-associated molecular pattern (PAMP)	

2.1. Cell Wall-Anchored Polypeptides

Among the cell wall-anchored polypeptides produced by oral Streptococci, antigen I/II acts as a mediator on the adherence of Streptococci to salivary glycoproteins called pellicles coated on the surfaces of teeth as well as collagen, fibronectin and laminin in the tissues, and is also engaged in biofilm formation by interacting with other oral microorganisms, such as *Actinomyces naeslundii*, *Porphyromonas gingivalis*, and *Candida albicans*, platelet aggregation, and tissue invasion [22,23]. Antigen I/II is conserved in oral Streptococcus species including *S. pyogenes*, *S. suis* and *S. agalactiae*. Spy1325, a member of the antigen I/II family and cell surface-anchored molecule produced by oral Streptococci, is very well conserved in group A Streptococcus (GAS) strains. Interestingly, the immunization of mice with recombinant Spy1325 fragments conferred protection against GAS-mediated mortality, suggesting that Spy1325 may represent a shared virulence factor among GAS, GBS, and oral Streptococci [24]. Therefore, these adhesion factors are considered as a candidate molecule for preventive and therapeutic measures against Streptococcal infections, including dental caries.

Fibronectin-binding protein expressed in all Streptococci plays the role of providing a bridge between Streptococci and host cells by attachment to the extracellular matrix, fibronectin [23,25]. Fibronectin binding proteins can be divided into two types: one type contains fibronectin binding repeats and another type has no repeats [26,27]. This kind of adhesion is different between the binding activity and structure. Some can bind soluble fibronectin and others attach to immobilized fibronectin expressed on the surface of host cells. Moreover, most of these adhesins are anchored to the bacterial cell wall, but some are not. In addition to the role of adhesins mediating attachment, fibronectin-binding protein has been identified as invasins invading epithelial and endothelial cells, which have contributed to evasion from host's innate immune defense mechanisms, such as the complement system and phagocytosis [27].

As another cell wall-anchored protein, collagen binding proteins adhere to collagen-rich tissues for colonization of oral and extra-oral tissues [28] and also bind complement C1 recognition protein, C1q, as inhibitors of the classical complement defense. Therefore, this function confers the ability of immune evasion on oral Streptococci [20].

Serine-rich repeat glycoproteins expressed in wide range of oral Streptococci has multiple serine-rich repeats, which are estimated as an approximately 75% of this protein [23]. After invading into bloodstream, oral Streptococci can bind to human platelets through this adhesion and are disseminated systemically [29]. Binding to platelets leads to form a thrombus, by which oral Streptococci can evade the host immune defense and antibiotics circulated in blood, and then cause infective endocarditis [30]. Therefore, this adhesin is considered as a major virulence factor of endocarditis.

Pili are filamentous apparatus typically extending 1–3 mm from the bacterial cell surface, and the genes encoding pili are identified in discrete loci called pilus islands flanked by mobile genetic elements [20,23]. Pili as virulent factors adhere to various host epithelial cells as well as extracellular matrix proteins such as collagen and fibrinogen, and then promotes Streptococcal colonization and biofilm formation on various sites in the host as well as non-biological surfaces [31]. In addition to adhesion, pili can facilitate bacterial invasion into human epithelial and endothelial cells and lead to Streptococcal dissemination in the host during the critical infection steps [32,33]. Moreover, pili have immunomodulatory abilities to evoke inflammatory cytokine responses and thwart the host innate immune defenses of resist phagocyte killing [34–36]. Therefore, pili have gotten much attention as potential vaccine candidates because of animal studies showing conferred protective immunity against Streptococcal infection [37].

M proteins expressed on a bacterial cell surface, α-helical coiled-coil dimers extending as hair like projections, bind host proteins such as immunoglobulins, fibronectin, and fibrinogen, complement factors such as albumin, and adhere to epithelial cells [38]. Interestingly, antigenically variable M proteins are considered as major virulence factors and immunogens in Streptococci by inducing pro-inflammatory responses and inhibiting phagocytic activities to assist Streptococci in evading host innate immune defenses [39,40]. Soluble M1 protein secreted from Streptococci has been also considered as a novel Streptococcal superantigen because it contributes to excess T cell activation and inflammatory response, such as the induction of T-cell proliferation and Th1 type cytokines production, during invasive Streptococcal infections [41]. Therefore, M proteins may be promising vaccine immunogens [39].

2.2. Cell Wall-Anchorless Polypeptides

Enolase, cell wall-anchorless adhesin and cytoplasmic glycolytic enzyme, is well conserved structurally in Streptococci [23,42]. α-enolase functionally binds to plasmin and plasminogen as well as laminin, fibronectin, and collagens, and also enhances plasminogen activation [43]. Plasmin cleaved from plasminogen by plasminogen activators can degrade extracellular matrix, in turn breakdown epithelial barriers and finally lead to bacterial invasion and infection. Therefore, this anchorless cell surface protein has been considered in promising vaccine candidates for the prevention of Streptococcal infection [42].

2.3. Proteases

Some proteases secreted from Streptococci have associated with their virulence. In addition to the role of adhesin to glycoprotein and laminin, Streptococcal pyrogenic exotoxin B (SpeB), predominant cysteine protease, has relatively indiscriminant specificity to degrade the extracellular matrix proteins, including fibronectin, cytokines, chemokines, compliment components, immunoglobulins, immune system components such as the antimicrobial peptide cathelicidin LL-37, and serum protease inhibitors. It also activates interleukin-1β [44,45]. This protease also degrades some proteins targeted by autophagy in the host cell cytosol, which is an important innate immune defense, and this proteolytic activity helps Streptococci to evade autophagy, to replicate in the cytoplasm of host cells, to colonize deep-seated tissues, and finally to lead to tissue destruction [46]. Moreover, SpeB increases the production of proapoptotic molecules, such as tumor necrosis factor (TNF)-α and Fas ligand, by activation of matrix metalloproteinase (MMP)- 9 and -2 and then induces apoptosis of host cells [45]. Based on the significant roles of SpeB as critical virulence factor, SpeB combined with inactive SpeA, Streptococcal pyrogenic endotoxin, has been considered as a potential vaccine candidate, which can produce neutralizing antibodies to prevent Streptococcal infection [47].

C5a peptidase, also called SCPA, is a cell wall-anchored immunogenic 125-kDa protein and a well-conserved antigen in Streptococci, and enzymatically cleaves the compliment component C5a to specifically inactivate [48–50]. As an adhesin, C5a peptidase binds directly integrin by the Arg-Gly-Asp (RGD) motifs and the extracellular matrix, fibronectin, with high affinity as well to epithelial cells [51]. This peptidase also inhibits neutrophil chemotaxis and the recruitment of phagocytes to the site of Streptococcal infection by cleavage of C5a and promotes invasion and colonization on damaged epithelium as invasin [26,51]. Therefore, C5a peptidase plays roles as a virulence factor through its multifunctional activities and is considered to be a promising vaccine candidate.

3. Pathogenic Factors Associated with Biofilm Formation

The characteristics of biofilm include high resistance to antibiotics and host immunity, as described above. Therefore, the Center for Disease Control (CDC) has warned that biofilm is involved in over 65% of human bacterial infections which are difficult to prevent, and that the emergence of multidrug-resistant bacteria and delays in biofilm measures is a serious problem in the entire medical field. Biofilm formed in the microbial immediate environment after their colonization creates a self-produced matrix consisting of extracellular polymeric substances (EPS), which are composed of polysaccharides, proteins, nucleic acids, and lipids [52]. EPS confers the adhesion ability and mechanical stability of biofilm, as well as embedded bacterial cells. Regarding the roles of biofilm in the etiology of systemic infectious diseases, the characteristic of resistance against abuse of a wider spectrum of antibiotics for biofilm infections has been focused on, and it has been considered that the ineffectiveness of the antimicrobial agent as a major feature of biofilm is greatly involved in the emergences of multidrug-resistant bacteria and higher toxic pathogens [7]. It has been also reported that the transformation is caused by frequent horizontal gene transfer, which occurs between bacteria in dental plaque biofilm. This leads to the acquisition of new resistance genes and high antibiotic resistance [53]. Moreover, microorganisms in biofilm share their metabolites and have an intercellular communication (cell-cell interaction) mechanism called quorum sensing (QS) that senses the cell density showing numbers of self and different species and synchronously regulates the expression of specific genes encoding virulent factors, such as enzymes and toxins. Therefore, solving these antibiotics-dependent problems requires the development of novel therapeutic methods to effectively suppress the biofilm formation without selective pressure, not using selective microorganisms based on the conventional antimicrobial sensitivity or the mechanism of antimicrobial action. Biofilm forms and matures through several stages (Figure 1). At each stage in the life style of biofilm, focusing on molecules common in bacteria involved in biofilm formation may lead to develop novel therapeutic agents. The first step of biofilm formation is that floating bacteria attaching to the biological surfaces, and this adhesion process is involved in various bacterial products and adhesins, including pili and surface proteins as described in the previous section.

3.1. Bis-(3′-5′)-Cyclic Dimeric Guanosine Monophosphate (Cyclic di-GMP) as a Bacterial Second Messenger

The attached bacteria grow and increase their number to form a microcolony, and subsequently produce extracellular matrix components consisting of polysaccharides, DNA, and proteins which connect the bacterial cells and strengthen the adhesion to the biological surface. The extracellular matrix of mature biofilm protects bacterial cells from the stresses, such as phagocytosis by host cells and oxidation, and bacterial communication in biofilm is more highly activated by the accumulation of signal substances and metabolites involved in QS. Some dispersal bacteria detached from the mature biofilm attach themselves to the new biological surface and then cause the infection to spread. Recently, it has been shown that an intracellular second messenger called bis-(3′-5′)-cyclic dimeric guanosine monophosphate (cyclic-di-GMP) plays an important role in the transition from reversible attachment to irreversible attachment and also regulates various genes expression through transcriptional factors [54]. With regard to the transition from the floating state to the biofilm state and vice versa, it has been reported that the change in the concentration of cyclic-di-GMP, the intracellular second messenger in bacterial cells, regulates the bacterial virulence, motility, the cell cycle and the synthesis of extracellular matrix, as well as biofilm formation [55]. Most cyclic-di-GMP-dependent signaling pathways also regulate the ability of bacteria to interact with other bacterial and eukaryotic cells. Therefore, cyclic di-GMP plays important roles in biofilm lifestyle including the multicellular bacterial biofilm development. Regarding these abilities, the modulation of bacterial cyclic-di-GMP signaling pathways might be a novel potential way to control biofilm formation in the medical area, and cyclic-di-GMP is considered to be a possible candidate for a vaccine adjuvant [56].

3.2. Extracellular DNA (eDNA)

In addition to polysaccharides and proteins, the extracellular matrix components in biofilm contain not only bacteria but also DNA derived from the host, and the interaction of eDNA in biofilm with other extracellular matrix components is also considered in terms of pathogenic factors in biofilm (Table 3). The roles of these eDNAs in the formation of biofilm have been also focused on as a target to replace or complement the use of antibiotics [57]. A previous study reported that the addition of DNase I suppresses biofilm formation and also degrades the mature biofilm, suggesting that eDNA is essential for biofilm formation and maturation as well as for its structural maintenance properties [58]. Therefore, it has been considered that enzymatic degradation of eDNA can prevent biofilm formation or sensitize biofilm to antimicrobials. Regarding oral bacterial biofilm, evidence showing eDNA plays a number of important roles in biofilm formation and maturation on oral soft and hard tissues and in its structural integrity has been accumulated [59]. The concentration of eDNA in Streptococcal biofilm is also involved in strength and rigidity of biofilm structure as well as biofilm formation and maturation. When the concentration of eDNA in Streptococcal biofilm is extremely high, biofilm maturation is suppressed and the bacteria in biofilm tends to detach [60]. This suggests that a high concentration of eDNA in formed or matured biofilm makes its structure fragile and makes bacteria easily disperse. In other words, when the concentration of eDNA in biofilm is increased and its concentration reaches a certain level, some bacteria in biofilm are detached and then attach to new sites to form biofilm, resulting in the spread of infection. Intriguingly, DNA derived from different bacteria, such as *Escherichia coli*, *Staphylococcus aureus*, and *Pseudomonas aeruginosa* in humans have also shown similar characteristics [60]. A recent interesting study has reported that calcium ion-regulated autolysin AtlA maturation mediates the release of eDNA by *S. mutans*, which contributes to its biofilm formation in infective endocarditis [61]. Therefore, all eDNAs present in biofilm, regardless of their origin, have been shown to be involved in biofilm formation, maturation, and structure, and an eDNA-targeting novel strategy may be applicable to novel treatments for bacterial biofilm-related infectious diseases.

Table 3. Interaction of eDNA with other pathogenic factors present in the extracellular matrix of biofilm.

Pathogenic Factors	Roles
1. DNA binding proteins	Binding to eDNA strand Present in the biofilm matrix and on the surface of bacterial cells Involvement in transformation ability
2. Toxins	Cross-linked with eDNA Secreted virulence factor Insoluble nuclear-protein complex formation
3. Pili	Binding to eDNA Involvement in motility Involvement in the structure of biofilm
4. Polysaccharides	Co-localization with eDNA
5. Membrane Vesicles	Interaction with eDNA Involvement in the secretion and transport of DNA, toxins and cell membrane components such as lipoproteins to outside of bacterial cells

3.3. DNA Binding Protein

The eukaryotic cell has a protein called histone, which plays a role of compactly housing its chromosomal DNA in the nucleus. Prokaryotes, such as bacteria, also have histone-like DNA binding protein (HLP) to compactly house their chromosomal DNA in small bacterial cells. The bacterial HLP equivalent to eukaryotic histone goes beyond the concept of the nucleoid-related protein which forms a DNA-protein complex, and involves itself in various intracellular processes, including the binding ability to DNA and mRNA, regulation of gene transcription and translation, replication, and rearrangement. To clarify the pathogenicity and roles of HLP in biofilm, we cloned the *hlp* gene of *S. intermedius* (*Si-hlp*) and sequenced its DNA. Through the homology analysis of the amino acid sequence predicted from its DNA sequence, it has been revealed that HLP has high homology (89–94%) at an amino acid sequence level and is structurally highly conserved in Streptococci [62,63]. Further functional analysis showed that *Si*-HLP forms homodimers outside of the cells and co-stimulation of *Si*-HLP with pathogen-associated molecular patterns (PAMPs) produced by bacteria synergistically or additively induces pro-inflammatory cytokines production in human monocytes, indicating that HLP itself has a possible role in causing inflammation at the site of bacterial infection [62]. Moreover, the knockdown of HLP expression with the antisense RNA expression system inhibits the growth of *S. intermedius* and suppresses its biofilm formation, suggesting that HLP is an essential protein for the viability and growth of *S. intermedius* as well as biofilm formation [63]. The knockdown of HLP reduced the hydrophobicity of the cell surface and suppressed the expression of its cytolytic toxin, intermedilysin, which is the main pathogenic factor of *S. intermedius*, suggesting that HLP also affects the regulation of pathogenic factors expression in addition to bacterial adhesion and aggregation [63]. As a bacterial pathogenic factor, HLP is not only involved in bacterial survival, growth, biofilm formation, and maturation, but also has the ability to directly induce pro-inflammatory responses in host cells and therefore HLP has huge roles in bacterial infection. Interestingly, fluorescence microscopic observation showed that eDNA and *Si*-HLP in biofilm were co-localized and uniformly distributed in biofilm (Figure 4). These findings suggest that HLP in addition to eDNA may also be a target as a novel treatment for biofilm infection control.

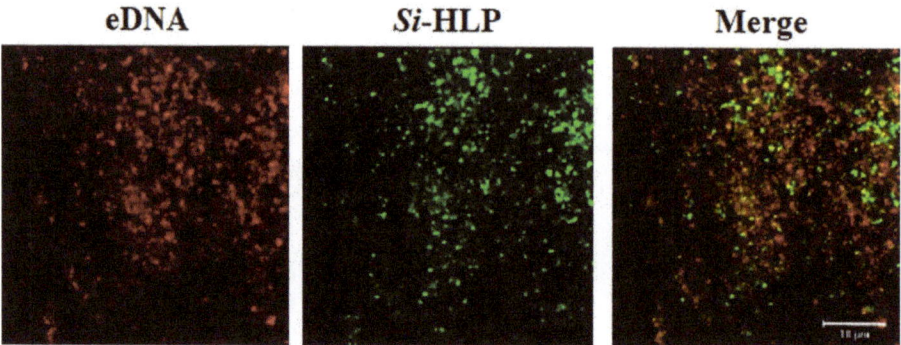

Figure 4. Co-localization and distribution of eDNA and *Si*-HLP in *S. intermedius* biofilm. eDNA in the formed *S. intermedius* biofilm was stained with propidium iodide (PI; red fluorescence), and *Si*-HLP was stained with anti-*Si*-HLP antibody and Alexafluor 488 (green fluorescence). Fluorescence microscopic observation showed that eDNA and HLP are co-localized (yellow fluorescence) and uniformly distributed in biofilm.

3.4. Membrane Vesicle

Membrane vesicles released from lots of bacterial species extracellularly contain proteins, nucleic acids such as DNA and RNA, and toxins. Lipoproteins, one of PAMPs, are also included as the cell membrane components of the surface of vesicles and released from the vesicles. Released PAMPs induce pro-inflammatory cytokines production after binding to the pattern recognition receptors (PRRs) expressed in host cells, suggesting that vesicles are involved in the exacerbation of inflammation [64]. Studies on membrane vesicles has been studied mainly using Gram-negative bacteria for a long time, but many research results on membrane vesicles of Gram-positive bacteria have been also shown increasingly in the last 10 years [65]. Membrane vesicles contained in the extracellular matrix of biofilm have various biological functions, such as intercellular communication, transport of toxins in vesicles, and horizontal gene transfer. Moreover, due to the similarity to liposomes, membrane vesicles is being tried in applications as drug delivery systems and vaccines using nanobiotechnology in the medical field [66].

As the second step following this bacterial adherence and biofilm formation, bacteria, which evaded antimicrobial peptides and host defense systems such as neutrophils and internalization by macrophages, invade the susceptible tissues to stimulate host cellular responses using capsule and PAMPs, such as lipoteichoic acid (LTA), in Streptococci. Neutrophils, key response cells recruited to the infectious site, release granule proteins and chromatin that together form extracellular fibers that bind bacteria. These neutrophil extracellular traps (NETs) are a form of innate response that binds microorganisms, prevents them from spreading, and degrade virulence factors and kill bacteria [67]. A recent intriguing study has shown that a nuclease, DeoC, in *S. mutans* degrades NETs and contributes to the escape of *S. mutans* from neutrophil killing and to the spread of *S. mutans* through biofilm dispersal [68]. After invasion into host cells and blood vessels of bacteria evaded from host innate defense system, bacteria are disseminated to tissues around the infection site and dispersed to colonize new sites through the blood stream.

4. Effects of Oral Streptococci on Systemic Diseases

The Viridans Group Streptococci is one of the most predominant bacterial groups in the oral bacterial flora, and has long been considered to be pathogens of severe infections such as infective endocarditis, sepsis, and meningitis (Table 1) [69]. In recent years, among the pathogenic factors possessed by the cariogenic bacterium *S. mutans*, a collagen binding protein (CBP, coding gene; *cnm*) has been focused for being associated with various systemic diseases. *S. mutans* expressing a CBP invade blood vessels, damage vascular endothelial cells, bind to collagen in the vascular endothelium to suppress platelet aggregation, and induce the expression of MMP-9, finally leading to the exacerbation of cerebral hemorrhage [70]. The epidemiological research also showed that the correlation between the occurrence of brain microbleeding and the high detection rate of CBP-positive *S. mutans* strains, suggesting that CBP-positive *S. mutans* is an independent risk for the onset and progression of cerebrovascular diseases [71]. Moreover, *S. mutans* expressing a CBP invade blood vessels, reach the liver and are then taken up into hepatic parenchymal cells to induce the production of cytokines such as interferon (IFN)-γ in the liver. It has also been reported that the imbalance of immune reactions and immune mechanisms caused by the infection of *cnm*-positive *S. mutans* leads to aggravation and deterioration of enteritis and ulcerative colitis in the digestive tracts [72]. Furthermore, the relationship between high DMFT (decayed, missing, and filled teeth) index and high urinary protein levels in patients with *cnm*-positive *S. mutans* has been shown and also suggests the association of its infection with renal diseases such as IgA nephropathy [73]. Recent study has reported that a 190-kDa protein antigen (PA), known as SpaP, P1 and antigen 1/2, of *S. mutans* affects the interaction with human serum, and the heart valves extirpated from rat infected with CBP-positive/PA-negative *S. mutans* strain showed prominent bacterial mass formation using in vivo infective endocarditis model, suggesting that CBP-positive/PA-negative *S. mutans* strain contribute to the pathogenicity in infective endocarditis [74].

5. Relationship Between Oral Streptococci and Autoimmune Diseases

Autoimmune diseases are types of chronic inflammation that occur in target organs as a result of the failure of immune tolerance to self-antigens and cellular immune responses by antibodies produced against self-antigens. In recent years, in addition to the reaction to the microorganisms which caused some types of infections, "molecular mimic" which cross-reacts with self-antigens has been considered to play roles in the mechanisms of onset and progression of autoimmune diseases. From this point of view, since the oral cavity is inhabited by lots of bacteria, it is always exposed to antigens derived from various bacteria, suggesting an association between the sensitization to antigens from resident bacteria and the onset of autoimmune diseases.

Regarding the association between oral bacteria, especially Gram-positive bacteria, and autoimmune diseases, some studies have focused on primary biliary cirrhosis (PBC) as autoimmune diseases. PBC is an autoimmune disease of unknown pathogenesis that often occurs in postmenopausal middle-aged women and its lesion is mainly composed of non-suppurative inflammation (chronic non-suppurative destructive cholangitis) around the intrahepatic small bile ducts. With progression of PBC to liver failure from liver cirrhosis, liver transplantation is the only way to treat the disease, and therefore it has been considered that PBC is an intractable disease. Laboratory findings of patients with PBC show that elevated biliary tract enzymes and high levels of IgM, and positive results for many autoantibodies, such as anti-mitochondrial antibody and anti-gp210, nuclear membrane protein, at a high rate (> 90%). Previous reports showed that LTA, a cell wall component of Gram-positive bacteria, was detected in the cytoplasm of lymphocytes and plasma cells infiltrating the site of chronic non-suppurative inflammation around interlobular bile ducts and in the serum of PBC patients, and it has been also reported that the levels of anti-LTA antibodies of IgM and IgA classes in PBC patients are higher than compared to those in healthy subjects and in patients with chronic hepatitis C, indicating that some Gram-positive bacteria might be involved in the onset and progression of PBC [75,76]. Moreover, the results of ELISA using whole cells of several Gram-positive Streptococci showed that the sera of PBC patients are highly reactive with these Streptococcal bacteria, especially *S. intermedius* and *Si*-HLP, compared to those of healthy subjects and patients with chronic hepatitis C, and HLP was detected in the lesion of PBC by immunohistochemical staining [77]. These results suggest that Streptococci and HLP may play important roles in the onset and progression of PBC. The administration of either live or heat-killed several Streptococci including *S. intermedius* twice a week for 8 weeks to the gingiva of BALB/c mice cause chronic non-suppurative inflammation around portal vein and the liver small bile ducts closely resembling PBC. Moreover, PBC-like clinical condition is observed even 20 months after the last administration and immunohistochemical staining showed that HLP was also detected in the non-suppurative inflammation area around the small bile duct of the liver, and inflammation was observed in the renal tubules [78]. Interestingly, although no bacteria were detected in the infected focal area, the depositions of LTA and HLP were observed around the small bile ducts similar to tissues from PBC patients, and the transplantation with the splenocytes (T cells) of this mouse into RAG2$^{-/-}$ immunodeficient mice caused similar chronic non-suppurative inflammation around the small bile ducts [79]. These findings also suggest the relationship between oral biofilm infection and autoimmune diseases. In patients with PBC, anti-gp210 autoantibodies are positive, and these positive patients progress to cirrhosis at a high rate compared to negative patients, and therefore anti-gp210 antibody levels are treated as a prognostic factor and are suggested to be deeply involved in the progression of PBC. More interestingly, a previous study reported that the epitope of gp210 was also found within the HLP sequence and the anti-HLP antibody cross-reacted with gp210 in mouse, indicating the sharing of the epitope [78]. Taken together, it has been suggested that Streptococci, especially dominant resident bacteria in the oral cavity and LTA, are strongly associated with the onset and progression of PBC.

6. Conclusions

The oral cavity is suggested as the reservoir of bacterial infection, and the oral and pharyngeal biofilms formed by oral bacterial flora have been found to be associated with various systemic diseases such as cardiovascular disease, arteriosclerosis, and diabetes. With the increasingly aging society, the rate of the elderly people with compromised immune function that are susceptible to infection is high and the onset and spread of infectious diseases among elderly people in nursing homes have become a major social problem. Therefore, the establishment of more effective prevention and treatment methods to reduce or minimize bacterial biofilm-related infectious diseases and their systemic complications is desired. However, even now, it has been pointed out that abuse of antibiotics for biofilm infections leads to the acquisition of antibiotic resistance and the emergence of higher toxic pathogens, such as emergence of multidrug resistant bacteria. In order to solve these problems, the development of therapeutic methods to effectively suppress the bacterial attachment, colonization, and biofilm formation without selective pressure, not for selective measures based on the conventional antimicrobial sensitivity or the mechanism of antimicrobial action, is expected. Regarding biofilm, which is the cause of bacterial infections, and considering its life cycle and its pathogenic factors, nucleic acids, such as DNAs that are commonly possessed by microorganisms, DNA binding proteins widely structurally conserved among microorganisms, and cyclic-di-GMP, intracellular second messenger involved in bacterial virulence and biofilm formation, may possibly be considered as target molecules to prevent and treat biofilm infections. Nucleic acids and their receptors are attracting attention as targets for the development of therapeutics not only for infectious diseases but also for other systemic diseases, such as autoimmune diseases and cancer. Therefore, the development of further research is expected.

Funding: This research received no external funding.

Conflicts of Interest: The authors declare no conflict of interest.

Abbreviations

LPS	Lipopolysaccharide
HSP	heat shock protein
GAS	group A Streptococcus
SpeB	Streptococcal pyrogenic exotoxin B
TNF	tumor necrosis factor
MMP	matrix metalloproteinase
RGD	Arg-Gly-Asp

EPS	extracellular polymeric substances
QS	quorum sensing
cyclic-di-GMP	bis-(3′-5′)-cyclic dimeric guanosine monophosphate
HLP	histone-like DNA binding protein
PAMPs	pathogen-associated molecular patterns
PRRs	pattern recognition receptors
LTA	lipoteichoic acid
NETs	neutrophil extracellular traps
CBP	collagen binding protein
DMFT	decayed, missing, and filled teeth
PA	190-kDa protein antigen
PBC	primary biliary cirrhosis

References

1. Dewhirst, F.E.; Chen, T.; Izard, J.; Paster, B.J.; Tanner, A.C.; Yu, W.H.; Lakshmanan, A.; Wade, W.G. The human oral microbiome. *J. Bacteriol.* **2010**, *192*, 5002–5017. [CrossRef] [PubMed]
2. Zbinden, A.; Bostanci, N.; Belibasakis, G.N. The novel species streptococcus tigurinus and its association with oral infection. *Virulence* **2015**, *6*, 177–182. [CrossRef] [PubMed]
3. Flemming, H.C.; Wingender, J.; Szewzyk, U.; Steinberg, P.; Rice, S.A.; Kjelleberg, S. Biofilms: An emergent form of bacterial life. *Nat. Rev. Microbiol.* **2016**, *14*, 563–575. [CrossRef] [PubMed]
4. Struzycka, I. The oral microbiome in dental caries. *Pol. J. Microbiol.* **2014**, *63*, 127–135. [PubMed]
5. Sitkiewicz, I. How to become a killer, or is it all accidental? Virulence strategies in oral streptococci. *Mol. Oral Microbiol.* **2018**, *33*, 1–12. [CrossRef] [PubMed]
6. Whiley, R.A.; Beighton, D. Current classification of the oral streptococci. *Oral Microbiol. Immunol.* **1998**, *13*, 195–216. [CrossRef] [PubMed]
7. Krzysciak, W.; Pluskwa, K.K.; Jurczak, A.; Koscielniak, D. The pathogenicity of the streptococcus genus. *Eur. J. Clin. Microbiol. Infect. Dis.* **2013**, *32*, 1361–1376. [CrossRef] [PubMed]
8. Richards, V.P.; Palmer, S.R.; Pavinski Bitar, P.D.; Qin, X.; Weinstock, G.M.; Highlander, S.K.; Town, C.D.; Burne, R.A.; Stanhope, M.J. Phylogenomics and the dynamic genome evolution of the genus streptococcus. *Genome Biol. Evol.* **2014**, *6*, 741–753. [CrossRef] [PubMed]
9. Frandsen, E.V.; Pedrazzoli, V.; Kilian, M. Ecology of viridans streptococci in the oral cavity and pharynx. *Oral Microbiol. Immunol.* **1991**, *6*, 129–133. [CrossRef] [PubMed]
10. Abranches, J.; Zeng, L.; Kajfasz, J.K.; Palmer, S.R.; Chakraborty, B.; Wen, Z.T.; Richards, V.P.; Brady, L.J.; Lemos, J.A. Biology of oral streptococci. *Microbiol. Spectr.* **2018**, *6*. [CrossRef]
11. Kim, S.L.; Gordon, S.M.; Shrestha, N.K. Distribution of streptococcal groups causing infective endocarditis: A descriptive study. *Diagn Microbiol. Infect. Dis.* **2018**, *91*, 269–272. [CrossRef] [PubMed]
12. Smith, E.G.; Spatafora, G.A. Gene regulation in s. Mutans: Complex control in a complex environment. *J. Dent. Res.* **2012**, *91*, 133–141. [CrossRef] [PubMed]
13. Ng, K.W.; Mukhopadhyay, A. Streptococcus constellatus bacteremia causing septic shock following tooth extraction: A case report. *Cases J.* **2009**, *2*, 6493. [CrossRef] [PubMed]
14. Tran, M.P.; Caldwell-McMillan, M.; Khalife, W.; Young, V.B. Streptococcus intermedius causing infective endocarditis and abscesses: A report of three cases and review of the literature. *BMC Infect. Dis.* **2008**, *8*, 154. [CrossRef] [PubMed]
15. Neumayr, A.; Kubitz, R.; Bode, J.G.; Bilk, B.; Haussinger, D. Multiple liver abscesses with isolation of streptococcus intermedius related to a pyogenic dental infection in an immuno-competent patient. *Eur J. Med. Res.* **2010**, *15*, 319–322. [CrossRef] [PubMed]
16. Whiley, R.A.; Beighton, D.; Winstanley, T.G.; Fraser, H.Y.; Hardie, J.M. Streptococcus intermedius, streptococcus constellatus, and streptococcus anginosus (the streptococcus milleri group): Association with different body sites and clinical infections. *J. Clin. Microbiol.* **1992**, *30*, 243–244.
17. Fisher, L.E.; Russell, R.R. The isolation and characterization of milleri group streptococci from dental periapical abscesses. *J. Dent. Res.* **1993**, *72*, 1191–1193. [CrossRef]
18. Socransky, S.S.; Haffajee, A.D.; Cugini, M.A.; Smith, C.; Kent, R.L., Jr. Microbial complexes in subgingival plaque. *J. Clin. Periodontol* **1998**, *25*, 134–144. [CrossRef]

19. Burton, J.P.; Drummond, B.K.; Chilcott, C.N.; Tagg, J.R.; Thomson, W.M.; Hale, J.D.; Wescombe, P.A. Influence of the probiotic streptococcus salivarius strain m18 on indices of dental health in children: A randomized double-blind, placebo-controlled trial. *J. Med. Microbiol.* **2013**, *62*, 875–884. [CrossRef]
20. Nobbs, A.H.; Jenkinson, H.F.; Everett, D.B. Generic determinants of streptococcus colonization and infection. *Infect. Genet. Evol.* **2015**, *33*, 361–370. [CrossRef]
21. Cunningham, M.W. Pathogenesis of group a streptococcal infections and their sequelae. *Adv. Exp. Med. Biol* **2008**, *609*, 29–42. [PubMed]
22. Brady, L.J.; Maddocks, S.E.; Larson, M.R.; Forsgren, N.; Persson, K.; Deivanayagam, C.C.; Jenkinson, H.F. The changing faces of streptococcus antigen i/ii polypeptide family adhesins. *Mol. Microbiol.* **2010**, *77*, 276–286. [CrossRef] [PubMed]
23. Nobbs, A.H.; Lamont, R.J.; Jenkinson, H.F. Streptococcus adherence and colonization. *Microbiol. Mol. Biol Rev.* **2009**, *73*, 407–450. [CrossRef] [PubMed]
24. Zhang, S.; Green, N.M.; Sitkiewicz, I.; Lefebvre, R.B.; Musser, J.M. Identification and characterization of an antigen i/ii family protein produced by group a streptococcus. *Infect. Immun.* **2006**, *74*, 4200–4213. [CrossRef] [PubMed]
25. Christie, J.; McNab, R.; Jenkinson, H.F. Expression of fibronectin-binding protein fbpa modulates adhesion in streptococcus gordonii. *Microbiology* **2002**, *148*, 1615–1625. [CrossRef] [PubMed]
26. Walker, M.J.; Barnett, T.C.; McArthur, J.D.; Cole, J.N.; Gillen, C.M.; Henningham, A.; Sriprakash, K.S.; Sanderson-Smith, M.L.; Nizet, V. Disease manifestations and pathogenic mechanisms of group a streptococcus. *Clin. Microbiol. Rev.* **2014**, *27*, 264–301. [CrossRef] [PubMed]
27. Yamaguchi, M.; Terao, Y.; Kawabata, S. Pleiotropic virulence factor-streptococcus pyogenes fibronectin-binding proteins. *Cell Microbiol.* **2013**, *15*, 503–511. [CrossRef]
28. Aviles-Reyes, A.; Miller, J.H.; Lemos, J.A.; Abranches, J. Collagen-binding proteins of streptococcus mutans and related streptococci. *Mol. Oral Microbiol.* **2017**, *32*, 89–106. [CrossRef]
29. Kahn, F.; Hurley, S.; Shannon, O. Platelets promote bacterial dissemination in a mouse model of streptococcal sepsis. *Microbes Infect.* **2013**, *15*, 669–676. [CrossRef]
30. Xiong, Y.Q.; Bensing, B.A.; Bayer, A.S.; Chambers, H.F.; Sullam, P.M. Role of the serine-rich surface glycoprotein gspb of streptococcus gordonii in the pathogenesis of infective endocarditis. *Microb. Pathog.* **2008**, *45*, 297–301. [CrossRef]
31. Kimura, K.R.; Nakata, M.; Sumitomo, T.; Kreikemeyer, B.; Podbielski, A.; Terao, Y.; Kawabata, S. Involvement of t6 pili in biofilm formation by serotype m6 streptococcus pyogenes. *J. Bacteriol.* **2012**, *194*, 804–812. [CrossRef] [PubMed]
32. Pezzicoli, A.; Santi, I.; Lauer, P.; Rosini, R.; Rinaudo, D.; Grandi, G.; Telford, J.L.; Soriani, M. Pilus backbone contributes to group b streptococcus paracellular translocation through epithelial cells. *J. Infect. Dis.* **2008**, *198*, 890–898. [CrossRef] [PubMed]
33. Maisey, H.C.; Hensler, M.; Nizet, V.; Doran, K.S. Group b streptococcal pilus proteins contribute to adherence to and invasion of brain microvascular endothelial cells. *J. Bacteriol.* **2007**, *189*, 1464–1467. [CrossRef] [PubMed]
34. Barocchi, M.A.; Ries, J.; Zogaj, X.; Hemsley, C.; Albiger, B.; Kanth, A.; Dahlberg, S.; Fernebro, J.; Moschioni, M.; Masignani, V.; et al. A pneumococcal pilus influences virulence and host inflammatory responses. *Proc. Natl. Acad. Sci. USA* **2006**, *103*, 2857–2862. [CrossRef] [PubMed]
35. Maisey, H.C.; Quach, D.; Hensler, M.E.; Liu, G.Y.; Gallo, R.L.; Nizet, V.; Doran, K.S. A group b streptococcal pilus protein promotes phagocyte resistance and systemic virulence. *FASEB J.* **2008**, *22*, 1715–1724. [CrossRef] [PubMed]
36. Jiang, S.; Park, S.E.; Yadav, P.; Paoletti, L.C.; Wessels, M.R. Regulation and function of pilus island 1 in group b streptococcus. *J. Bacteriol.* **2012**, *194*, 2479–2490. [CrossRef] [PubMed]
37. Gianfaldoni, C.; Censini, S.; Hilleringmann, M.; Moschioni, M.; Facciotti, C.; Pansegrau, W.; Masignani, V.; Covacci, A.; Rappuoli, R.; Barocchi, M.A.; et al. Streptococcus pneumoniae pilus subunits protect mice against lethal challenge. *Infect. Immun.* **2007**, *75*, 1059–1062. [CrossRef] [PubMed]
38. Nilson, B.H.; Frick, I.M.; Akesson, P.; Forsen, S.; Bjorck, L.; Akerstrom, B.; Wikstrom, M. Structure and stability of protein h and the m1 protein from streptococcus pyogenes. Implications for other surface proteins of gram-positive bacteria. *Biochemistry* **1995**, *34*, 13688–13698. [CrossRef]

39. McNamara, C.; Zinkernagel, A.S.; Macheboeuf, P.; Cunningham, M.W.; Nizet, V.; Ghosh, P. Coiled-coil irregularities and instabilities in group a streptococcus m1 are required for virulence. *Science* **2008**, *319*, 1405–1408. [CrossRef]
40. Smeesters, P.R.; McMillan, D.J.; Sriprakash, K.S. The streptococcal m protein: A highly versatile molecule. *Trends Microbiol.* **2010**, *18*, 275–282. [CrossRef]
41. Pahlman, L.I.; Olin, A.I.; Darenberg, J.; Morgelin, M.; Kotb, M.; Herwald, H.; Norrby-Teglund, A. Soluble m1 protein of streptococcus pyogenes triggers potent t cell activation. *Cell Microbiol.* **2008**, *10*, 404–414. [CrossRef] [PubMed]
42. Henningham, A.; Chiarot, E.; Gillen, C.M.; Cole, J.N.; Rohde, M.; Fulde, M.; Ramachandran, V.; Cork, A.J.; Hartas, J.; Magor, G.; et al. Conserved anchorless surface proteins as group a streptococcal vaccine candidates. *J. Mol. Med.* **2012**, *90*, 1197–1207. [CrossRef] [PubMed]
43. Antikainen, J.; Kuparinen, V.; Lahteenmaki, K.; Korhonen, T.K. Enolases from gram-positive bacterial pathogens and commensal lactobacilli share functional similarity in virulence-associated traits. *FEMS Immunol. Med. Microbiol.* **2007**, *51*, 526–534. [CrossRef] [PubMed]
44. Nelson, D.C.; Garbe, J.; Collin, M. Cysteine proteinase speb from streptococcus pyogenes-a potent modifier of immunologically important host and bacterial proteins. *Biol Chem.* **2011**, *392*, 1077–1088. [CrossRef] [PubMed]
45. Tamura, F.; Nakagawa, R.; Akuta, T.; Okamoto, S.; Hamada, S.; Maeda, H.; Kawabata, S.; Akaike, T. Proapoptotic effect of proteolytic activation of matrix metalloproteinases by streptococcus pyogenes thiol proteinase (streptococcus pyrogenic exotoxin b). *Infect. Immun.* **2004**, *72*, 4836–4847. [CrossRef] [PubMed]
46. Barnett, T.C.; Liebl, D.; Seymour, L.M.; Gillen, C.M.; Lim, J.Y.; Larock, C.N.; Davies, M.R.; Schulz, B.L.; Nizet, V.; Teasdale, R.D.; et al. The globally disseminated m1t1 clone of group a streptococcus evades autophagy for intracellular replication. *Cell Host Microbe* **2013**, *14*, 675–682. [CrossRef]
47. Morefield, G.; Touhey, G.; Lu, F.; Dunham, A.; HogenEsch, H. Development of a recombinant fusion protein vaccine formulation to protect against streptococcus pyogenes. *Vaccine* **2014**, *32*, 3810–3815. [CrossRef]
48. Brown, C.K.; Gu, Z.Y.; Matsuka, Y.V.; Purushothaman, S.S.; Winter, L.A.; Cleary, P.P.; Olmsted, S.B.; Ohlendorf, D.H.; Earhart, C.A. Structure of the streptococcal cell wall c5a peptidase. *Proc. Natl. Acad. Sci. USA* **2005**, *102*, 18391–18396. [CrossRef]
49. Sagar, V.; Bergmann, R.; Nerlich, A.; McMillan, D.J.; Nitsche Schmitz, D.P.; Chhatwal, G.S. Variability in the distribution of genes encoding virulence factors and putative extracellular proteins of streptococcus pyogenes in india, a region with high streptococcal disease burden, and implication for development of a regional multisubunit vaccine. *Clin. Vaccine Immunol.* **2012**, *19*, 1818–1825. [CrossRef]
50. Tamura, G.S.; Hull, J.R.; Oberg, M.D.; Castner, D.G. High-affinity interaction between fibronectin and the group b streptococcal c5a peptidase is unaffected by a naturally occurring four-amino-acid deletion that eliminates peptidase activity. *Infect. Immun.* **2006**, *74*, 5739–5746. [CrossRef]
51. Cheng, Q.; Stafslien, D.; Purushothaman, S.S.; Cleary, P. The group b streptococcal c5a peptidase is both a specific protease and an invasin. *Infect. Immun.* **2002**, *70*, 2408–2413. [CrossRef] [PubMed]
52. Flemming, H.C.; Wingender, J. The biofilm matrix. *Nat. Rev. Microbiol.* **2010**, *8*, 623–633. [CrossRef] [PubMed]
53. Li, Y.H.; Lau, P.C.; Lee, J.H.; Ellen, R.P.; Cvitkovitch, D.G. Natural genetic transformation of streptococcus mutans growing in biofilms. *J. Bacteriol.* **2001**, *183*, 897–908. [CrossRef] [PubMed]
54. Jakobsen, T.H.; Tolker-Nielsen, T.; Givskov, M. Bacterial biofilm control by perturbation of bacterial signaling processes. *Int J. Mol. Sci.* **2017**, *18*, 1970. [CrossRef] [PubMed]
55. McDougald, D.; Rice, S.A.; Barraud, N.; Steinberg, P.D.; Kjelleberg, S. Should we stay or should we go: Mechanisms and ecological consequences for biofilm dispersal. *Nat. Rev. Microbiol.* **2011**, *10*, 39–50. [CrossRef] [PubMed]
56. Romling, U.; Galperin, M.Y.; Gomelsky, M. Cyclic di-gmp: The first 25 years of a universal bacterial second messenger. *Microbiol. Mol. Biol Rev.* **2013**, *77*, 1–52. [CrossRef] [PubMed]
57. Okshevsky, M.; Regina, V.R.; Meyer, R.L. Extracellular DNA as a target for biofilm control. *Curr. Opin. Biotechnol.* **2015**, *33*, 73–80. [CrossRef]
58. Whitchurch, C.B.; Tolker-Nielsen, T.; Ragas, P.C.; Mattick, J.S. Extracellular DNA required for bacterial biofilm formation. *Science* **2002**, *295*, 1487. [CrossRef]
59. Jakubovics, N.S.; Burgess, J.G. Extracellular DNA in oral microbial biofilms. *Microbes Infect.* **2015**, *17*, 531–537. [CrossRef]

60. Nur, A.; Hirota, K.; Yumoto, H.; Hirao, K.; Liu, D.; Takahashi, K.; Murakami, K.; Matsuo, T.; Shu, R.; Miyake, Y. Effects of extracellular DNA and DNA-binding protein on the development of a streptococcus intermedius biofilm. *J. Appl. Microbiol.* **2013**, *115*, 260–270. [CrossRef]
61. Jung, C.J.; Hsu, R.B.; Shun, C.T.; Hsu, C.C.; Chia, J.S. Atla mediates extracellular DNA release, which contributes to streptococcus mutans biofilm formation in an experimental rat model of infective endocarditis. *Infect. Immun.* **2017**, *85*, e00252-17. [CrossRef]
62. Liu, D.; Yumoto, H.; Hirota, K.; Murakami, K.; Takahashi, K.; Hirao, K.; Matsuo, T.; Ohkura, K.; Nagamune, H.; Miyake, Y. Histone-like DNA binding protein of streptococcus intermedius induces the expression of pro-inflammatory cytokines in human monocytes via activation of erk1/2 and jnk pathways. *Cell Microbiol.* **2008**, *10*, 262–276. [CrossRef]
63. Liu, D.; Yumoto, H.; Murakami, K.; Hirota, K.; Ono, T.; Nagamune, H.; Kayama, S.; Matsuo, T.; Miyake, Y. The essentiality and involvement of streptococcus intermedius histone-like DNA-binding protein in bacterial viability and normal growth. *Mol. Microbiol.* **2008**, *68*, 1268–1282. [CrossRef] [PubMed]
64. Brown, L.; Wolf, J.M.; Prados-Rosales, R.; Casadevall, A. Through the wall: Extracellular vesicles in gram-positive bacteria, mycobacteria and fungi. *Nat. Rev. Microbiol.* **2015**, *13*, 620–630. [CrossRef] [PubMed]
65. Kim, J.H.; Lee, J.; Park, J.; Gho, Y.S. Gram-negative and gram-positive bacterial extracellular vesicles. *Semin Cell Dev. Biol* **2015**, *40*, 97–104. [CrossRef]
66. Toyofuku, M.; Tashiro, Y.; Hasegawa, Y.; Kurosawa, M.; Nomura, N. Bacterial membrane vesicles, an overlooked environmental colloid: Biology, environmental perspectives and applications. *Adv. Colloid Interface Sci.* **2015**, *226*, 65–77. [CrossRef]
67. Brinkmann, V.; Reichard, U.; Goosmann, C.; Fauler, B.; Uhlemann, Y.; Weiss, D.S.; Weinrauch, Y.; Zychlinsky, A. Neutrophil extracellular traps kill bacteria. *Science* **2004**, *303*, 1532–1535. [CrossRef] [PubMed]
68. Liu, J.; Sun, L.; Liu, W.; Guo, L.; Liu, Z.; Wei, X.; Ling, J. A nuclease from streptococcus mutans facilitates biofilm dispersal and escape from killing by neutrophil extracellular traps. *Front. Cell Infect. Microbiol.* **2017**, *7*, 97. [CrossRef] [PubMed]
69. Mitchell, T.J. The pathogenesis of streptococcal infections: From tooth decay to meningitis. *Nat. Rev. Microbiol.* **2003**, *1*, 219–230. [CrossRef] [PubMed]
70. Nakano, K.; Hokamura, K.; Taniguchi, N.; Wada, K.; Kudo, C.; Nomura, R.; Kojima, A.; Naka, S.; Muranaka, Y.; Thura, M.; et al. The collagen-binding protein of streptococcus mutans is involved in haemorrhagic stroke. *Nat. Commun* **2011**, *2*, 485. [CrossRef] [PubMed]
71. Miyatani, F.; Kuriyama, N.; Watanabe, I.; Nomura, R.; Nakano, K.; Matsui, D.; Ozaki, E.; Koyama, T.; Nishigaki, M.; Yamamoto, T.; et al. Relationship between cnm-positive streptococcus mutans and cerebral microbleeds in humans. *Oral Dis* **2015**, *21*, 886–893. [CrossRef] [PubMed]
72. Kojima, A.; Nakano, K.; Wada, K.; Takahashi, H.; Katayama, K.; Yoneda, M.; Higurashi, T.; Nomura, R.; Hokamura, K.; Muranaka, Y.; et al. Infection of specific strains of streptococcus mutans, oral bacteria, confers a risk of ulcerative colitis. *Sci. Rep.* **2012**, *2*, 332. [CrossRef] [PubMed]
73. Misaki, T.; Naka, S.; Hatakeyama, R.; Fukunaga, A.; Nomura, R.; Isozaki, T.; Nakano, K. Presence of streptococcus mutans strains harbouring the cnm gene correlates with dental caries status and iga nephropathy conditions. *Sci. Rep.* **2016**, *6*, 36455. [CrossRef] [PubMed]
74. Otsugu, M.; Nomura, R.; Matayoshi, S.; Teramoto, N.; Nakano, K. Contribution of streptococcus mutans strains with collagen-binding proteins in the presence of serum to the pathogenesis of infective endocarditis. *Infect. Immun.* **2017**, *85*, e00401-17. [CrossRef]
75. Tsuneyama, K.; Harada, K.; Kono, N.; Hiramatsu, K.; Zen, Y.; Sudo, Y.; Gershwin, M.E.; Ikemoto, M.; Arai, H.; Nakanuma, Y. Scavenger cells with gram-positive bacterial lipoteichoic acid infiltrate around the damaged interlobular bile ducts of primary biliary cirrhosis. *J. Hepatol.* **2001**, *35*, 156–163. [CrossRef]
76. Haruta, I.; Hashimoto, E.; Kato, Y.; Kikuchi, K.; Kato, H.; Yagi, J.; Uchiyama, T.; Kobayash, M.; Shiratori, K. Lipoteichoic acid may affect the pathogenesis of bile duct damage in primary biliary cirrhosis. *Autoimmunity* **2006**, *39*, 129–135. [CrossRef] [PubMed]
77. Haruta, I.; Kikuchi, K.; Hashimoto, E.; Kato, H.; Hirota, K.; Kobayashi, M.; Miyake, Y.; Uchiyama, T.; Yagi, J.; Shiratori, K. A possible role of histone-like DNA-binding protein of streptococcus intermedius in the pathogenesis of bile duct damage in primary biliary cirrhosis. *Clin. Immunol.* **2008**, *127*, 245–251. [CrossRef]

78. Haruta, I.; Kikuchi, K.; Hashimoto, E.; Nakamura, M.; Miyakawa, H.; Hirota, K.; Shibata, N.; Kato, H.; Arimura, Y.; Kato, Y.; et al. Long-term bacterial exposure can trigger nonsuppurative destructive cholangitis associated with multifocal epithelial inflammation. *Lab. Invest.* **2010**, *90*, 577–588. [CrossRef]
79. Haruta, I.; Kikuchi, K.; Nakamura, M.; Hirota, K.; Kato, H.; Miyakawa, H.; Shibata, N.; Miyake, Y.; Hashimoto, E.; Shiratori, K.; et al. Involvement of commensal bacteria may lead to dysregulated inflammatory and autoimmune responses in a mouse model for chronic nonsuppurative destructive cholangitis. *J. Clin. Immunol.* **2012**, *32*, 1026–1037. [CrossRef]

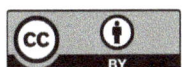

© 2019 by the authors. Licensee MDPI, Basel, Switzerland. This article is an open access article distributed under the terms and conditions of the Creative Commons Attribution (CC BY) license (http://creativecommons.org/licenses/by/4.0/).

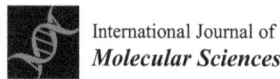

Review

T and B Cells in Periodontal Disease: New Functions in A Complex Scenario

C.M. Figueredo [1,2,*], R. Lira-Junior [3] and R.M. Love [1]

1. School of Dentistry and Oral Health, Griffith University, Queensland 4222, Australia
2. Menzies Health Institute Queensland, Griffith University, Gold Coast, QLD 4222, Australia
3. Division of Oral Diseases, Department of Dental Medicine, Karolinska Institutet, 141 04 Stockholm, Sweden
* Correspondence: c.dasilvafigueredo@griffith.edu.au; Tel.: +61-7-5678-0767

Received: 29 July 2019; Accepted: 13 August 2019; Published: 14 August 2019

Abstract: Periodontal disease is characterised by a dense inflammatory infiltrate in the connective tissue. When the resolution is not achieved, the activation of T and B cells is crucial in controlling chronic inflammation through constitutive cytokine secretion and modulation of osteoclastogenesis. The present narrative review aims to overview the recent findings of the importance of T and B cell subsets, as well as their cytokine expression, in the pathogenesis of the periodontal disease. T regulatory (Treg), $CD8^+$ T, and tissue-resident $\gamma\delta$ T cells are important to the maintenance of gingival homeostasis. In inflamed gingiva, however, the secretion of IL-17 and secreted osteoclastogenic factor of activated T cells (SOFAT) by activated T cells is crucial to induce osteoclastogenesis via RANKL activation. Moreover, the capacity of mucosal-associated invariant T cells (MAIT cells) to produce cytokines, such as IFN-γ, TNF-α, and IL-17, might indicate a critical role of such cells in the disease pathogenesis. Regarding B cells, low levels of memory B cells in clinically healthy periodontium seem to be important to avoid bone loss due to the subclinical inflammation that occurs. On the other hand, they can exacerbate alveolar bone loss in a receptor activator of nuclear factor kappa-B ligand (RANKL)-dependent manner and affect the severity of periodontitis. In conclusion, several new functions have been discovered and added to the complex knowledge about T and B cells, such as possible new functions for Tregs, the role of SOFAT, and MAIT cells, as well as B cells activating RANKL. The activation of distinct T and B cell subtypes is decisive in defining whether the inflammatory lesion will stabilise as chronic gingivitis or will progress to a tissue destructive periodontitis.

Keywords: lymphocyte; T cells; B cells; cytokine; periodontal disease

1. Introduction

Periodontal disease is an inflammatory response to bacterial biofilm accumulation around teeth. This host inflammatory response is mediated mainly by neutrophils, monocytes/macrophages, and T and B lymphocytes (T and B cells). The development of the disease is characterised by a dense inflammatory infiltrate in the connective tissue, in which polymorphonuclear leukocytes and macrophages are abundant immune cells that firstly respond to the bacterial insult. When inflammation is not resolved, antigen-presenting cells (APCs) are activated by bacterial products and interact with naive T helper cells (Th0), driving their differentiation into several subsets, such as Th1, Th2, Th9, Th17, T-follicular helper (Tfh), and regulatory T cells (Treg) [1]).

Overexpression of the Th17/Treg axis is seen in disease initiation, followed by persistence of the Th17 response in periodontitis progression in a non-human primate model of periodontitis [2]. Tregs are required to keep periodontal health homeostasis, where their presence is essential to ensure a controlled response that minimises collateral tissue damage [3]. However, recent evidence suggested Th17 might not be the main source of interleukin (IL)-17A in periodontal tissues, suggesting Tregs may have a more prominent role in the pathogenesis of the periodontal disease [4]. These findings might change our understanding of the current literature. More recently, a new cell type named mucosal-associated invariant T (MAIT) cells has been associated with autoimmune and other inflammatory diseases in humans [5] and its role in the periodontal disease pathogenesis should be taken into consideration.

B cells, on the other hand, are part of the adaptive humoral immunity specialised in secreting antibodies and cytokines, as well as presenting antigens, and have been strongly associated with periodontal homeostasis and disease [5]. A minimal presence of B cells in healthy gingiva has been reported [6,7], which might be important to avoid bone loss due to the subclinical inflammation that occurs in the clinically healthy periodontium. B cells in periodontitis patients may contribute to chronic systemic inflammation through cytokine secretion [8]. Memory B cells can induce bone loss in rheumatoid arthritis [9], which led to the hypothesis that they express RANKL and regulate alveolar bone homeostasis during periodontitis [10]. The present narrative review aims to overview the recent findings of the importance of T and B cell subsets, as well as their cytokine expression, in the pathogenesis of the periodontal disease.

2. T and B Lymphocytes

2.1. T Lymphocytes

T lymphocytes (T cells) are immune cells involved in host defence and control of immune-mediated inflammatory disease development. They can be distinguished from other lymphocytes by the presence of a T-cell receptor (TCR) on the cell surface. Most T cells are composed of two glycoprotein chains named α (alpha) and β (beta) TCR chains. However, a smaller group of T cells, named γδ T cells, presents a gamma/delta composition. They are an important subset of T cells as they can recognise a broad range of antigens without the presence of major histocompatibility complex (MHC) molecules [11]. T cells are subdivided into Th, Treg, T cytotoxic ($CD8^+$), natural killer, and memory cells. Also, T cell anergy has been defined as a mechanism of peripheral tolerance that determines the functional inactivation of T cells following antigen recognition under non-optimal conditions [12].

Naive $CD4^+$ T cells are activated after interaction with antigen-MHC complex and differentiate into specific subtypes depending on the cytokine microenvironment [13]. After such interactions, they become activated and differentiated into effector T cells, which are responsible for the production of effector molecules, such as pro-/anti-inflammatory cytokines and cytotoxic molecules. Most of the effector T cells undergo programmed cell death after the antigen clearance. The ones that survive differentiate into memory T cells. Th cells are classified as Th1, Th2, Th17, and Treg subpopulations based on their unique cytokine properties [14].

Besides the classical Th cell subpopulations, Tfh, Th9, and Th22 cells have recently been defined as new subpopulations that produce IL-21, IL-9, and IL-22, respectively [14,15]. Tfh is a specialised $CD4^+$ T-cell subset that provides survival, proliferation, and selection signals by engaging in cognate interactions with B cells [16]. Th9 cells have been shown to present both beneficial and detrimental functions. Among the beneficial functions is their ability to initiate antitumor immunity and immune response to helminth parasites [17]. Detrimental functions of Th9 cells include the promotion of allergic inflammation and the mediation of some types of autoimmunity [17]. Duhen et al. [18] showed that memory T cells with skin-homing properties from healthy donors are characterised by the production of IL-22 in the absence of IL-17 and IFN-γ. The authors found that several T cell clones isolated from psoriatic lesions were Th22. Their function is the specific production of IL-22, which has been linked to skin homeostasis and inflammation [14].

Cytotoxic T lymphocytes ($CD8^+$ T cells) are generated in the thymus and express a dimeric co-receptor, usually composed of one CD8α and one CD8β chain, and they recognise peptides presented by MHC class I molecules. $CD8^+$ T cells present three major mechanisms to kill infected or malignant cells: (a) secretion of cytokines, primarily TNF-α and IFN-γ, which have anti-tumor, anti-viral, and anti-microbial effects, (b) production and release of cytotoxic granules (also found in

NK cells), which contain two families of proteins, perforin and granzymes, and (c) destruction of infected cells via Fas/FasL interactions which can result in apoptosis of the target cell. Besides cytotoxic activities, $CD8^+$ T cells also have regulatory/suppressor functions ($CD8^+$ Treg), since they can control other leukocytes to avoid excessive immune activation and its pathological consequences [19].

Besides the T cells subgroups mentioned above, mucosal-associated invariant T (MAIT) cells represent a unique subset of innate-like T cells described in the late 1990s [20]. MAIT cells represent the most abundant innate-like T-cell population within human beings, comprising up to ~5% of the total T-cell population [21]. Characterisation of the MAIT cells in the buccal mucosa showed that the major subset displayed a tissue-resident and activated profile with high expression of CD69, CD103, HLA-DR, and PD-1. These tissue-resident MAIT cells produced higher IL-17 levels than tissue non-resident and circulating populations [22]. New research projects should be stimulated to better understanding the role of tissue-resident MAIT cells in the osteoclastogenesis activation in periodontal diseases.

2.2. B Lymphocytes

B lymphocytes (B cells) are part of the humoral component of the adaptive immune system and specialised in secreting antibodies. B cells can also present antigens and secrete cytokines. In mammals, B cells mature in the bone marrow, and B cell receptors (BCRs) mature on their cell membranes, which allow B cells to bind specific antigens initiating an antibody response. Such antigen recognition can happen through either low- or high-affinity binding modes [23]. After maturation, multiple subsets of B-cells co-expressing IgM and IgD emerge from the bone marrow and colonise compartments of secondary lymphoid organs [24].

B cell subpopulations can be distinguished in peripheral blood based on surface-marker expression, which mainly represents different developmental stages of the cell. Alterations in some of these populations have been associated with clinical phenotypes in immunodeficiency and autoimmune diseases. The second phase of B-cell development occurs after the antigen-dependent phase. Depending on various contacts and cytokine stimuli received by the activated cell, it will become either a memory cell to be activated once again in the future or it will become a plasma cell producing large amounts of antibodies [25].

Didactically, B cells can be subdivided as follows: plasmablasts (the immature precursor of plasmacytes), plasma cells (antibody-secreting cells arising from B cell differentiation), memory B cells (B2 cells and synonymous with classical B cells), marginal zone (MZ) B cells (specialized population of B cells that are located in the marginal zone of the spleen), B1 cells (subtype of B cells that are distinct from classical B cells with respect to their phenotype, distribution in the body, and function). Unlike classical B cells, B-1 cells are considered functionally to be part of the innate immune response [26]. Regulatory B cells (Breg) negatively regulate the immune response by producing regulatory cytokines and directly interacting with pathogenic T cells via cell-to-cell contact [27].

Abnormal B-cell recognition of self-antigens may lead to autoimmunity, which results in autoantibody production. Autoantibodies produced by B-cell-derived plasma cells provide diagnostic markers for autoimmunity, and also contribute significantly to disease pathogenesis [28]. Autoimmune diseases where B-cell functions are closely correlated with disease activity include systemic lupus erythematosus, rheumatoid arthritis, scleroderma, type 1 diabetes, and multiple sclerosis [28].

2.3. T and B Lymphocytes in Periodontal Homeostasis

2.3.1. T Lymphocytes

The characterisation of T lymphocytes in healthy gingiva has shown a dominance of $CD4^+$ helper T cells [6]. These cells play fundamental roles in the adaptive immune responses, and their cytokine production in response to specific immunological challenges led to the classical framework of distinct Th cell subsets [29]. $CD8^+$ T cells were the second most abundant T lymphocyte in healthy gingiva, followed by a small percentage of γδT cells. Gingival CD8+ T cells seem to have regulatory/suppressor properties important to the maintenance of gingival tissue integrity by downregulating inflammation under homeostatic conditions. These cells can produce IL-10 and TGF-β, which then suppress osteoclastogenesis [30]. Tissue-resident epithelial γδ T cells have been reported to be the major T cell population in the epithelial tissues and are important in carrying out barrier surveillance and helping to keep tissue homeostasis, and to some extent, epithelial repair [31]. Gingival γδ T cells accumulate after birth in response to barrier damage and are crucial for immune homeostasis. These cells produce amphiregulin, a wound healing-associated cytokine, which limits the development of periodontitis [32]. γδ T cells are also the major source of IL-17 in homeostasis. Interestingly, ablation of γδT cells resulted in increased gingival inflammation and alterations in the microbial diversity [33]. Within the CD4 compartment, about 15% are presumed to be Treg cells, which are crucial for periodontal homeostasis. Increased numbers of Tregs are associated with bone homeostasis, even in the presence of local inflammation [34] and may be related to the non-progression of gingivitis lesions in some patients, even after a long period of oral biofilm exposure. The new roles of γδT cells and Tregs in periodontal tissue homeostasis are crucial to the understanding of periodontal disease initiation and progression.

Dutzan et al. [6] characterised memory and naive T-cell subsets in the gingiva, showing that approximately 80% of CD4+ and 50% of CD8+ T cells had a CD45RO+ (activated T cell) memory phenotype. The CD4+ cell compartment in gingiva had a minimal CD45RA+ (naive T cell) population, but the CD8+ T cell compartment had a substantial population of CD45RA+/CCR7− cells (terminally differentiated effector T cells, T_{EMRA}) alongside a smaller population of naive CD45RA+CCR7+ cells [6,35]. CCR7 is a chemokine receptor that divides human memory T cells into two functionally distinct subsets. CCR7− memory cells express receptors for migration to inflamed tissues and display immediate effector function; CCR7+ memory cells lack immediate effector function, but efficiently stimulate dendritic cells and differentiate into CCR7− effector cells upon secondary stimulation [36].

The combination of CD45RO and CCR7 (memory subset markers) with CD69 (a stimulatory receptor expressed at sites of chronic inflammation) was performed by Dutzan et al. [6] to analyse circulating and tissue-resident memory CD4+ and CD8+ T cell subsets. Their results showed that the majority of CD4 memory T cells in gingiva were CCR7−CD69+ (resident effector memory, rT_{EM} cells), followed almost equally by resident memory, effector memory (T_{EM}), and central memory (rT_{CM}; CCR7+CD69+) cells. Regarding CD8, memory CD45RO+ cells were also rT_{EM} in their majority, followed by a large population of T_{EM} and a small population of central memory cells (T_{CM}). Increased proportions of resident memory T cells are common at barrier sites, where they have been reported to support early/immediate defence mechanisms, providing site-specific protection from pathogen challenges [37]. Resident memory T cells would then have special importance to protect the connective tissue form the bacterial products released in the periodontal sulcus.

Besides the T-cell characterisation, it is important to understand how these cells behave under physiological conditions. Having clinically healthy gingiva does not ensure that T cells are not being activated. Dutzan et al. [38], demonstrated in mouse gingiva that gingiva-resident Th17 cells developed via a commensal colonisation-independent mechanism. Th17 cells might accumulate at the gingiva in response to the physiological barrier damage that occurs, for instance, during mastication. The authors showed that physiological mechanical damage could induce the expression of IL-6 from epithelial cells, promoting an increase in gingival Th17 cell numbers.

2.3.2. B Lymphocytes

The characterisation of B cell subsets in gingival tissues was recently described by Mahanonda et al. [39]. The authors reported very few naïve B cells (<8%) in all stages of healthy and diseased tissues. Additionally, memory B cells (CD19+CD27+CD38−) represented the majority of the B cell population in the clinically healthy gingiva and were detected in the connective tissue subjacent to the apical region of the junctional epithelium, which could be due to the local low-grade inflammatory response to a constant challenge of the biofilm. The authors highlighted the importance of detecting memory B cells in clinically healthy human gingiva since very little is known about memory B cells residing in human nonlymphoid tissues. The minimal presence of B cells in healthy gingiva was also reported by others [6,7,35,40]. Such low levels might be important to avoid bone loss around teeth due to the subclinical inflammation that occurs in the clinically healthy periodontium.

Another aspect of the B cell biology that is relevant for gingival homeostasis is the production of antibodies against periodontal pathogens, which can contribute to host protection [41,42]. Page et al. [43] demonstrated that immunisation using *P. gingivalis* as antigen could reduce the onset and progression of alveolar bone loss in non-human primates. Also, Shelburne et al. [41] suggested that anti-*P. gingivalis* HtpG antibodies predict health in patients susceptible to periodontal disease. The potential role of B cell humoral immunity in maintaining homeostasis needs further investigations. A description of the main functions of T and B cells' subsets in the periodontal tissues is presented in the Table 1.

2.4. Changes with Age

Furthermore, age is also a variable that needs to be considered when evaluating the lymphocyte function in healthy periodontium. The effects of aging on periodontal tissues are thought to intensify alveolar bone resorption in elderly individuals [44]. Witkowski et al. [45] reviewed the proteodynamics in aging human T cells and reported that the proteolytic elimination of altered proteins, as well as modulation of the activity of those remaining, leads to the dynamic change of proteome composition and function in aging lymphocytes. Ebersole et al. [44] reported that several B cell and plasmacyte genes are altered in aging healthy gingival tissues, which are mainly associated with antigen-dependent activation and B cell differentiation/maturation processes. Aging T and B cell dynamics requires further comprehensive analysis and may influence the pathophysiology of periodontal disease.

2.5. T and B Lymphocytes in Periodontal Inflammation

In 1983, Okada et al. [46] published a very elegant paper characterising the immunocompetent cells on histological sections from diseased human gingiva. According to the authors, human periodontitis contains numerous sets of infiltrating cells which are organized unusually, with a region rich in T lymphocytes and monocytes/macrophages just subjacent to the pocket or sulcular epithelium; and a region in the central lamina propria, located farther away from the microbial agent, which is rich in B cells and plasma cells and poor in T lymphocytes. Furthermore, the same group characterised the T lymphocyte subsets (T4+ and T8+) in the inflamed gingiva from human periodontitis and showed the ratio T4+/T8+ was lower in gingival tissue than in peripheral blood [47]. Dutzan et al. [6] evaluated the major cell subsets and revealed that the lymphocytic compartment, CD3+T cells remained the dominant population in both health and disease, yet in disease the total number of T cells is much greater, reflecting a 10 fold increase in total inflammatory cells [6].

The role of T cells in the immune dysregulation of periodontitis has been consistently revised by Campbell et al. [1]. Activated Th1, Th2, and Th17 cells can produce a variety of pro-inflammatory cytokines, such as IL-1β, IL-17E (IL-25) and IL-17, that activate other immune cells such as dendritic cells, neutrophils, and B cells. Activation of both T cells and subsequently, B cells can cause the production of the receptor activator of nuclear factor κ B -Ligand (RANKL), which leads to alveolar bone resorption by osteoclasts, resulting in tooth loss. Moreover, the activation of B cells by Tfh in either peripheral lymph nodes or tertiary lymph organs can result in clonal activation of B cells, which produce antibodies to recognise bacterial components; however, production of autoantibodies to collagen, fibronectin and laminin can contribute to local destruction of the gingival tissue. Finally, a lack of Treg cells or an inability of those present to reduce local inflammatory responses by other immune cells may play a role in the chronic inflammation associated with periodontitis [1].

Table 1. A summary of the main functions of mentioned T and B cells in periodontal health and disease.

Cell	Subtype	Function in the Periodontal Tissues
T cells	Treg	Periodontal homeostasis by producing IL-10 and TGF-β.
	MAIT	Largely unknown.
	Th	Specific immunological challenges lead to distinct cells' subsets; Th1, Th2, and Th17 cells can produce a variety of pro-inflammatory cytokines that activate other immune cells such as dendritic cells, neutrophils, and B cells. Th17 can also be produced in response to biological barrier damage in healthy tissue.
	Tissue-resident epithelial γδ	Barrier surveillance, tissue homeostasis, and epithelial repair; Major source of IL-17 in homeostasis.
	CD8+	Downregulate inflammation and suppress osteoclastogenesis. IL-10 and TGF-β production.
	Tfh	Activation of B cells; IL-21 production.
	SOFAT	Induce osteoclastogenesis in a RANKL-independent manner.
	Activated	Activation and expression of RANKL in the gingiva; promote osteoclastogenesis.
	Memory	To prevent bone loss due to subclinical inflammation in clinically healthy periodontium.
B cells	Immunoglobulin-bearing lymphocytes; plasma cells	Production of antibodies against periodontal pathogens. Clinical progression of the periodontal lesion; Stimulate the expression of RANKL in the gingiva.
	B1	Associated with regulatory functions and the numbers might be decreased in periodontitis patients; produces antibodies against antigens and act as antigen-presenting cells.
	Breg/B10	Negatively regulates the inflammatory responses via IL-10.
	CD138+ plasma cells	Association with the advancing front of the periodontal lesion.

Treg: regulatory T cells; MAIT cells: mucosal-associated invariant T cells; Th: helper T cells; CD: cluster of differentiation; SOFAT: secreted osteoclastogenic factor of activated T cells; Tfh: T-follicular helper; Breg: regulatory B cel.

T cells have a crucial role in the tissue secretion of IL-17, a cytokine strongly associated with bone loss around teeth. Chen et al. [48] reported that IL-17 and IFN-γ levels in biopsy specimens of gingival lesions from chronic periodontitis patients were higher than those in the healthy controls. Moreover, relative IFN-γ, IL-17A, and T-bet mRNA levels were also significantly higher in patients with chronic periodontitis compared to controls, suggesting that Th17 and Th1 cells might be involved in the pathogenesis of chronic periodontitis. Dutzan et al. [6,35] characterised IL-17-secreting cells within the hematopoietic compartment in healthy and periodontitis gingival samples and found a significant increase in IL-17$^+$ cells in diseased sites. The major source of IL-17 was CD4$^+$ T cells, with minimal contribution from CD8, γδT, and non-T-cell sources.

Moreover, the percentage of CD4$^+$ T cells producing IL-17 significantly increased in periodontitis. CD4$^+$ T cells preferentially upregulated IL-17 and not IFN-γ in gingival tissue from periodontitis patients. The same group also reported that Th17 cells in periodontitis are dependent on the local dysbiotic microbiota, and both IL-6 and IL-23 are required for their accumulation. Also, pharmacologically targeting RORγt, a transcription factor relevant for Th17 differentiation, reduces alveolar bone loss in a murine model of periodontitis [49]. On the other hand, Parachuru et al. [4] presented an interesting paper that compared healthy/gingivitis tissues with chronic periodontitis tissues. Among other goals, they aimed to determine the identity of FoxP3 and IL-17A positive cells in periodontal tissues. The authors reported that Th17 cells either do not exist in periodontal disease or are present in small numbers and that, as with other chronic inflammatory lesions, the source of the relatively small amounts of IL-17 may be mast cells. Moreover, they also suggested that Tregs may have an important role in the pathogenesis of the chronic inflammatory periodontal disease. Such a statement needs to be better investigated since it might affect our present understanding of the Th17/Treg imbalance that leads to periodontal disease progression.

Besides the importance of IL-17 secreted by CD4$^+$ T cell or mast cells, a novel T cell-secreted cytokine, called secreted osteoclastogenic factor of activated T cells (SOFAT), that can induce osteoclastogenesis in a RANKL-independent manner, has been described in periodontal tissues [50]. The authors showed that the mRNA and protein levels of SOFAT were significantly higher in the gingival tissue of periodontitis patients compared to controls. More recently, Jarry et al. [51] demonstrated that B-lineage cells, including plasma cells, also exhibited strong staining for SOFAT in diseased periodontal tissue. Therefore, SOFAT might have an important role in periodontal disease by activating RANKL related osteoclastogenesis.

The characterisation and identification of interstitial T cells are relevant to understanding the immunopathogenesis of periodontitis. Bittner-Eddy et al. [52] have made an important contribution to this subject by describing a flow cytometry assay that distinguishes interstitial leukocytes in the oral mucosa of mice from those circulating within the vasculature or in post-dissection contaminating blood. They reported that, unlike circulating CD4 T cells, interstitial CD4 T cells were almost exclusively antigen-experienced cells (CD44^{hi}). The authors reported the presence of antigen-experienced *P. gingivalis*-specific CD4 T cells in nasal-associated lymphoid tissues following oral feeding of mice with *P. gingivalis*. Such differentiation might be critical for future understanding of the players driving alveolar bone destruction.

B cells infiltrate and dominate sites showing progressive chronic inflammatory periodontal disease in humans [53]. It has been shown that periodontitis lesions contain significant numbers of immunoglobulin-bearing lymphocytes and plasma cells, suggesting that the clinical progression of the periodontal lesion is followed by a shift in cellular infiltrates from predominantly immunoglobulin-negative lymphocytes to IgG and IgM-bearing lymphocytes and plasma cells [54]. Oliver-Bell et al. [55] demonstrated that B cells make a substantial contribution to alveolar bone loss in murine periodontitis, probably due to B-cell activation and expression of RANKL in the gingiva. Abe et al. [56] reported that ligature-induced periodontitis resulted in significantly less bone loss in B cell-deficient mice compared with wild-type controls, supporting the importance of B cells in periodontal bone loss. The authors also suggested that two cytokines of the TNF ligand superfamily, a proliferation-inducing ligand (APRIL) and B-lymphocyte stimulator (BLyS), might be potential therapeutic targets in periodontitis [56].

Mahanonda et al. [39] have characterised B cell subsets in gingivitis and periodontitis. The density of memory B cells in periodontitis lesions was significantly lower than in healthy and gingivitis tissues. On the other hand, Ab-secreting cells were the major cell type in the $CD19^+$ B cell population, with the mean percentage of Ab-secreting cells being significantly higher than that of memory B cells. Moreover, an abundance of $CD138^+$ plasma cells was observed in periodontitis tissues. The authors reported that plasma cells were arranged in clusters detected at the base of the periodontal pocket area and scattered throughout the gingival connective tissue, especially apically toward the advancing front of the lesion [39].

B cells in patients with periodontal disease may contribute to chronic systemic inflammation through constitutive secretion of IL-8 and IL-1β [8], but the in situ impact of such cytokine production should be elucidated. Kawai et al. [57] have demonstrated that B cells can be the cellular source of RANKL for bone resorption in homogenised gingival tissue from sites showing periodontal disease. Moreover, Malcolm et al. [58] have shown that the percentage of B cells expressing RANKL was elevated following *P. gingivalis* infection in gingival tissues. Oliver-Bell et al. [55] have also investigated the impact of *P. gingivalis* infection in the RANKL expression of B cells, showing that mice infected with *P. gingivalis* presented a significant increase in B-cell RANKL expression in the gingiva. Moreover, B-cell-deficient mice did not show *P. gingivalis*-induced alveolar bone loss. Recently, Kanzaki et al. [59] demonstrated that sRANKL and TNF-α cleaved from activated tumour necrosis factor-α-converting enzyme-bearing B cells might be important as an osteoclastogenic factor in periodontitis lesions.

Han et al. [10] suggested that B cells affect alveolar bone homeostasis in a murine model of periodontitis through antibody-independent and RANKL-dependent mechanisms. They reported that gingival memory B cells promote osteoclastogenesis and that this potential was increased by the development of periodontitis. Demoersman et al. [60] reported that a significantly higher percentage of $CD27^+$ memory B cells was observed in patients with severe periodontitis. At the same time, human B1 cells, which were previously associated with a regulatory function, decreased in such patients. The authors also reported that the RANKL expression increased in every B cell subset from severe periodontitis patients and was significantly greater in activated B cells than in the subjects without periodontitis. Moreover, an interesting literature review published by Zouali [54] supports that B cells are key participants in RANKL-mediated bone resorption. Activated RANKL-positive B cells can exacerbate alveolar bone loss in a RANKL-dependent manner in animal models. On the other hand, blocking RANKL, B-cell-activating factor (BAFF), and a proliferation-inducing ligand (APRIL) reduces alveolar bone loss in experimental models of periodontitis. Coat et al. [61] reported that periodontal parameters could be significantly improved after treatment with rituximab, concluding that anti-B lymphocyte therapy could be beneficial in improving de clinical conditions of patients with periodontitis.

Besides the fact that B cells positively activate immune responses, functioning as APCs and producing antibodies, regulatory B cells (Bregs) have been shown to exert a suppressive role in immune response [62]. B10 cells are a Breg cell subset that produces IL-10 and therefore, negatively regulates the inflammatory responses [63]. B10 cells are present in gingival tissues of patients with and without periodontal disease, but in significantly higher levels in periodontal disease lesions (5.89 ± 2.02) when compared to healthy tissues (0.1 ± 0.3, $p < 0.01$) [64]. Yu et al. [65] demonstrated that the local induction of IL-10 competency of B10 cells was associated with the inhibition of both inflammation and bone loss in ligature-induced experimental periodontitis. Wang et al. [66] also reported that the adoptive transfer of B10 cells significantly inhibited inflammation and bone loss in a mouse model of experimental periodontitis, suggesting a potential novel principle of treatment for periodontal diseases. It has been suggested that the in vitro treatment of B10 cells with a combination of IL-21, anti-Tim1, and CD40L might inhibit periodontal bone loss in ligature-induced experimental periodontitis [65]. A schematic of the lymphocyte subsets and their possible contribution to periodontal homeostasis and inflammation is presented in the Figure 1.

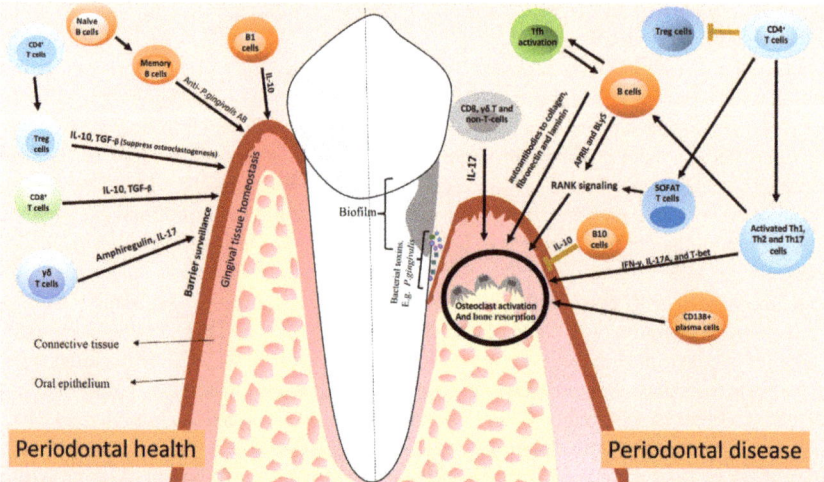

Figure 1. A summary of how mentioned T and B cells can contribute to periodontal health and disease. In periodontal health, Treg and CD8+ T cells contribute to periodontal homeostasis through the production of IL-10 and TGF-β. γδ T cells produce amphiregulin and IL-17 to promote periodontal homeostasis. B cells produce antibodies against periodontal pathogens, limiting the development of periodontal inflammation. In periodontal disease, activated Th1, Th2, and Th17 cells produce pro-inflammatory cytokines that contribute to tissue damage. Both T and B cells produce RANKL, which leads to osteoclast activation and alveolar bone resorption. Clonal activation of B cells by Tfh cells can lead to the production of autoantibodies to collagen, fibronectin and laminin, contributing to local tissue destruction. Lack of Treg cells or an impaired function probably impact on the development of periodontitis. IL-17 produced by other cells can also contribute to tissue damage via osteoclast activation. The figure was adapted from Lira-Junior & Figueredo [67].

The increased knowledge in T and B cells' biology, as well as their functions during gingival tissue homeostasis and inflammation might help in designing novel therapeutic strategies for bone disorders where these cells are a crucial part of the local tissue inflammation, such as periodontitis.

3. Conclusions

Several new roles have been discovered and added to the complex knowledge about T and B cells. These include different functions of Tregs, the role of γδ T cells in gingival homeostasis, the role of SOFAT in osteoclastogenesis, and the possible pathogenic role of MAIT cells. Also, the importance of B cells activating RANKL-mediated bone resorption adds to this complex scenario. During periodontal inflammation, the activation of distinct T and B-cell subtypes, as well as their cytokine production, are crucial in defining whether the inflammatory lesion will stabilise as chronic gingivitis or progress to tissue-destructive periodontitis.

Funding: This research received no external funding.

Conflicts of Interest: The authors declare no conflict of interest.

References

1. Campbell, L.; Millhouse, E.; Malcolm, J.; Culshaw, S. T cells, teeth and tissue destruction—what do T cells do in periodontal disease? *Mol. Oral. Microbiol.* **2016**, *31*, 445–456. [CrossRef] [PubMed]

2. Ebersole, J.L.; Kirakodu, S.; Novak, M.J.; Stromberg, A.J.; Shen, S.; Orraca, L.; Orraca, L.; Gonzalez-Martinez, J.; Burgos, A.; Gonzalez, O.A. Cytokine gene expression profiles during initiation, progression and resolution of periodontitis. *J Clin Periodontol.* **2014**, *41*, 853–861. [CrossRef] [PubMed]
3. Alvarez, C.; Rojas, C.; Rojas, L.; Cafferata, E.A.; Monasterio, G.; Vernal, R. Regulatory T Lymphocytes in Periodontitis: A Translational View. *Mediators Inflamm.* **2018**, *2018*, 7806912. [CrossRef] [PubMed]
4. Parachuru, V.P.B.; Coates, D.E.; Milne, T.J.; Rich, A.M.; Seymour, G.J. FoxP3(+) regulatory T cells, interleukin 17 and mast cells in chronic inflammatory periodontal disease. *J. Periodontal Res.* **2018**, *53*, 622–635. [CrossRef] [PubMed]
5. Berglundh, T.; Liljenberg, B.; Tarkowski, A.; Lindhe, J. The presence of local and circulating autoreactive B cells in patients with advanced periodontitis. *J. Clin. Periodontol.* **2002**, *29*, 281–286. [CrossRef] [PubMed]
6. Dutzan, N.; Konkel, J.E.; Greenwell-Wild, T.; Moutsopoulos, N.M. Characterization of the human immune cell network at the gingival barrier. *Mucosal Immunol.* **2016**, *9*, 1163–1172. [CrossRef] [PubMed]
7. Artese, L.; Simon, M.J.; Piattelli, A.; Ferrari, D.S.; Cardoso, L.A.; Faveri, M.; Onuma, T.; Piccirilli, M.; Perrotti, V.; Shibli, J.A. Immunohistochemical analysis of inflammatory infiltrate in aggressive and chronic periodontitis: A comparative study. *Clin. Oral Investig.* **2011**, *15*, 233–240. [CrossRef] [PubMed]
8. Jagannathan, M.; Hasturk, H.; Liang, Y.; Shin, H.; Hetzel, J.T.; Kantarci, A.; Rubin, D.; McDonnell, M.E.; Van Dyke, T.E.; Ganley-Leal, L.M.; et al. TLR cross-talk specifically regulates cytokine production by B cells from chronic inflammatory disease patients. *J. Immunol.* **2009**, *183*, 7461–7470. [CrossRef]
9. Zundler, S.; Neurath, M.F. Interleukin-12: Functional activities and implications for disease. *Cytokine Growth Factor Rev.* **2015**, *26*, 559–568. [CrossRef]
10. Han, Y.K.; Jin, Y.; Miao, Y.B.; Shi, T.; Lin, X.P. Improved RANKL production by memory B cells: A way for B cells promote alveolar bone destruction during periodontitis. *Int. Immunopharmacol.* **2018**, *64*, 232–237. [CrossRef]
11. Bonneville, M.; O'Brien, R.L.; Born, W.K. Gammadelta T cell effector functions: A blend of innate programming and acquired plasticity. *Nat. Rev. Immunol.* **2010**, *10*, 467–478. [CrossRef] [PubMed]
12. Valdor, R.; Macian, F. Induction and stability of the anergic phenotype in T cells. *Semin Immunol.* **2013**, *25*, 313–320. [CrossRef] [PubMed]
13. Luckheeram, R.V.; Zhou, R.; Verma, A.D.; Xia, B. CD4(+)T cells: Differentiation and functions. *Clin. Dev. Immunol.* **2012**, *2012*, 925135. [CrossRef] [PubMed]
14. Jia, L.; Wu, C. The biology and functions of Th22 cells. *Adv. Exp. Med. Biol.* **2014**, *841*, 209–230. [PubMed]
15. Lee, N.; Kim, W.U. Microbiota in T-cell homeostasis and inflammatory diseases. *Exp. Mol. Med.* **2017**, *49*, e340. [CrossRef] [PubMed]
16. Crotty, S. Follicular helper CD4 T cells (TFH). *Annu. Rev. Immunol.* **2011**, *29*, 621–663. [CrossRef] [PubMed]
17. Kaplan, M.H.; Hufford, M.M.; Olson, M.R. The development and in vivo function of T helper 9 cells. *Nat. Rev. Immunol.* **2015**, *15*, 295–307. [CrossRef] [PubMed]
18. Duhen, T.; Geiger, R.; Jarrossay, D.; Lanzavecchia, A.; Sallusto, F. Production of interleukin 22 but not interleukin 17 by a subset of human skin-homing memory T cells. *Nat. Immunol.* **2009**, *10*, 857–863. [CrossRef]
19. Xu, Z.; Ho, S.; Chang, C.C.; Zhang, Q.Y.; Vasilescu, E.R.; Vlad, G.; Suciu-Foca, N. Molecular and Cellular Characterization of Human CD8 T Suppressor Cells. *Front. Immunol.* **2016**, *7*, 549. [CrossRef]
20. Tilloy, F.; Treiner, E.; Park, S.H.; Garcia, C.; Lemonnier, F.; de la Salle, H.; Bendelac, A.; Bonneville, M.; Lantz, O. An invariant T cell receptor alpha chain defines a novel TAP-independent major histocompatibility complex class Ib-restricted alpha/beta T cell subpopulation in mammals. *J. Exp. Med.* **1999**, *189*, 1907–1921. [CrossRef]
21. Treiner, E.; Lantz, O. CD1d- and MR1-restricted invariant T cells: Of mice and men. *Curr. Opin. Immunol.* **2006**, *18*, 519–526. [CrossRef]
22. Sobkowiak, M.J.; Davanian, H.; Heymann, R.; Gibbs, A.; Emgard, J.; Dias, J.; Aleman, S.; Krüger-Weiner, C.; Moll, M.; Tjernlund, A.; et al. Tissue-resident MAIT cell populations in human oral mucosa exhibit an activated profile and produce IL-17. *Eur. J. Immunol.* **2018**. [CrossRef]
23. Cerutti, A.; Cols, M.; Puga, I. Activation of B cells by non-canonical helper signals. *EMBO Rep.* **2012**, *13*, 798–810. [CrossRef]
24. Cerutti, A.; Puga, I.; Cols, M. New helping friends for B cells. *Eur. J. Immunol.* **2012**, *42*, 1956–1968. [CrossRef]
25. Bonilla, F.A.; Oettgen, H.C. Adaptive immunity. *J. Allergy Clin. Immunol.* **2010**, *125*, S33–S40. [CrossRef]
26. Smith, F.L.; Baumgarth, N. B-1 cell responses to infections. *Curr. Opin. Immunol.* **2019**, *5*, 23–31. [CrossRef]

27. Yang, M.; Rui, K.; Wang, S.; Lu, L. Regulatory B cells in autoimmune diseases. *Cell Mol. Immunol.* **2013**, *10*, 122–132. [CrossRef]
28. Yanaba, K.; Bouaziz, J.D.; Matsushita, T.; Magro, C.M.; St Clair, E.W.; Tedder, T.F. B-lymphocyte contributions to human autoimmune disease. *Immunol. Rev.* **2008**, *223*, 284–299. [CrossRef]
29. Zhu, J.; Paul, W.E. CD4 T cells: Fates, functions, and faults. *Blood* **2008**, *112*, 1557–1569. [CrossRef]
30. Cardoso, E.M.; Arosa, F.A. CD8(+) T Cells in Chronic Periodontitis: Roles and Rules. *Front. Immunol.* **2017**, *8*, 145. [CrossRef]
31. Nielsen, M.M.; Witherden, D.A.; Havran, W.L. Gammadelta T cells in homeostasis and host defence of epithelial barrier tissues. *Nat. Rev. Immunol.* **2017**, *17*, 733–745. [CrossRef]
32. Krishnan, S.; Prise, I.E.; Wemyss, K.; Schenck, L.P.; Bridgeman, H.M.; McClure, F.A.; Zangerle-Murray, T.; O'Boyle, C.; Barbera, T.A.; Mahmood, F.; et al. Amphiregulin-producing gammadelta T cells are vital for safeguarding oral barrier immune homeostasis. *Proc. Natl. Acad. Sci. USA* **2018**, *115*, 10738–10743. [CrossRef]
33. Wilharm, A.; Tabib, Y.; Nassar, M.; Reinhardt, A.; Mizraji, G.; Sandrock, I.; Heyman, O.; Barros-Martins, J.; Aizenbud, Y.; Khalaileh, A.; et al. Mutual interplay between IL-17-producing gammadeltaT cells and microbiota orchestrates oral mucosal homeostasis. *Proc. Natl. Acad. Sci. USA* **2019**, *116*, 2652–2661. [CrossRef]
34. Arizon, M.; Nudel, I.; Segev, H.; Mizraji, G.; Elnekave, M.; Furmanov, K.; Eli-Berchoer, L.; Clausen, B.E.; Shapira, L.; Wilensky, A.; et al. Langerhans cells down-regulate inflammation-driven alveolar bone loss. *Proc. Natl. Acad. Sci. USA* **2012**, *109*, 7043–7048. [CrossRef]
35. Dutzan, N.; Abusleme, L.; Konkel, J.E.; Moutsopoulos, N.M. Isolation, Characterization and Functional Examination of the Gingival Immune Cell Network. *J. Vis. Exp.* **2016**, *108*, 53736. [CrossRef]
36. Sallusto, F.; Lenig, D.; Forster, R.; Lipp, M.; Lanzavecchia, A. Two subsets of memory T lymphocytes with distinct homing potentials and effector functions. *Nature* **1999**, *401*, 708–712. [CrossRef]
37. Sheridan, B.S.; Lefrancois, L. Regional and mucosal memory T cells. *Nat. Immunol.* **2011**, *12*, 485–491. [CrossRef]
38. Dutzan, N.; Abusleme, L.; Bridgeman, H.; Greenwell-Wild, T.; Zangerle-Murray, T.; Fife, M.E.; Bouladoux, N.; Linley, H.; Brenchley, L.; Wemyss, K.; et al. On-going Mechanical Damage from Mastication Drives Homeostatic Th17 Cell Responses at the Oral Barrier. *Immunity* **2017**, *46*, 133–147. [CrossRef]
39. Mahanonda, R.; Champaiboon, C.; Subbalekha, K.; Sa-Ard-Iam, N.; Rattanathammatada, W.; Thawanaphong, S.; Rerkyen, P.; Yoshimura, F.; Nagano, K.; Lang, N.P.; et al. Human Memory B Cells in Healthy Gingiva, Gingivitis, and Periodontitis. *J. Immunol.* **2016**, *197*, 715–725. [CrossRef]
40. Kim, Y.C.; Ko, Y.; Hong, S.D.; Kim, K.Y.; Lee, Y.H.; Chae, C.; Choi, Y. Presence of Porphyromonas gingivalis and plasma cell dominance in gingival tissues with periodontitis. *Oral Dis.* **2010**, *16*, 375–381. [CrossRef]
41. Shelburne, C.E.; Shelburne, P.S.; Dhople, V.M.; Sweier, D.G.; Giannobile, W.V.; Kinney, J.S.; Coulter, W.A.; Mullally, B.H.; Lopatin, D.E. Serum antibodies to Porphyromonas gingivalis chaperone HtpG predict health in periodontitis susceptible patients. *PLoS ONE* **2008**, *3*, e1984. [CrossRef]
42. Garlet, G.P. Destructive and protective roles of cytokines in periodontitis: A re-appraisal from host defense and tissue destruction viewpoints. *J. Dent. Res.* **2010**, *89*, 1349–1363. [CrossRef]
43. Page, R.C.; Lantz, M.S.; Darveau, R.; Jeffcoat, M.; Mancl, L.; Houston, L.; Braham, P.; Persson, G.R. Immunization of Macaca fascicularis against experimental periodontitis using a vaccine containing cysteine proteases purified from Porphyromonas gingivalis. *Oral Microbiol. Immunol.* **2007**, *22*, 162–168. [CrossRef]
44. Ebersole, J.L.; Kirakodu, S.S.; Novak, M.J.; Orraca, L.; Martinez, J.G.; Cunningham, L.L.; Thomas, M.V.; Stromberg, A.; Pandruvada, S.N.; Gonzalez, O.A. Transcriptome Analysis of B Cell Immune Functions in Periodontitis: Mucosal Tissue Responses to the Oral Microbiome in Aging. *Front. Immunol.* **2016**, *7*, 272. [CrossRef]
45. Witkowski, J.M.; Mikosik, A.; Bryl, E.; Fulop, T. Proteodynamics in aging human T cells—The need for its comprehensive study to understand the fine regulation of T lymphocyte functions. *Exp. Gerontol.* **2018**, *107*, 161–168. [CrossRef]
46. Okada, H.; Kida, T.; Yamagami, H. Identification and distribution of immunocompetent cells in inflamed gingiva of human chronic periodontitis. *Infect. Immun.* **1983**, *41*, 365–374.
47. Okada, H.; Kassai, Y.; Kida, T. T lymphocyte subsets in the inflamed gingiva of human adult periodontitis. *J. Periodontal Res.* **1984**, *19*, 595–598. [CrossRef]

48. Chen, M.L.; Sundrud, M.S. Cytokine Networks and T-Cell Subsets in Inflammatory Bowel Diseases. *Inflamm. Bowel Dis.* **2016**, *22*, 1157–1167. [CrossRef]
49. Dutzan, N.K.T.; Abusleme, L.; Greenwell-Wild, T.; Zuazo, C.E.; Ikeuchi, T.; Brenchley, L.; Abe, T.; Hurabielle, C.; Martin, D.; Morell, R.J.; et al. A dysbiotic microbiome triggers TH17 cells to mediate oral mucosal immunopathology in mice and humans. *Sci. Transl. Med.* **2018**, *10*, eaat0797. [CrossRef]
50. Jarry, C.R.; Duarte, P.M.; Freitas, F.F.; de Macedo, C.G.; Clemente-Napimoga, J.T.; Saba-Chujfi, E.; Passador-Santos, F.; de Araújo, V.C.; Napimoga, M.H. Secreted osteoclastogenic factor of activated T cells (SOFAT), a novel osteoclast activator, in chronic periodontitis. *Hum Immunol.* **2013**, *74*, 861–866. [CrossRef]
51. Jarry, C.R.; Martinez, E.F.; Peruzzo, D.C.; Carregaro, V.; Sacramento, L.A.; Araujo, V.C.; Weitzmann, M.N.; Napimoga, M.H. Expression of SOFAT by T- and B-lineage cells may contribute to bone loss. *Mol. Med. Rep.* **2016**, *13*, 4252–4258. [CrossRef]
52. Bittner-Eddy, P.D.; Fischer, L.A.; Tu, A.A.; Allman, D.A.; Costalonga, M. Discriminating between Interstitial and Circulating Leukocytes in Tissues of the Murine Oral Mucosa Avoiding Nasal-Associated Lymphoid Tissue Contamination. *Front. Immunol.* **2017**, *8*, 1398. [CrossRef]
53. Seymour, G.J.; Powell, R.N.; Davies, W.I. The immunopathogenesis of progressive chronic inflammatory periodontal disease. *J. Oral Pathol.* **1979**, *8*, 249–265. [CrossRef]
54. Zouali, M. The emerging roles of B cells as partners and targets in periodontitis. *Autoimmunity.* **2017**, *50*, 61–70. [CrossRef]
55. Oliver-Bell, J.; Butcher, J.P.; Malcolm, J.; MacLeod, M.K.; Adrados Planell, A.; Campbell, L.; Nibbs, R.J.; Garside, P.; McInnes, I.B.; Culshaw, S. Periodontitis in the absence of B cells and specific anti-bacterial antibody. *Mol. Oral Microbiol.* **2015**, *30*, 160–169. [CrossRef]
56. Abe, T.; AlSarhan, M.; Benakanakere, M.R.; Maekawa, T.; Kinane, D.F.; Cancro, M.P.; Korostoff, J.M.; Hajishengallis, G. The B Cell-Stimulatory Cytokines BLyS and APRIL Are Elevated in Human Periodontitis and Are Required for B Cell-Dependent Bone Loss in Experimental Murine Periodontitis. *J. Immunol.* **2015**, *195*, 1427–1435. [CrossRef]
57. Kawai, T.; Matsuyama, T.; Hosokawa, Y.; Makihira, S.; Seki, M.; Karimbux, N.Y.; Goncalves, R.B.; Valverde, P.; Dibart, S.; Li, Y.P.; et al. B and T lymphocytes are the primary sources of RANKL in the bone resorptive lesion of periodontal disease. *Am. J. Pathol.* **2006**, *169*, 987–998. [CrossRef]
58. Malcolm, J.; Awang, R.A.; Oliver-Bell, J.; Butcher, J.P.; Campbell, L.; Adrados Planell, A.; Lappin, D.F.; Fukada, S.Y.; Nile, C.J.; Liew, F.Y.; et al. IL-33 Exacerbates Periodontal Disease through Induction of RANKL. *J. Dent. Res.* **2015**, *94*, 968–975. [CrossRef]
59. Kanzaki, H.; Makihira, S.; Suzuki, M.; Ishii, T.; Movila, A.; Hirschfeld, J.; Mawardi, H.; Lin, X.; Han, X.; Taubman, M.A.; et al. Soluble RANKL Cleaved from Activated Lymphocytes by TNF-alpha-Converting Enzyme Contributes to Osteoclastogenesis in Periodontitis. *J. Immunol.* **2016**, *197*, 3871–3883. [CrossRef]
60. Demoersman, J.; Pochard, P.; Framery, C.; Simon, Q.; Boisrame, S.; Soueidan, A.; Pers, J.O. B cell subset distribution is altered in patients with severe periodontitis. *PLoS ONE.* **2018**, *13*, e0192986. [CrossRef]
61. Coat, J.; Demoersman, J.; Beuzit, S.; Cornec, D.; Devauchelle-Pensec, V.; Saraux, A.; Pers, J.O. Anti-B lymphocyte immunotherapy is associated with improvement of periodontal status in subjects with rheumatoid arthritis. *J. Clin. Periodontol.* **2015**, *42*, 817–823. [CrossRef]
62. Kalampokis, I.; Yoshizaki, A.; Tedder, T.F. IL-10-producing regulatory B cells (B10 cells) in autoimmune disease. *Arthritis Res. Ther.* **2013**, *15*, S1. [CrossRef]
63. Yanaba, K.; Yoshizaki, A.; Asano, Y.; Kadono, T.; Tedder, T.F.; Sato, S. IL-10-producing regulatory B10 cells inhibit intestinal injury in a mouse model. *Am. J. Pathol.* **2011**, *178*, 735–743. [CrossRef]
64. Dai, J.; Bi, L.; Lin, J.; Qi, F. Evaluation of interleukin-10 producing CD19(+) B cells in human gingival tissue. *Arch. Oral Biol.* **2017**, *84*, 112–117. [CrossRef]
65. Hu, Y.; Yu, P.; Yu, X.; Hu, X.; Kawai, T.; Han, X. IL-21/anti-Tim1/CD40 ligand promotes B10 activity in vitro and alleviates bone loss in experimental periodontitis in vivo. *Biochim. Biophys Acta Mol. Basis Dis.* **2017**, *1863*, 2149–2157. [CrossRef]

66. Wang, Y.; Yu, X.; Lin, J.; Hu, Y.; Zhao, Q.; Kawai, T.; Taubman, M.A.; Han, X. B10 Cells Alleviate Periodontal Bone Loss in Experimental Periodontitis. *Infect Immun.* **2017**, *85*, e00335-17. [CrossRef]
67. Lira-Junior, R.; Figueredo, C.M. Periodontal and inflammatory bowel diseases: Is there evidence of complex pathogenic interactions? *World J. Gastroenterol.* **2016**, *22*, 7963. [CrossRef]

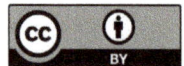

© 2019 by the authors. Licensee MDPI, Basel, Switzerland. This article is an open access article distributed under the terms and conditions of the Creative Commons Attribution (CC BY) license (http://creativecommons.org/licenses/by/4.0/).

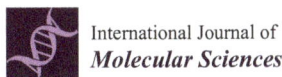

Review

Periodontal Therapy for Improving Lipid Profiles in Patients with Type 2 Diabetes Mellitus: A Systematic Review and Meta-Analysis

Siddharth Garde [1], Rahena Akhter [1], Mai Anh Nguyen [1], Clara K. Chow [2] and Joerg Eberhard [1,*]

1 The University of Sydney School of Dentistry, Faculty of Medicine and Health, The University of Sydney, Camperdown 2006, Australia
2 Westmead Applied Research Centre, Sydney Medical School, Westmead 2145, Australia
* Correspondence: joerg.eberhard@sydney.edu.au

Received: 13 June 2019; Accepted: 31 July 2019; Published: 5 August 2019

Abstract: Periodontitis is a chronic inflammatory disorder often seen in patients with diabetes mellitus (DM). Individuals with diabetes are at a greater risk of developing cardiovascular complications and this may be related, in part, to lipid abnormalities observed in these individuals. The objective of this systematic review is to compile the current scientific evidence of the effects of periodontal treatment on lipid profiles in patients with type 2 diabetes mellitus. Through a systematic search using MEDLINE, EMBASE, PubMed, and Web of Science, 313 articles were identified. Of these, seven clinical trials which met all inclusion criteria were chosen for analysis. Between baseline and 3-month follow-up, there was a statistically significant reduction in the levels of total cholesterol (mean differences (MD) −0.47 mmol/L (95% confidence interval (CI), −0.75, −0.18, $p = 0.001$)), triglycerides (MD −0.20 mmol/L (95% CI −0.24, −0.16, $p < 0.00001$)) favouring the intervention arm, and a statistically significant reduction in levels of high density lipoprotein (HDL) (MD 0.06 mmol/L (95% CI 0.03, 0.08, $p < 0.00001$)) favouring the control arm. No significant differences were observed between baseline and 6-month follow-up levels for any lipid analysed. The heterogeneity between studies was high. This review foreshadows a potential benefit of periodontal therapy for lipid profiles in patients suffering from type 2 DM, however, well designed clinical trials using lipid profiles as primary outcome measures are warranted.

Keywords: periodontal therapy; type 2 diabetes mellitus; lipid profiles; inflammation

1. Introduction

Periodontal diseases are a group of inflammatory conditions affecting the connective tissues surrounding teeth. Periodontitis, a specific type of periodontal disease, is a major cause of tooth loss and the prevalence of its moderate to severe forms in adult Western populations is approximately 50% [1,2]. Periodontitis is caused by gram-negative bacteria which induce a host inflammatory response, resulting in the destruction of tissues that supports the teeth and also has adverse systemic effects [3].

Type 2 diabetes mellitus (type 2 DM) is a metabolic disorder ranging from insulin resistance to insulin deficiency, with poor glycaemic control presenting as a predominant feature [3]. Diabetes is also a major risk factor for periodontitis, and the risk of developing periodontitis is increased approximately three times in patients with diabetes compared with non-diabetic individuals [4]. There is an increasing prevalence of type 2 DM worldwide, and this is expected to contribute to an increase in diabetes-related complications [5].

Cardiovascular disease (CVD) is also one of the major complications associated with diabetes, and there is a high prevalence of cardiovascular risk factors and markers of cardiovascular organ injury in patients with type 2 DM. Ninety-seven percent of patients with diabetes are dyslipidaemic, with a characteristic pattern of increased plasma triglycerides and decreased high density lipoprotein (HDL) cholesterol. In a large clinical study with an average follow-up period of 3.9 years, low density lipoprotein (LDL) cholesterol, non-HDL cholesterol, apolipoprotein B, triglyceride, and homocysteine levels all increased over time, with most participants also having low HDL levels [6]. The downregulation of the enzyme lipoprotein lipase due to low insulin levels may be the cause of the dyslipidaemic profiles noted in diabetic individuals [7]. Other mechanisms involved linking diabetes to higher CVD risk involve chronic oxidative stress in diabetics, purportedly related to the metabolism of excess substrates (glucose and fatty acids [8]) and a state of chronic, low-level inflammation [9] in diabetes.

Recent intervention trials have demonstrated that anti-inflammatory periodontitis therapy may reduce serum levels of glycated haemoglobin (HbA1c) and high sensitivity C-reactive protein (hsCRP) [10–16], demonstrating the capacity to modulate glucose control and cardiovascular risk. However, little attention has been paid to the potential effects of periodontitis therapy in patients with diabetes to improve lipid profiles. This systematic review aims to evaluate the scientific evidence of the impact of periodontal therapy on lipid profiles in patients with type 2 DM.

2. Results

2.1. Selection of Studies

Six hundred and eighty-two studies were retrieved from the electronic databases PubMed, MEDLINE via Ovid, EMBASE via Ovid, and Web of Science. Three hundred and sixty-nine duplicates were removed, and the remaining abstracts were screened for eligibility, resulting in sixty-eight studies being further excluded. Two hundred and forty-five studies were then selected for full-text analysis. After reading of the full texts, seven studies [10–16] were included in the systematic review (Figure 1). Full text studies were excluded if they did not report lipid levels as an outcome or studies did not have appropriate intervention and control arms.

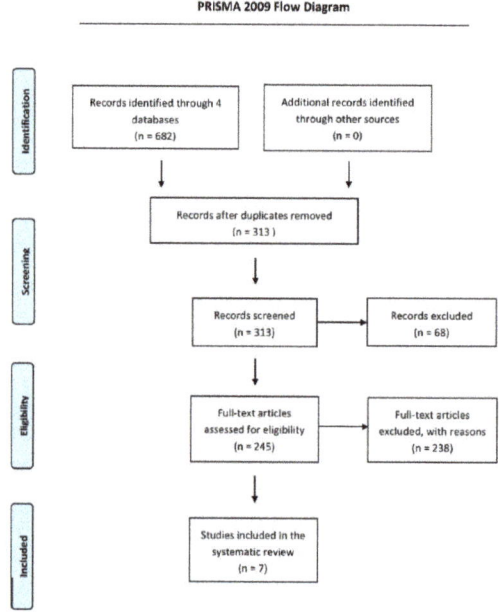

Figure 1. Study selection flow diagram.

2.2. Characteristics of Studies

The characteristics of the included studies are described in Table 1. In total, there were 411 individuals who underwent periodontal treatment (intervention arm) and 341 individuals who did not or received post-trial intervention (control arm). The total number of participants in each study ranged from 40 to 264. The follow-up times for the studies ranged from 3 to 12 months, however, for this review only the 3- and 6-month follow-up data has been analysed. Among seven studies, five studies reported 3-month follow-up [10,12,13,15,16] and three studies reported 6-month follow-up data [10,11,14].

The mean age of individuals in the studies ranged from 45.5 to 63.2 years old. Three out of seven studies [11,12,16] excluded patients with cardiovascular disease. Three studies [10,14,15] excluded patients with uncontrolled systemic diseases, however, did not specify whether cardiovascular disease was amongst this exclusion criteria. One study [13] did not specify whether participants with any uncontrolled systemic diseases were excluded or not. Two studies [11,14] specified that participants taking anti-hypertensive/cholesterol medications were included whereas five studies [10,12,13,15,16] did not specify whether patients taking anti-hypertensive/cholesterol medications were included or not. Six out of the seven studies [10–12,14–16] presented periodontal inclusion criteria and, among them, four different criteria were identified. All studies [10–16] reported diabetes inclusion criteria, and seven different criteria were identified (Table 1).

Table 1. Characteristics of included studies.

Author	Country	Intervention/ Control	Participants at Baseline (n)	Follow Up TIME (months)	Diabetes Inclusion Criteria	Periodontal Inclusion Criteria
D'Aiuto et al. 2018 [11]	United Kingdom	SPT + NSPT	133	12	Type 2 DM for >6 months (WHO diagnostic criteria)	>20 periodontal pockets with PD > 4mm and alveolar bone loss > 30%
		Supragingival SRP	131			
Masi et al. 2018 [14]	United Kingdom	NSPT	27	6	Diagnosed type 2 DM (WHO criteria)	>15 remaining teeth and >20 sites with PD >5mm
		Supragingival SRP	24			
Kapellas et al. 2017 [12]	Australia	NSPT	35	3	HbA1c > 6.5% or >47.5 mmol/mol	Joint Centers for Disease Control and Prevention and American Academy of Periodontology case definition
		No treatment	27			
Chen et al. 2012 [10]	China	NSPT	45	6	Type 2 DM for >12 months	American Academy of Periodontology criteria
		No treatment	44			
Moeintaghavi et al. 2012 [15]	Iran	NSPT	22	3	HbA1c > 7%	Mild-moderate periodontitis- American Academy of Periodontology criteria
		No treatment	18			
Sun et al. 2011 [16]	China	NSPT	82	3	Diagnosed type 2 DM for >12 months and HbA1c 7.5–9.5%	>20 remaining teeth, PD > 5 mm, more than 30% teeth CAL over 4 mm, or over 60% teeth with PD > 4 mm and CAL > 3 mm
		No treatment	75			
Kiran et al. 2005 [13]	Turkey	NSPT	22	3	HbA1c 6–8%	Not specified
		No treatment	22			

SPT: surgical periodontal treatment; NSPT: non-surgical periodontal treatment; SRP: scaling and root planing; DM: diabetes mellitus; HbA1c: glycated haemoglobin; WHO: World Health Organization; PD: pocket depth; CAL: clinical attachment loss.

2.3. Risk of Bias within Studies

The Cochrane Collaboration's tool for assessing risk of bias [17] was used to assess the risk of bias within the included studies which have been summarized in Figure 2. Of the seven clinical trials included [10–16], five studies described the methods of randomisation [10–12,14,15]. Three studies [11,12,14] used a computer-generated table for allocation concealment, two studies [10,15] assigned an independent individual to allocate participants, and two studies [13,16] did not specify allocation concealment. Blinding of patients and personnel was not possible due to the nature of the periodontal treatment. Blinding of investigators was conducted in four studies [10–12,14], two did not specify whether investigators were blinded [13,15], and one study was non-blinded [16]. Four studies had minimal/no participant drop out or the data for the participants who dropped out was excluded [13–16], two studies had a moderate number of participants drop out [10,11] and one study [12] had a high participant dropout rate indicating attrition bias. There was no evidence of selective reporting or any other form of bias in any of the studies.

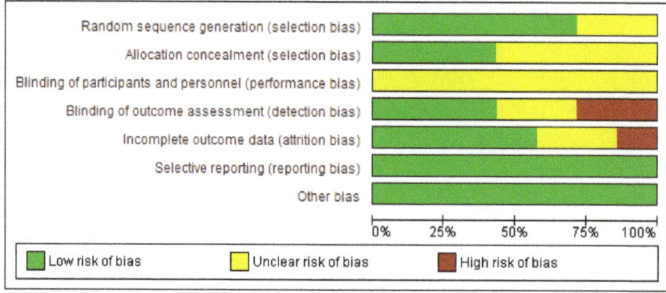

Figure 2. Risk of bias analysis of individual studies.

2.4. Lipid Profiles

Changes in lipid profiles between baseline and the 3- and 6-month follow-ups have been depicted in Table 2.

Table 2. Lipid profiles at baseline, 3 months, and 6 months in mmol/L.

Author	Groups		Baseline								3 Month Follow Up								6 Month Follow Up							
			TC		TG		LDL		HDL		TC		TG		LDL		HDL		TC		TG		LDL		HDL	
			Mean	SD	Mean	SD	Mean	SD	Mean	SD	Mean	SD	Mean	SD	Mean	SD	Mean	SD	Mean	SD	Mean	SD	Mean	SD	Mean	SD
D'Aiuto et al. 2018 [11]	Intervention	SPT+NSPT	4.2	1*	1.6	1.2*	2.2	0.9*	1.2	0.4*									4.3	0.1*	1.7	0.1*	2.3	0.1*	1.3	0.0*
	Control	SG SRP	4.3	1.1*	1.6	1.1*	2.4	0.9*	1.3	0.4*									4.2	0.1*	1.5	0.1*	2.3	0.1*	1.2	0.0*
Masi et al. 2018 [14]	Intervention	NSPT	4.3	1.1	1.48	1.13	2.3	0.9	1.3	0.4									4.2	0.9	1.4	0.9	2.2	0.7	1.4	0.4
	Control	SG SRP	4.3	1	2.3	2.6	2	0.9	1.3	0.4									4.1	1.1	2.2	1.9	2	0.8	1.2	0.5
Kapellas et al. 2017 [12]	Intervention	NSPT	4.8	1.1							4.5	1					1	0.3								
	Control	No tx	4.6	0.8							4.4	0.9					0.9	0.2								
Chen et al. 2012 [10]	Intervention	NSPT	2.63	1.32	6.02	1.57	3.5	1.3	1.31	0.46	2.2	1.33	5.61	1.41	3.37	1.3	1.23	0.39	2.15	1.93	5.26	1.41	3.04	1.23	1.14	0.39
	Control	No tx	2.35	1.78	6.37	1.87	3.79	1.48	1.44	0.53	2.3	2.16	5.94	1.22	3.5	1.17	1.36	0.49	2.25	1.98	5.81	1.61	1.26	0.5	3.25	1.27
Moeintaghavi et al. 2012 [5]	Intervention	NSPT	10.66	1.5	7.66	4.54	6.6	1.38	2.55	0.51	10.31	1.72	7.22	3.22	6.26	1.76	2.45	0.37								
	Control	No tx	10.69	1.5	8.4	1.51	6.51	1.9	2.57	0.69	10.95	1.51	8.19	1.62	6.36	2.12	2.44	0.54								
Sun et al. 2011 [16]	Intervention	NSPT			2.07	0.69	3.32	0.71	1.17	0.29	1.85		1.85	0.64	3.21	0.76	1.23	0.33								
	Control	No tx			2.1	0.68	3.37	0.74	1.15	0.28	2.08		2.08	0.66	3.31	0.75	1.16	0.3								
Kiran et al. 2005 [13]	Intervention	NSPT	10.4	2.13	7.6	5.5	6.31	1.35	2.87	0.77	10.17	1.73	6.82	3.1	6.15	1.73	2.94	0.85								
	Control	No tx	9.95	1.95	7.26	3.8	5.96	1.81	2.54	0.73	10.57	2.07	9.17	5.95	5.94	2.16	2.85	0.79								

TC: total cholesterol; TG: triglyceride; LDL: low-density lipoprotein; HDL: high-density lipoprotein; SD: standard deviation; *: standard error; NSPT: non-surgical periodontal treatment; SG SRP: supragingival scaling and root planning; tx: treatment.

2.4.1. Baseline vs. 3-Month Follow-Up

After a 3 month observation period data from five studies [10,12,13,15,16] were included in the meta-analysis (Figure 3). A total of 235 participants in four studies [10,12,13,15] were analysed for changes in their total cholesterol levels and there was a statistically significant differences in favour of the intervention group ($p = 0.001$, mean difference −0.47 mmol/L (95% CI, −0.75 mmol/L to −0.18 mmol/L)) with evidence of high heterogeneity (Chi^2 = 35.22, 3 df, $p < 0.00001$, I^2 = 91%). A total of 330 patients in four studies [10,13,15,16] were analysed for changes in triglycerides, and there was a statistically significant difference in favour of the intervention treatment ($p < 0.00001$, mean difference −0.20 mmol/L (95% CI −0.24 mmol/L to −0.16 mmol/L, Chi^2 = 179.34, 3 df, $p < 0.00001$, I^2 = 98%)), with evidence of high heterogeneity. A total of 330 patients in four studies [10,13,15,16] compared changes in LDL levels, and there was no significant difference between the intervention and the control treatment ($p = 0.21$, mean difference −0.02 mmol/L (95% CI −0.06 mmol/L to 0.01 mmol/L, Chi^2 = 16.64, 3 df, $p = 0.0008$, I^2 = 82%)). A total of 392 patients in five studies [10,12,13,15,16] compared changes in HDL levels, and there was a statistically significant difference in favour of the control treatment ($p < 0.00001$, mean difference 0.06 mmol/L (95% CI 0.03 mmol/L to 0.08 mmol/L, Chi^2 = 37.06, 4 df, $p < 0.00001$, I^2 = 89%)), with evidence of high heterogeneity.

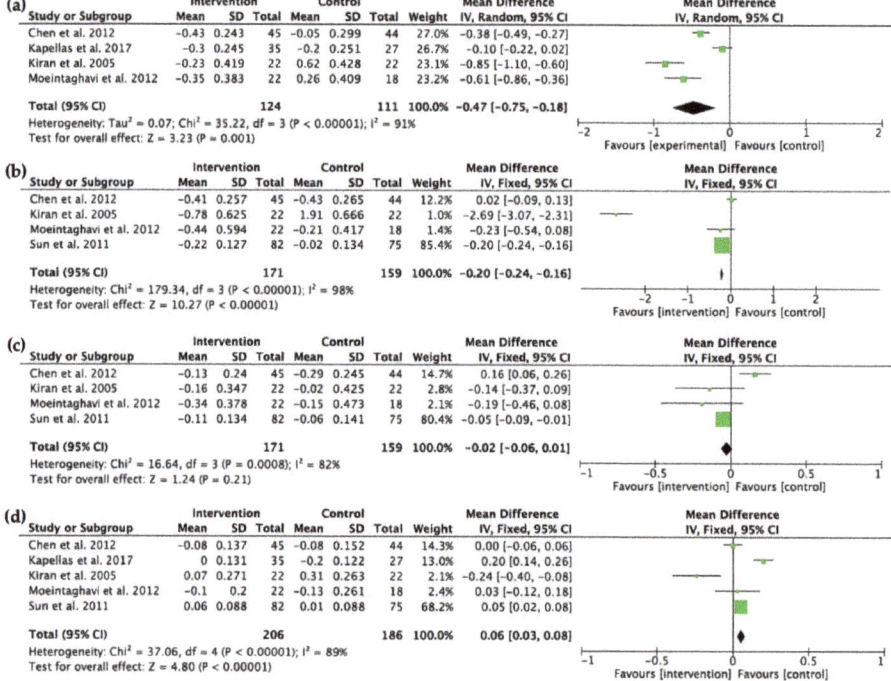

Figure 3. Forest plots depicting the changes of (**a**) total cholesterol, (**b**) triglycerides, (**c**) LDL, and (**d**) HDL (all in mmol/L) between the intervention and control groups at baseline and the 3-month follow-up.

2.4.2. Baseline vs. 6-Month Follow-Up

After 6 months, three studies [10,11,14] were included in a meta-analysis of total cholesterol, triglycerides, LDL and HDL. There were no statistically significant differences found for any lipid levels (Figure 4).

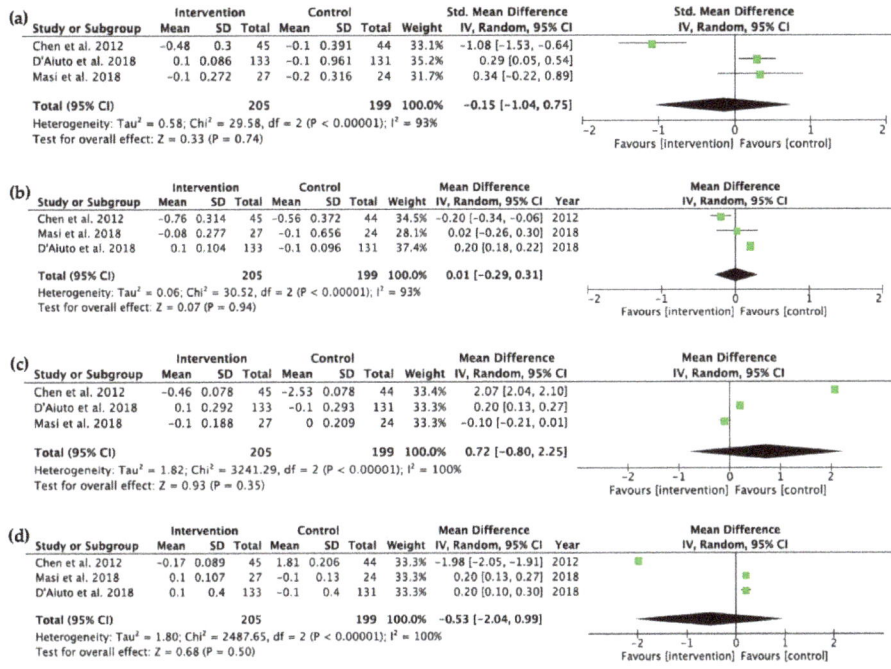

Figure 4. Forest plots depicting the changes of (**a**) total cholesterol, (**b**) triglycerides, (**c**) LDL, and (**d**) HDL (all in mmol/L) between the intervention and control groups at baseline and the 6-month follow-up.

2.5. Periodontal Outcomes

The periodontal parameters at baseline, 3 months, and 6 months are outlined in Table 3. At baseline, four studies [10,13,15,16] reported a mean periodontal probing depth of 2.93 mm for the intervention groups, compared to 2.82 mm in the control groups. Three months after therapy a mean PD of 2.30 mm was reported in the intervention groups (PD reduction of 0.63 mm), compared to 2.81 mm in the control groups (PD reduction of 0.1 mm). For the comparison between baseline vs. 6 months, three studies [10,11,14] reported a mean baseline PD of 3.46 mm in the intervention group and of 3.99 mm in the control group. After 6 months, a mean PD of 2.63 mm in the intervention group (PD reduction 0.83 mm) and a mean PD of 3.14 mm in the control groups (PD reduction 0.18 mm) was reported.

Two studies [10,13] reported changes in bleeding on probing (BOP) between baseline and 3-month follow-up. For the intervention group a mean BOP of 43.4% was calculated at baseline and of 18.0% at 3-month follow-up. For the control group the mean BOP at baseline was 42.2%, compared to 40.2% at 3-month follow-up. Three studies [10,11,14] reported BOP values for baseline and 6-month follow-up. For the intervention group a mean BOP of 56.5% was calculated at baseline and of 27.0% at the 6-month follow-up assessment. For the control group, the mean BOP at baseline was 56.3%, compared to 47.8% at 6-month follow-up.

Table 3. Periodontal parameters at baseline, and 3 and 6 months.

Author	Groups		Baseline				3-month Follow Up				6-month Follow Up			
			PD		BOP		PD		BOP		PD		BOP	
			Mean	SD	Mean	SD	Mean	SD	Mean	SD	Mean	SD	Mean	SD
D'Aiuto et al. 2018 [11]	Intervention	SPT + NSPT	3.9	0.1*	65	2.0*					2.9	0.1*	33.0	2.0*
	Control	SG SRP	3.9	0.1*	63	2.0*					3.7	0.1*	57.0	2.0*
Masi et al. 2018 [14]	Intervention	NSPT	3.9	0.8	70.0	20.0								
	Control	SG SRP	3.6	0.7	72.0	15.0								
Kapellas et al. 2017 [12]	Intervention	NSPT												
	Control	No treatment												
Chen et al. 2012 [10]	Intervention	NSPT	2.57	0.66	32.42	16.63	2.2	0.39	12.13	8.24	2.1	0.39	12.02	8.99
	Control	No treatment	2.47	0.57	34.01	18.91	2.38	0.47	28.53	14.42	2.42	0.5	28.37	13.5
Moeintaghavi et al. 2012 [15]	Intervention	NSPT	2.31	0.65			2.21	0.6						
	Control	No treatment	2.06	0.24			2.33	0.3						
Sun et al. 2011 [16]	Intervention	NSPT	4.53	0.83			2.97	0.78						
	Control	No treatment	4.49	0.85			4.28	0.81						
Kiran et al. 2005 [13]	Intervention	NSPT	2.29	0.49	54.38	18.75	1.8	0.25	23.9	12.73				
	Control	No treatment	2.24	0.7	50.48	26.1	2.26	0.63	51.91	27.38				
Total	Intervention		3.3	0.6	55.5	16.1	2.3	0.5	18.0	10.7	2.6	0.5	27.0	13.1
	Control		3.1	0.6	54.9	17.8	2.8	0.3	40.2	21.9	3.1	0.5	47.8	13.0

SPT: surgical periodontal treatment; NSPT: non-surgical periodontal treatment; SG SRP: supragingival scaling and root planing; PD: pocket depth (mm); SD: standard deviation; *: standard error; BOP: bleeding on probing (%).

3. Discussion

This is the first meta-analysis aimed to evaluate the effect of anti-inflammatory periodontal therapy on changes of lipid levels in patients with type 2 DM. Periodontal therapy involves the mechanical removal of dental plaque associated with periodontitis. The majority of the studies used non-surgical periodontal treatment as the intervention, however one study [11] used surgical periodontal treatment for select individuals in the intervention arm as well. The analyses demonstrated that total cholesterol and triglycerides were significantly reduced in the intervention arm 3 months after therapy to lower levels, while HDL levels were reduced in the control group. However, no significant differences were observed after 6 months. The studies included in this review showed considerable heterogeneity, which has to be recognized before any conclusion can be drawn. However, this systematic review highlighted the potential benefits of periodontitis therapy to reduce total cholesterol and triglycerides levels. These positive effects may reduce the risk for cardiovascular complications in patients with type 2 DM.

The studies included were selected using stringent selection criteria described in the methods section, however, none of the studies included were designed to analyse lipid profiles as primary outcome measures. This may contribute to the high heterogeneity of the outcomes, as well as factors affecting lipid levels in general, including how long the individuals have had type 2 DM, lifestyle factors, and diet, which have not been assessed or reported in the included studies. All studies demonstrated a substantial reduction of clinical parameters of periodontal disease, including PD and BOP in the intervention groups 3 and 6 months after therapy, indicative of a successful treatment of the inflammatory reaction involved in periodontal disease. By contrast, the control groups did not show obvious changes in assessed oral health parameters. The mean levels of investigated total cholesterol and triglycerides decreased 3 months after periodontitis therapy, however, no differences were observed after 6 months. A possible explanation for this fading effect on lipid profiles after prolonged observation periods is recolonization by the subgingival microbiota and subsequent inflammation [18] if supportive periodontal treatment is not provided. Even though the periodontal parameters were significantly improved at the 6-month follow-up relative to baseline, five out of the seven included studies [10,12,13,15,16] did not provide supportive periodontal therapy to participants in the intervention arm after the initial treatment. In these participants, it is very likely that the recolonization of the microflora re-induced the inflammatory reaction which may have adversely affected lipid parameters. It should also be noted that average periodontal probing depths and bleeding on probing percentages are lower at the 3-month follow-up compared to the 6-month follow-up. This observation indicates the necessity of a regular periodontal maintenance program aimed to minimise the recolonization of tooth surfaces with periodontal pathogens and the concordant inflammation of the adjacent tissues.

Three out of the seven studies included in the current review [14–16] showed a significant reduction in levels of glycated haemoglobin and four studies [10–13] did not show significant changes between baseline and follow-up. In those studies reporting a significant reduction of glycated haemoglobin after periodontal treatment, one study [15] showed improved levels of total cholesterol, one study [16] showed an improvement in levels of HDL, whereas in both studies, other lipid parameters showed no significant changes. The third study [16] did not find any difference in lipid parameters between baseline and follow-up despite the reduction in levels of glycated haemoglobin. Within the limitations of this comparison, a reduction in glycated haemoglobin may not necessarily be accompanied by changes in lipid levels.

Individuals with periodontitis have been noted to have an increased risk of hyperlipidaemia and hypercholesterolaemia [19]. As mentioned previously, periodontitis is a chronic infection of the tooth supporting structures [1], and local chronic infections have been shown to alter concentrations of cytokines and hormones which can result in changes in lipid metabolism [20]. Specifically, systemic exposure to infectious challenges such as bacterial lipopolysaccharide can result in the release of inflammatory cytokines including interleukin-1 (IL-1) and tumour necrosis factor alpha (TNF-α) that alter fat metabolism and promote hyperlipidaemia. Both TNF-α and IL-1 inhibit the production of lipoprotein lipase, which causes disturbances of lipid metabolism, including increased amounts of serum cholesterol and LDL [21]. A second mechanism by which bacterial lipopolysaccharides contribute to the development of atherosclerosis is by oxidative modification of increased LDL caused by macrophage activation. Oxidized LDL is taken up by macrophage scavengers, which leads to transformation of macrophages into foam cells, the hallmark of the atherosclerotic process. Oxidized LDL is also cytotoxic to endothelial cells and a potent chemoattractant for circulating human monocytes [22]. Conversely, it has also been demonstrated that a short-term high-fat diet results in prolonged impairment in the antibacterial function of polymorphonuclear leukocytes, which may cause damage of periodontal tissues [23]. Thus, a chronic hyperlipidaemic state may impair the host resistance to bacterial infection.

Cardiovascular disease is a major complication of type 2 DM and lipid abnormalities seen in diabetics are a serious contributor to this complication [6]. Glycaemic control via maintaining adequate levels of HbA1c is considered as an essential way to lower patients' risk of having diabetic complications and each 1% drop in HbA1c levels is associated with a risk reduction of 21% for diabetes-related deaths, 14% for myocardial infarction, and 37% for microvascular complications [24]. Several studies have indicated that periodontal infection caused by gram-negative bacteria had adverse effects on diabetic patients' glycaemic control [25,26]. By contrast, improved periodontal conditions following periodontal treatment can significantly improve HbA1c levels [11,27]. A lipid-lowering management in type 2 DM patients is also aimed at reducing the incidence of cardiovascular complications, and statins can be very effective in improving the lipid profile and are therefore the first line class of drugs [28]. In general, different statins have varying abilities to improve lipid profiles in patients, e.g., HDL cholesterol levels increase between 5% and 10% with statin therapy, LDL levels reduce, ranging from 27% to 60%, and triglycerides levels reduce between 11% and 40% [29]. The current analysis demonstrated a mean reduction of triglyceride levels by approximately 8% achieved by periodontitis treatment. Within the limitations of the available study data and the heterogeneity of studies, this will not be sufficient to annotate periodontitis treatment as an adjunct to a lipid-lowering management in patients suffering from type 2 DM. However, it may stimulate the interest in further exploring the benefits of good oral health for the prevention of diabetes complications and especially to setup well designed clinical trials with lipid profiles as the primary outcome.

4. Materials and Methods

4.1. Types of Studies

Randomized control trials of 3- or 6-month follow-ups were considered for this review.

4.2. Types of Participants

The participants of the included studies had a diagnosis of type 2 DM and periodontitis. Patients with type I diabetes were excluded.

4.3. Types of Intervention

All periodontal treatments using mechanical debridement (surgical and non-surgical, with and without adjunctive treatment) were included.

4.4. Types of Outcome Measures

Primary outcome measures were total cholesterol, triglycerides, LDL cholesterol, and HDL cholesterol between baseline and 3- or 6-month follow-ups. Secondary outcome measures were periodontal probing depths, clinical attachment loss, and bleeding on probing.

4.5. Search Methods

The search attempted to identify all relevant trials in English. The electronic databases searched were (date of most recent search 19 May 2019) PubMed, MEDLINE via Ovid, EMBASE via Ovid and Web of Science. A sensitive search strategy was developed following the PICO process for the question: Does periodontal treatment improve lipid profiles in individuals with type 2 DM?

- Patients = individuals with type 2 DM
- Intervention = anti-inflammatory surgical or non-surgical periodontal treatment
- Comparison = no periodontal treatment or only supragingival scaling and polishing
- Outcome = lipid profiles

The search strategy for PubMed is given as an example: ("periodontal treatment" OR "periodontitis treatment" OR "periodontal therapy" OR "periodontitis therapy" AND "diabet*"). Incomplete information and ambiguous data were researched further by contacting the author and/or researcher responsible for the study directly. If the corresponding author failed to reply, the studies were excluded. Cross-sectional studies, retrospective studies, literature reviews, systematic reviews, editors'/authors'/reviewers' comments, articles not in English, studies where the intervention was not periodontal treatment, studies which did not have an appropriate control arm, studies where lipids were not analysed both pre and post-trial, and trials involving individuals with diabetes other than type 2 DM were excluded.

4.6. Selection of Studies

Titles and abstracts were managed by downloading to Endnote X8 software. The selection of papers, the decision about eligibility, and data extraction were carried out independently, in duplicate, by three reviewers (S.G., J.E. and M.A.N.). Any disagreement was resolved by discussion. The full text of the included studies was evaluated by two authors (S.G. and M.A.N.). Data entry to a computer and data extraction was carried out by one reviewer (S.G.).

4.7. Data Extraction

The following data was extracted:

- General study characteristics: authors, year of study, country of origin, intervention/control, number of participants at baseline, follow-up period, diabetes and periodontal inclusion criteria
- Primary outcomes: lipid profiles (total cholesterol, triglycerides, LDL, HDL)
- Secondary outcomes: probing depth and bleeding on probing at baseline and 3- or 6-month follow-ups.

4.8. Quality Assessment

Quality assessment was done according to the guidelines of the Cochrane Handbook for Systematic Reviews of Interventions [17].

4.9. Data Synthesis

For continuous outcomes, mean differences (MD) and 95% CI were used to summarize the data for each group. All statistical analyses were conducted with Review Manager 5.3. Heterogeneity was assessed with Cochran's test for heterogeneity undertaken prior to each meta-analysis, and I^2 statistics.

Author Contributions: Conceptualization, S.G., C.K.C. and J.E.; methodology, S.G.; software, J.E.; validation, S.G. and M.A.N.; formal analysis, J.E.; investigation, S.G. and J.E.; resources, J.E.; data curation, S.G.; writing—original draft preparation, S.G., J.E. and R.A.; writing—review and editing, J.E., C.K.C. and R.A.; visualization, M.A.N.; supervision, J.E. and R.A.; project administration, J.E.

Funding: This research received no external funding.

Conflicts of Interest: The authors declare no conflict of interest.

References

1. Ericsson, J.S.; Abrahamsson, K.H.; Ostberg, A.L.; Hellström, M.K.; Jönsson, K.; Wennström, J.L. Periodontal health status in Swedish adolescents: An epidemiological, cross-sectional study. *Swed. Dent. J.* **2009**, *33*, 131–139. [PubMed]
2. Li, Y.; Lee, S.; Hujoel, P.; Su, M.; Zhang, W.; Kim, J.; Zhang, Y.P.; De Vizio, W. Prevalence and severity of gingivitis in American adults. *Am. J. Dent.* **2010**, *23*, 9. [PubMed]
3. Negrato, C.A.; Tarzia, O.; Jovanovič, L.; Chinellato, L.E.M. Periodontal disease and diabetes mellitus. *J. Appl. Oral Sci.* **2013**, *21*, 1. [CrossRef] [PubMed]
4. Preshaw, P.; Alba, A.; Herrera, D.; Jepsen, S.; Konstantinidis, A.; Makrilakis, K.; Taylor, R. Periodontitis and diabetes: A two-way relationship. *Diabetologia* **2012**, *55*, 21–31. [CrossRef] [PubMed]
5. Capewell, S.; Buchan, I. Why have sustained increases in obesity and type 2 diabetes not offset declines in cardiovascular mortality over recent decades in Western countries? *Nutr. Metab. Cardiovasc. Dis. NMCD* **2012**, *22*, 307–311. [CrossRef] [PubMed]
6. Fagot-campagna, A.; Rolka, D.B.; Beckles, G.L.; Gregg, E.W.; Narayan, K. Prevalence of lipid abnormalities, awareness, and treatment in US adults with diabetes. *Diabetes* **2000**, *49*, A78.
7. Shen, G.X. Lipid disorders in diabetes mellitus and current management. *Curr. Pharm. Anal.* **2007**, *3*, 17–24. [CrossRef]
8. Nourooz-Zadeh, J.; Rahimi, A.; Tajaddini-Sarmadi, J.; Tritschler, H.; Rosen, P.; Halliwell, B.; Betteridge, D. Relationships between plasma measures of oxidative stress and metabolic control in NIDDM. *Diabetologia* **1997**, *40*, 647–653. [CrossRef]
9. Pickup, J.; Mattock, M.; Chusney, G.; Burt, D. NIDDM as a disease of the innate immune system: association of acute-phase reactants and interleukin-6 with metabolic syndrome X. *Diabetologia* **1997**, *40*, 1286. [CrossRef]
10. Chen, L.; Luo, G.; Xuan, D.; Wei, B.; Liu, F.; Li, J.; Zhang, J. Effects of non-surgical periodontal treatment on clinical response, serum inflammatory parameters, and metabolic control in patients with type 2 diabetes: A randomized study. *J. Periodontol.* **2012**, *83*, 435–443. [CrossRef]
11. D'Aiuto, F.; Gkranias, N.; Bhowruth, D.; Khan, T.; Orlandi, M.; Suvan, J.; Masi, S.; Tsakos, G.; Hurel, S.; Hingorani, A.D.; et al. Systemic effects of periodontitis treatment in patients with type 2 diabetes: A 12 month, single-centre, investigator-masked, randomised trial. *Lancet Diabetes Endocrinol.* **2018**, *6*, 954–965. [CrossRef]
12. Kapellas, K.; Mejia, G.; Bartold, P.M.; Skilton, M.R.; Maple-Brown, L.J.; Slade, G.D.; O'Dea, K.; Brown, A.; Celermajer, D.S.; Jamieson, L.M. Periodontal therapy and glycaemic control among individuals with type 2 diabetes: Reflections from the PerioCardio study. *Int. J. Dent. Hyg.* **2017**, *15*, e42–e51. [CrossRef] [PubMed]
13. Kiran, M.; Arpak, N.; Unsal, E.; Erdogan, M.F. The effect of improved periodontal health on metabolic control in type 2 diabetes mellitus. *J. Clin. Periodontol.* **2005**, *32*, 266–272. [CrossRef] [PubMed]
14. Masi, S.; Orlandi, M.; Parkar, M.; Bhowruth, D.; Kingston, I.; O'Rourke, C.; Virdis, A.; Hingorani, A.; Hurel, S.J.; Donos, N.; et al. Mitochondrial oxidative stress, endothelial function and metabolic control in patients with type II diabetes and periodontitis: A randomised controlled clinical trial. *Int. J. Cardiol.* **2018**, *271*, 263–268. [CrossRef] [PubMed]
15. Moeintaghavi, A.; Arab, H.R.; Bozorgnia, Y.; Kianoush, K.; Alizadeh, M. Non-surgical periodontal therapy affects metabolic control in diabetics: A randomized controlled clinical trial. *Aust. Dent. J.* **2012**, *57*, 31–37. [CrossRef]
16. Sun, W.L.; Chen, L.L.; Zhang, S.Z.; Wu, Y.M.; Ren, Y.Z.; Qin, G.M. Inflammatory cytokines, adiponectin, insulin resistance and metabolic control after periodontal intervention in patients with type 2 diabetes and chronic periodontitis. *Intern. Med. (Tokyo, Japan)* **2011**, *50*, 1569–1574. [CrossRef]
17. Higgins, J.P.; Green, S. *Cochrane Handbook for Systematic Reviews of Interventions*; John Wiley & Sons: Hoboken, NJ, USA, 2008.
18. Sbordone, L.; Ramaglia, L.; Gulletta, E.; Iacono, V. Recolonization of the subgingival microflora after scaling and root planing in human periodontitis. *J. Periodontol.* **1990**, *61*, 579–584. [CrossRef]
19. Pejcic, A.; Kesic, L.; Brkic, Z.; Pesic, Z.; Mirkovic, D. Effect of periodontal treatment on lipoproteins levels in plasma in patients with periodontitis. *South. Med. J.* **2011**, *104*, 547–552. [CrossRef]

20. Oz, S.G.; Fentoglu, O.; Kilicarslan, A.; Guven, G.S.; Tanriover, M.D.; Aykac, Y.; Sozen, T. Beneficial effects of periodontal treatment on metabolic control of hypercholesterolemia. *South. Med. J.* **2007**, *100*, 686–692. [CrossRef]
21. Feingold, K.R.; Staprans, I.; Memon, R.; Moser, A.; Shigenaga, J.; Doerrler, W.; Dinarello, C.; Grunfeld, C. Endotoxin rapidly induces changes in lipid metabolism that produce hypertriglyceridemia: low doses stimulate hepatic triglyceride production while high doses inhibit clearance. *J. Lipid Res.* **1992**, *33*, 1765–1776.
22. Fentoglu, O.; Bozkurt, F.Y. The bi-directional relationship between periodontal disease and hyperlipidemia. *Eur. J. Dent.* **2008**, *2*, 142.
23. Cutler, C.W.; Eke, P.; Arnold, R.R.; Van Dyke, T.E. Defective neutrophil function in an insulin-dependent diabetes mellitus patient. A case report. *J. Periodontol.* **1991**, *62*, 394–401. [CrossRef]
24. Stratton, I.M.; Adler, A.I.; Neil, H.A.W.; Matthews, D.R.; Manley, S.E.; Cull, C.A.; Hadden, D.; Turner, R.C.; Holman, R.R. Association of glycaemia with macrovascular and microvascular complications of type 2 diabetes (UKPDS 35): Prospective observational study. *BMJ* **2000**, *321*, 405–412. [CrossRef]
25. Borgnakke, W.S. Does treatment of periodontal disease influence systemic disease? *Dent. Clin.* **2015**, *59*, 885–917. [CrossRef]
26. Teeuw, W.J.; Gerdes, V.E.; Loos, B.G. Effect of periodontal treatment on glycemic control of diabetic patients: A systematic review and meta-analysis. *Diabetes Care* **2010**, *33*, 421–427. [CrossRef]
27. Iwamoto, Y.; Nishimura, F.; Nakagawa, M.; Sugimoto, H.; Shikata, K.; Makino, H.; Fukuda, T.; Tsuji, T.; Iwamoto, M.; Murayama, Y. The effect of antimicrobial periodontal treatment on circulating tumor necrosis factor-alpha and glycated hemoglobin level in patients with type 2 diabetes. *J. Periodontol.* **2001**, *72*, 774–778. [CrossRef]
28. Thompson, P.D.; Panza, G.; Zaleski, A.; Taylor, B. Statin-associated side effects. *J. Am. Coll. Cardiol.* **2016**, *67*, 2395–2410. [CrossRef]
29. Feingold, K.R.; Grunfeld, C. Cholesterol Lowering Drugs. *MDText* **2000**.

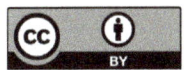

© 2019 by the authors. Licensee MDPI, Basel, Switzerland. This article is an open access article distributed under the terms and conditions of the Creative Commons Attribution (CC BY) license (http://creativecommons.org/licenses/by/4.0/).

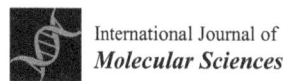

Review

Periodontal Disease in Patients Receiving Dialysis

Yasuyoshi Miyata [1,*], Yoko Obata [2], Yasushi Mochizuki [1,3], Mineaki Kitamura [2,3], Kensuke Mitsunari [1], Tomohiro Matsuo [1], Kojiro Ohba [1], Hiroshi Mukae [4], Tomoya Nishino [2], Atsutoshi Yoshimura [5] and Hideki Sakai [1,3]

[1] Department of Urology, Nagasaki University Graduate School of Biomedical Sciences, Nagasaki 852-8501, Japan
[2] Department of Nephrology, Nagasaki University Hospital, Nagasaki 852-8501, Japan
[3] Division of Blood Purification, Nagasaki University Hospital, Nagasaki 852-8501, Japan
[4] Department of Respiratory Medicine, Unit of Basic Medical Sciences, Nagasaki University Graduate School of Biomedical Sciences, Nagasaki 852-8591, Japan
[5] Department of Periodontology and Endodontology, Nagasaki University Graduate School of Biomedical Sciences, Nagasaki 852-8501, Japan
* Correspondence: yasu-myt@nagasaki-u.ac.jp; Tel.: +81-95-819-7340; Fax: +81-95-819-7343

Received: 9 June 2019; Accepted: 1 August 2019; Published: 3 August 2019

Abstract: Chronic kidney disease (CKD) is characterized by kidney damage with proteinuria, hematuria, and progressive loss of kidney function. The final stage of CKD is known as end-stage renal disease, which usually indicates that approximately 90% of normal renal function is lost, and necessitates renal replacement therapy for survival. The most widespread renal replacement therapy is dialysis, which includes peritoneal dialysis (PD) and hemodialysis (HD). However, despite the development of novel medical instruments and agents, both dialysis procedures have complications and disadvantages, such as cardiovascular disease due to excessive blood fluid and infections caused by impaired immunity. Periodontal disease is chronic inflammation induced by various pathogens and its frequency and severity in patients undergoing dialysis are higher compared to those in healthy individuals. Therefore, several investigators have paid special attention to the impact of periodontal disease on inflammation-, nutrient-, and bone metabolism-related markers; the immune system; and complications in patients undergoing dialysis. Furthermore, the influence of diabetes on the prevalence and severity of manifestations of periodontal disease, and the properties of saliva in HD patients with periodontitis have been reported. Conversely, there are few reviews discussing periodontal disease in patients with dialysis. In this review, we discuss the available studies and review the pathological roles and clinical significance of periodontal disease in patients receiving PD or HD. In addition, this review underlines the importance of oral health and adequate periodontal treatment to maintain quality of life and prolong survival in these patients.

Keywords: periodontal disease; peritoneal dialysis; hemodialysis; immune response; diabetes

1. Introduction

Chronic kidney disease (CKD) is defined as a specific, irreversible loss of functional nephrons characterized by progression towards end-stage renal disease (ESRD). The loss of renal function is the most severe form of CKD. In general, when renal function decreases below approximately 10% of normal efficiency, renal replacement therapy is necessary to maintain survival.

Dialytic therapy, mainly peritoneal dialysis (PD) and hemodialysis (HD), are common renal replacement therapies that are used worldwide. Both techniques are performed to remove excessive fluids, electrolytes, and uremic toxins. PD uses the peritoneum as the membrane through which fluids and substances are exchanged with the blood. Solute clearance occurs by solute diffusion from the plasma into a dialysate or ultrafiltration is driven by the osmotic gradient between the hyperosmotic dialysate and the plasma. In contrast, in HD, the transfer between blood and dialysis fluid is performed using a dialyzer membrane. Furthermore, PD has been reported to have the advantage of maintaining residual renal function (RRF) and achieving better outcomes than HD during the first few years of treatment [1]. Other benefits include greater effectiveness in improving quality of life (QoL) and better tolerability in patients with decreased cardiac function. However, PD is less efficient at removing wastes from the body than HD, and the presence of the catheter presents a risk of peritonitis due to the possibility of microbial entry into the abdomen.

Periodontal disease is an oral, chronic infectious, and inflammatory disease caused predominantly by gram-negative anaerobic bacteria, and is characterized by the destruction of tooth-supporting tissues, including the alveolar bone and connective tissues of the periodontium [2,3]. Currently, there is a general agreement that the prevalence of periodontal disease in patients undergoing dialysis is higher than that in healthy individuals. In fact, Borawski et al. [4] reported a marked increase in periodontitis in CKD patients, including patients undergoing predialysis, PD, and HD, compared with the general population. Conversely, when the prevalence and severity of periodontal disease are stratified according to PD or HD treatment, the observed rate was as high as 42.6% in continuous ambulatory PD (CAPD) patients [5]. Moreover, Cengiz et al. [6] reported that the prevalence of moderate to severe periodontitis was 67.3% in CAPD patients. However, in contrast to these results, there have been several reports indicating that PD patients and healthy individuals show a similar prevalence of periodontitis [7,8]. Surprisingly, a recent report suggested that 106 of 107 HD patients (99.1%) exhibit some form of periodontitis [9], and another study also showed that only one of 103 HD patients evaluated had a healthy periodontium [10]. Even if such reports are excluded, many studies have reported that over half of HD patients exhibit periodontitis [11–14]. Furthermore, most periodontal parameters in HD patients were reported to be significantly higher than those in age-matched control subjects and healthy individuals [15–17]. Thus, many investigators have shown that periodontal disease is an important issue in patients with PD and HD.

In this review, we searched for the literature on "periodontal disease" or "periodontitis" and "peritoneal dialysis" or "hemodialysis" using PubMed. We subsequently excluded studies without clinical and laboratory data, and prioritized the most recent studies and those with comparative analyses. We also discuss periodontal indices, the biochemical profile of the blood, and the molecular mechanisms involved in periodontal disease in patients with PD. We focus on the impact of periodontal disease on pathological mechanisms including inflammation, the immune response, and bone metabolism in HD patients. In addition, we compare the severity of periodontal disease, periodontal parameters, and oral health-related conditions in HD patients with diabetic and non-diabetic nephropathies.

2. Peritoneal Dialysis

2.1. Impact of Periodontal Disease

In this review, different measures of the severity of periodontal disease are discussed. These measures and their criteria are familiar essentially to dentists. Therefore, we present a summary of some representative measures Table 1 [4].

There have been several studies to date indicating that longer duration of CAPD is associated with the severity of periodontitis [5,6]. In addition, the severity of periodontitis correlated positively with levels of inflammatory parameters (high-sensitivity C-reactive protein (hs-CRP), serum ferritin, and white blood cell count) and atherosclerotic risk factors (serum low-density lipoprotein cholesterol, lipoprotein (a), and homocysteine) [5,6]. Conversely, periodontal health status showed a significant negative correlation with serum albumin and blood urea nitrogen (BUN) levels, which suggest poor nutritional status [6]. In contrast to HD, the timing of blood sampling did not have a significant impact in CAPD. Therefore, we believe that periodontal conditions affect the inflammatory and nutritional parameters in PD patients' blood samples.

Table 1. Criteria for representative periodontal measures.

Plaque Index	
0	No plaque in the gingival area
1	A film of plaque adhering to the free gingival margin and adjacent area of the tooth; may be recognized only by running a probe across the tooth surface
2	Moderate accumulation of soft deposits within the gingival pocket and on the gingival margin and/or adjacent tooth surface; can be seen by the naked eye
3	Abundance of soft material within the gingival pocket and/or on the gingival margin and adjacent tooth surface
Papillary Bleeding Index	
0	No bleeding on probing
1	Single ecchymosis of the gingiva on probing
2	Multiple ecchymoses or minor single spot extravasation from the gingiva on probing
3	Bleeding into the pocket immediately after probe insertion
4	Intensive extra pocket bleeding on probing
Gingival Index	
0	Normal gingiva
1	Mild inflammation, slight change in color, slight edema, no bleeding on palpation
2	Moderate inflammation, redness, edema, glazing, bleeding on palpation
3	Severe inflammation, marked redness and edema, ulceration, tendency to spontaneous bleeding
Community Periodontal Index	
0	Healthy gingiva
1	Bleeding observed, directly or by using mouth mirror, after probing
2	Calculus detected during probing, but all the black band on the probe visible
3	Pocket 4–5 mm (gingival margin within the black band on the probe)
4	Pocket 6 mm or more (black band on the probe not visible)
X	Excluded sextant (less than two teeth present)

Hepatocyte growth factor (HGF) is known to play important roles in embryogenesis, morphogenesis, wound repair, and tissue regeneration [18]. Oshima et al. reported that these pleiotropic properties of HGF might be involved in the development and progression of periodontal diseases [19–21]. Previously, Wilczynska-Borawska et al. [22] showed that there was no difference in HGF levels in the saliva of HD, PD, and chronic renal failure patients, although the levels in the saliva of periodontitis patients were higher than those in the healthy population. In PD patients specifically, significant and positive correlations between HGF levels in the saliva and plaque index (PI), papillary bleeding index (PBI), and gingival index (GI) have been reported. Similar to blood sampling, the timing of saliva collection may not be a factor influencing HGF levels in patients on PD. Thus, HGF might contribute to the development of periodontal disease in PD patients. However, the molecular mechanism involved in the pathogenesis of periodontal disease in PD patients remains to be clarified. Herein, we hoped to clarify the precise mechanisms of pathogenesis and progression of periodontal diseases.

2.2. Impact of Periodontal Care and Treatment

Several studies have investigated the effects of periodontal therapy in PD patients [5,22]. Briefly, treatment of periodontal disease improved periodontal status, inflammatory markers, and nutrition status [5]. Tasdemir et al. [23] investigated the effects of periodontal therapy on inflammation markers in PD patients with diabetic nephropathy, diabetic patients without CKD, and in the healthy population, since it has been reported that diabetes mellitus (DM) is one of the risk factors of periodontitis, and that periodontal inflammation causes poor glycemic control. The authors demonstrated that all inflammatory markers including tumor necrosis factor (TNF)-α, pentraxin-3 (PTX-3), interleukin (IL)-6, and hs-CRP in blood samples were significantly higher in PD patients with diabetic nephropathy than in the other two groups, and TNF-α was reduced after 3 months of periodontal treatment in all patients [23]. Conversely, PTX-3, IL-6, and hs-CRP levels were decreased after periodontal treatment only in PD patients with diabetic nephropathy [23]. Thus, the authors speculated that periodontal disease is a major source of inflammation in CAPD patients with diabetes [23]. Conversely, in a study evaluating the clinical impact of PD on oral health, Keles et al. [23] reported that the degree of halitosis was significantly reduced by PD therapy. As a potential underlying mechanism, the authors speculated that a decrease in BUN levels and an increase in salivary flow rates (SFR) resulting from adequate PD treatment might be associated with the improvement of halitosis, as high BUN levels and low SFRs have been reported to play important roles in the severity of halitosis [24]. Thus, periodontal care and treatment are useful for ameliorating a variety of the inflammatory manifestations in diabetic nephropathy patients, and for partially relieving symptoms caused by periodontal diseases. However, further studies in non-diabetic patients, with a focus on periodontal disease-related symptoms, are necessary before drawing definitive conclusions.

3. Hemodialysis

3.1. Correlations with Blood Test Indices

As mentioned above, HD is a form of renal replacement therapy, whereby toxins, waste, and excessive proteins and electrolytes, such as urea, potassium, and excess fluids are removed from the blood. This enables HD to improve QoL and prolong survival in patients with ESRD. Unfortunately, bacterial infection is common in patients with HD, and is a major cause of death because of the suppression of immunological function, increasing incidence of diabetes, and deterioration of nutritional status [25–27]. In HD patients, periodontal disease induces not only local inflammation but also systematic inflammatory responses [28–30]. In a QoL analysis of HD patients, 5 of 8 indices of the SF-36 health scale (physical functioning, role physical, vitality, social functioning, and mental health) were significantly lower in patients with severe periodontitis ($p < 0.05$) compared to those with no/mild periodontitis [14]. Thus, many studies have investigated the relationships between the prevalence and/or severity of periodontal disease and serum levels of inflammation-related factors in HD patients. Moreover, periodontal disease may also affect nutritional and bone loss parameters in HD patients [10,31]. Based on these reports, several researchers and clinicians have paid special attention to the relationship between periodontal disease and changes in systemic conditions, including inflammation, nutrition, and bone metabolism, resulting from HD. Therefore, we have reviewed the data on serum levels of CRP, albumin, calcium, phosphorus, parathyroid hormone (PTH), and other hematological parameters in HD patients. However, we should note the fact that the timing of blood sampling is not clearly defined in almost all of the previous reports. In general, routine blood sampling is performed at the initiation of HD. However, if it is performed at the time of a dental consultation, sampling at the initiation of HD is not possible. In real-world settings, the overall management of patients and supervision of HD is performed by nephrologists or urologists. Therefore, blood sampling can be assumed to have been performed at the initiation of HD.

3.1.1. Serum CRP Levels

Serum CRP levels in HD patients with advanced periodontitis have been reported to be significantly higher ($p < 0.05$) than in those without periodontitis [32]. Furthermore, other investigators have shown that serum CRP levels were decreased following periodontal therapy ($p = 0.001$) in HD patients with periodontal disease [30]. Moreover, the number of teeth was negatively associated with serum CRP level in patients with HD ($r = -0.23$, $p < 0.05$) [10]. These results support the notion that serum CRP levels may reflect the inflammatory status of periodontal tissues, and that the serum CRP level is a useful marker of treatment success in HD patients with periodontal disease. In contrast to these findings, in 154 patients on HD, the mean serum CRP level in those with severe periodontitis was reported to be similar to that in those without periodontitis (9.27 and 11.90 mg/dL, respectively; $p = 0.28$) [33]. In addition, the same study found no significant difference in serum CRP levels ($p = 0.23$) between HD patients with no/mild periodontitis ($n = 100$) and moderate/severe periodontitis ($n = 68$). This non-significant relationship between serum CRP levels and severity of periodontal disease was supported by other investigators [10,12]. Moreover, salivary CRP levels in HD patients were reported to be significantly higher compared to both controls and patients with CKD not receiving HD [34]. Thus, there are contrasting opinions regarding the pathological significance of serum CRP levels in HD patients with periodontal disease.

Conversely, a study measuring hs-CRP levels showed that the median (interquartile range) serum level in HD patients with no, mild, moderate, and severe periodontitis was 1.96 (0.79–8.17), 2.72 (0.87–6.91), 4.19 (1.92–10.47), and 4.42 (2.46–13.4), respectively, showing a significant positive correlation (p = 0.008) [35]. Likewise, serum hs-CRP levels have been reported to be a significant and independent predictor for the development of periodontal disease in a multivariate model that included DM, frequency of teeth brushing, and various serum markers in HD patients [36]. Based on these results, we felt that hs-CRP was a better marker of the severity of periodontal disease and progression of the disease in HD patients than CRP.

Regarding changes in serum CRP level following treatment of periodontal disease in HD patients, conflicting results have been reported. For example, one report showed that serum CRP levels were significantly decreased (p = 0.001) after periodontal treatment in 41 patients receiving HD [30]. Similar results have also been reported in 77 HD patients treated with non-surgical methods [12]. In contrast, other investigators have reported that serum CRP levels in HD patients with treated chronic periodontitis (n = 43) were similar (p = 0.634) to untreated patients (n = 30) [37]. Conversely, a study measuring hs-CRP showed that serum levels were significantly decreased (p < 0.001) by the treatment of periodontal diseases, including non-surgical and surgical methods (mean/SD: 3.8/21.9 to 0.6/5.9 mg/L) [38]. As mentioned above, there is the possibility that hs-CRP levels are a better indicator of the inflammatory status caused by periodontal disease in HD patients. However, it should be noted that not only periodontal diseases but also other factors are recognizable as sources of inflammation in patients with HD [39,40]. Further studies with more detailed analyses and larger populations are necessary to determine the pathological significance and value of CRP or hs-CRP levels as biomarkers in HD patients with periodontal disease. A summary of these results is shown in Table 2.

Table 2. Relationships between serum C-reactive protein level and periodontal disease.

n	Correlation with Periodontal Disease and Its Severity	Author/Year/Ref
253 *	Positively correlated with periodontitis severity	Chen/2006/[35]
44	Higher in advanced periodontitis versus non-cases	Franek/2006/[32]
154	Not different between non-cases and periodontitis	Kshirsagar/2007/[33]
253 *	Positively correlated with periodontitis severity	Chen/2011/[11]
77	Not correlated with periodontitis severity	Yazdi/2013/[12]
136 *	Higher in periodontal disease versus non-cases	Hou/2017/[36]
128	Not different between healthy/gingivitis and periodontitis	Cholewa/2018/[10]
211	Higher in periodontal disease versus non-cases	Iwasaki/2018/[41]

* High-sensitive C-reactive protein; Ref: Reference.

3.1.2. Serum Albumin Levels

Evaluation of nutritional status in HD patients is important because hypo-albuminemia is known as a predictive factor of worse mobility and mortality [42,43]. Many investigators have paid special attention to the relationship between periodontal disease and serum albumin levels. Kshirsagar et al. reported that the mean/SD serum albumin levels in HD patients with and without periodontitis (n = 35 and 119, respectively) were 3.83/0.41 and 3.99/0.53 mg/dL, respectively, although this difference did not reach statistical significance (p = 0.06) [33]. However, their study also showed that severe periodontitis was significantly associated with low serum albumin levels in univariate logistic regression analysis (odds ratio = 3.23, 95% confidential interval [CI]; 1.16–8.96, p = 0.02) [33]. In addition, the same significant correlation was confirmed by multivariate analysis models including clinical features and laboratory data [33]. A positive association between periodontitis and hypo-albuminemia was confirmed by other investigators [13]. Furthermore, several reports have demonstrated that serum albumin levels were negatively associated with representative parameters of periodontal health status including plaque index ($r = -0.26$, $p < 0.01$), ($r = -0.28$, $p < 0.01$), periodontal disease index ($r = -0.29$, $p < 0.01$), and pocket depth ($r = -0.20$, $p < 0.05$) [10,35], and a multivariate analysis showed that the serum albumin level is an independent predictor of the periodontal disease index (relative ratio = -0.47, CI = -0.91 to 0.03, $p = 0.036$) [35]. Moreover, serum albumin levels in HD patients with treated chronic periodontitis were significantly lower ($p = 0.023$) than in untreated patients [37]. Thus, periodontal disease seems to decrease serum albumin level in patients with HD. This negative correlation can be explained by various reasons, including protein energy malnutrition, consistent inflammation, and reduced oral intake [33]. However, in patients with HD, there is no general agreement on this relationship, and the detailed mechanism is not fully understood. In fact, a recent report indicated that serum albumin levels were not significantly different between dentate HD patients and edentulous patients ($p = 0.761$), or patients with healthy periodontium or gingivitis and those with periodontitis ($p = 0.601$) [10].

In contrast to these findings, HD patients with moderate-severe periodontitis exhibited higher serum albumin levels (mean/SD; none or mild periodontitis: 3.7/0.4 g/dL and moderate or severe periodontitis: 3.9/0.4 g/dL) [44]. In addition, another report suggested that serum albumin levels increased following treatment of periodontal diseases (mean/SD: 3.15/0.30 to 3.38/0.37 g/dL) in 30 patients with HD [38]. We have no clear answer for these differing findings. However, besides nutritional status, serum albumin levels are regulated by various pathological conditions including aortic calcification, peptic ulcer diseases, and body fat mass [45–47]. Furthermore, we should note the method of statistical analysis used for each study. Briefly, one study showed that the frequency of patients with hypo-albuminemia (<3.6 g/dL) was not significantly associated with periodontitis in HD patients [14,41], the same group also showed that serum albumin levels in HD patients with periodontitis was significantly lower ($p = 0.01$) compared to patients without periodontitis [41]. This information is shown in Table 3.

Table 3. Relationships between serum albumin levels and periodontal disease.

n	Correlation with Periodontal Disease and Its Severity	Author/Year/Ref
253	Negatively correlated with periodontitis severity	Chen/2006/[35]
154	No difference between non-patients and periodontitis patients	Kshirsagar/2007/[33]
154	Lower in severe periodontitis versus no periodontitis	Kshirsagar/2007/[33]
253	Negatively correlated with periodontitis severity	Chen/2011/[11]
96	Lower in periodontal disease versus no periodontal disease	Rodrigues/2014/[13]
188	Not correlated with periodontitis severity	Iwasaki/2016/[14]
1355	Positively correlated with periodontitis severity	Ruospo/2017/[44]
57	Lower in periodontitis versus gingivitis cases	Naghsh/2017/[48]
128	No difference between healthy/gingivitis and periodontitis	Cholewa/2018/[10]

3.1.3. Calcium, Phosphorus, Alkaline Phosphatase, and PTH

Secondary hyper-parathyroidism and 1,25-dihydroxy vitamin D3 deficiency are common and important complications in HD patients. Furthermore, they can lead to bone fracture and arthropathy via the reduction in bone density, and changes in serum calcium, and phosphorus, while PTH levels play important roles in pathogenesis and progression of HD-related complications. However, there is a report indicating that alkaline phosphatase is a useful marker for the diagnosis of periodontal disease [49]. Therefore, we will discuss the relationship between periodontal disease and serum levels of calcium, phosphorus, alkaline phosphatase, and PTH in patients with HD.

As shown in Table 3, to our knowledge, all reports that have investigated changes in serum calcium levels by periodontitis in HD patients showed no significant difference [10,13,36,48]. In contrast, a cross-sectional study reported that higher calcium intake (584.5–1478.5 mg/day) was inversely associated with probing pocket depth (PPD) > 4 mm (adjusted odds ratio; 0.53, 95% CI; 0.30–0.94, $p = 0.03$) compared to a lower intake group (230.7–393.4 mg/day) [50]. Based on this result, supplementation with calcium might be useful to prevent periodontal disease in HD patients [36].

However, we must consider the fact that the study population comprised young women with a mean age of 31.5 years and normal renal function [50].

Regarding phosphorus in HD patients, the mean/SD serum levels in healthy/gingivitis patients (5.87/1.59 mg/dL) showed a trend towards being higher than in moderate/severe periodontitis (5.29/1.68 mg/dL) patients; however, this difference did not reach statistical significance ($p = 0.084$) [10]. In addition, several investigators have shown that serum phosphorus levels in periodontal disease are not significantly different compared to non-gingivitis groups [36,48]. However, in contrast to these results, other investigators showed that serum phosphorus levels in HD patients with periodontitis (mean/SD; 5.02/1.19 mg/dL) were significantly lower ($p = 0.024$) than in patients without periodontitis (6.25/1.72 mg/dL) [13]. In addition, serum phosphorus levels have been reported to be positively correlated with clinical attachment loss (CAL; $r = 0.47$, $p = 0.037$) [48]. However, the above study also showed that serum phosphorus levels were not associated with other periodontal parameters, such as PD, PI, GI, or bleeding on probing [48]. Conversely, serum phosphorus levels in patients with untreated chronic periodontitis (6.1/1.2 mg/dL) have been reported to be similar ($p = 0.221$) to those of treated patients (6.5/1.2 mg/dL) [37]. Although further studies are necessary, it appears that serum phosphorus levels might not influence periodontal disease in HD patients based on the calcium and PTH levels observed (see below).

Several studies have reported that periodontal disease had no significant correlation with serum PTH levels in HD patients [10,35,36,51]. In addition, alveolar bone loss was not correlated to serum PTH level in 35 HD patients with secondary hyper-parathyroidism [51]. Finally, the authors speculated that secondary hyper-parathyroidism and increased serum PTH levels played minimal roles in periodontal disease and periodontal indices in HD patients, a speculation that we also find plausible.

Conversely, as shown in Table 3, several reports have shown no significant correlation between serum levels of alkaline phosphatase and periodontal diseases [10,13]. In addition, serum alkaline phosphatase levels in HD patients with untreated chronic periodontitis (mean/SD: 134/145 mg/dL) showed a trend towards higher levels than in treated patients (117/70 mg/dL); however, this difference was not statistically significant ($p = 0.687$) [37]. Thus, there is no evidence that periodontal disease affects serum alkaline phosphatase levels. Unfortunately, there is little information on changes in serum bone-specific alkaline phosphatase levels related to periodontal disease in HD patients. In an animal model, experimental periodontitis was reported to affect serum levels of bone-specific alkaline phosphatase [52]. Thus, there is a possibility that bone-specific alkaline phosphatase reflects periodontal bone loss and/or its metabolism in patients with HD. These results are shown in Table 4.

Table 4. Correlations of alkaline phosphatase, calcium, parathyroid hormone, and phosphorous with periodontal disease in patients receiving hemodialysis.

	n	Correlation with Periodontal Disease or Its Severity	Author/Year/Ref
ALP	96	Not different between no disease and periodontal disease	Rodrigues/2014/[13]
	128	Not different between no disease and periodontal disease	Cholewa/2018/[10]
Ca	96	Not different between no disease and periodontal disease	Rodrigues/2014/[13]
	136	Not different between no disease and periodontal disease	Hou/2017/[36]
	57	Not different between gingivitis and periodontitis	Naghsh/2017/[48]
	128	Not different between healthy/gingivitis and periodontitis	Cholewa/2018/[10]
PTH	35	Not correlated with periodontal indices	Frankenthal/2002/[51]
	253	Not correlated with periodontitis severity	Chen/2006/[35]
	136	Not different between no disease and periodontal disease	Hou/2017/[36]
	128	Not different between healthy/gingivitis and periodontitis	Cholewa/2018/[10]
P	96	Lower in periodontal disease versus no disease	Rodrigues/2014/[13]
	136	Not different between no disease and periodontal disease	Hou/2017/[36]
	57	Not different between gingivitis and periodontitis	Naghsh/2017/[48]
	128	Not different between healthy/gingivitis and periodontitis	Cholewa/2018/[10]

ALP; alkaline phosphatase, Ca; calcium, PTH; parathyroid hormone, P; phosphorous.

3.1.4. Hematological Data

Several investigators have reported that there was no significant correlation between periodontitis and hematological data, such as white blood cell and platelet counts, and hematocrit [11,13,28,35,48]. However, others have found that the presence of periodontal disease was positively correlated with white blood cell count ($p < 0.001$), but not with hemoglobin levels or platelet count [36]. Such increases in white blood cell count might be due to local and/or systematic inflammation. However, to our knowledge, a significant correlation between periodontal disease and white blood cell counts was found in only one study [36]. In addition, the number of white blood cells in the gingival crevicular fluid of HD patients with periodontal disease (mean/SD: 6.05/1.81 k/µL) was significantly lower ($p < 0.001$) than that in a control group (7.02/1.30 k/µL) [53]. Based on these findings, the impact of inflammation on circulating white blood cell counts in HD patients with periodontal disease can be considered minimal.

Periodontal treatment has also been reported to significantly increase hemoglobin levels, from 9.4 g/dL to 10.6 g/dL ($p = 0.009$) [30]. In addition, hemoglobin levels in HD patients receiving periodontal treatment (11.7/1.5 mg/dL) were significantly higher ($p = 0.039$) when compared to untreated patients (10.9/1.6 mg/dL) [37]. Thus, anemia might be associated with periodontal disease in HD patients. In general, various factors can affect the anemic status of HD patients, including administration of recombinant erythropoietin and iron, nutrition, inflammation, and dialysis dose. Regarding iron deficiency-related markers, serum ferritin levels have been reported to be positively associated with periodontitis severity in 253 HD patients [35]. However, interpretation of this finding is difficult because serum ferritin levels are recognized to be not only a marker of bone marrow iron stores but also inflammation [54,55]. In addition, the role of inflammation and serum ferritin levels in HD patients also depends on iron sufficiency [56]. Conversely, other reports have shown that serum transferrin levels in HD patients with periodontitis (mean/SD; 211.7/68.2 mg/dL) were similar ($p = 0.11$) to those without periodontitis (263.8/81.4 mg/dL) [13]. Thus, the impact of iron metabolism and storage on anemia caused by periodontal disease in HD patients is not fully understood and we believe that further studies are necessary to reach a definitive conclusion [48].

3.2. Correlation with Duration of HD

Various physiological functions and pathological conditions are mediated by long term HD [56–60]. Regarding periodontitis, the lack of a significant correlation between severity of the disease and the duration of HD has been reported in 103 HD patients [10]. Likewise, no significant relationships between HD duration and the prevalence and/or severity of periodontal disease have been reported by other investigators [9,11,14,41,61]. Furthermore, one report indicated that periodontal indices, such as PI, GI, and PPD, in HD patients were similar to those in healthy controls, and these values showed no variation during the first 5 years of HD [16]. However, that study also demonstrated that a significant increase in these values was detected during the second 5-year period, and a significantly greater increase was observed after 10 years [16]. In short, their results showed that these periodontal indices worsened with longer duration of HD. In addition, another report showed that GI and PPD scores were significantly higher in subgroups receiving HD for 3 or more years ($p \leq 0.001$ and < 0.001, respectively), and were positively correlated with HD duration ($r = 0.48$; $p < 0.001$ and $r = 0.48$; $p < 0.001$, respectively) [15]. Furthermore, another study confirmed the correlation between duration of HD and GI or PPD ($r = 0.27$; $p = 0.008$ or $r = 0.39$, $p < 0.001$, respectively) [62]. Thus, several reports have indicated a positive correlation between longer dialysis duration and periodontal disease-related parameters in HD patients [15,16,35,44], and a multivariate analysis model including age, DM, smoking status, and serum albumin level confirmed these findings [35].

Conversely, there have been conflicting results regarding the relationship between HD duration and decayed, missing, and filled teeth (DMFT). In short, although Bayrakter et al. reported that HD duration was positively correlated with missing ($r = 0.26$, $p = 0.024$), but not with decayed, filled teeth, or the DMFT index, Sekiguchi et al. found that HD duration was correlated with decayed teeth ($r = 0.42$, $p < 0.001$) and the DMFT index ($r = 0.28$, $p = 0.006$), but not with missing and filled teeth [15,62]. Thus, the relationship between the prevalence and/or severity of periodontitis and duration of HD is still under debate. This discrepancy may be due to differences in patient backgrounds and lifestyle habits, as various factors including age, diabetes, and smoking status, may have affected the pathogenesis and progression of periodontitis [35]. Furthermore, negligence of oral hygiene and a period of pre-dialysis with CKD are the main causes of higher prevalence and severity of periodontitis in HD patients rather than uremic conditions [10]. Conversely, a study has also reported that the duration of HD was not associated with specific microbiota or biofilms in 52 HD patients [63]. In this review, we would like to emphasize that duration of HD is one of the most powerful predictors of HD-induced complications and survival. Finally, more detailed investigations considering factors such as patient background, lifestyle habits, microbiota, complications, quantity, and method of HD are important to further clarify this issue.

3.3. Correlation with an Immune Response

A variety of immune cells, such as monocytes and dendritic cells, in periodontal tissues recognize and/or phagocytose bacteria, and subsequently secret various inflammatory mediators including ILs, TNF-α, vascular endothelial growth factor, and matrix metalloproteinase [33,64,65]. Furthermore, intervention studies have shown that treatment of periodontal disease decreased systemic levels of IL-6 and CRP [29]. Thus, the above evidence suggests that periodontal disease may mediate the immune response in patients receiving HD.

It has been suggested that a weak immune response underlies the increased incidence and rapid progression of periodontitis in patients with HD [66]. In short, the immune system in HD patients, especially those with DM-induced ESRD, might be unable to fend off the bacteria. In addition to this immune vulnerability, deteriorated dental and oral status due to greater plaque accumulation, dental calculus, salivary urea concentration, and salivary pH levels have been suggested to be related the high frequency of periodontal diseases [66,67]. Furthermore, poor oral hygiene due to gingival bleeding and decreased SFR compared to healthy persons is likely to be associated with persistent inflammation of periodontal tissues in HD patients [61,63,66,68,69]. In fact, a study with a large population (n = 4205 adults) showed that poorer dental health was positively associated with early all-cause death and cardiovascular diseases [70]. Finally, this chronic inflammation and consistent bacterial infection under weak immune responses is speculated to contribute to spreading of bacteria from the focal periodontal tissues into the bloodstream, and to the subsequent systematic inflammation in patients with HD.

The cytokine levels in the periodontium of HD patients have been previously investigated [53]. In that study, TNF-α and IL-8 were measured in the gingival fluids of 43 HD patients. The results showed that gingival fluid levels of TNF-α in HD patients (31.4/1.41 pg/mL) was nearly ten times as high as those in healthy controls (3.06/0.15; p < 0.001) [53]. A similar significant difference in IL-8 levels was also detected (90.98/94.03 and 35.05/16.86 pg/mL, respectively; p < 0.001) [53]. Furthermore, TNF-α levels in the gingival crevicular fluids were positively associated with PI, GI, and PPD (p < 0.001) in HD patients, and similar positive correlations were also detected between IL-8, and PI (p = 0.002), GI (p = 0.002), and PPD (p = 0.012) [53]. Based on these observations, TNF-α and IL-8 expression in the periodontal pocket is speculated to play crucial roles in the pathogenesis, development, and immune response to periodontal disease in HD patients. Nevertheless, there is no general agreement on the relationship between periodontal disease and gingival crevicular fluid levels of TNF-α and IL-8 in patients with normal renal function. In short, the levels of these cytokines in patients with periodontal disease were significantly higher than in healthy controls [71]; however, other investigators have shown that gingival crevicular fluid levels of TNF-α and IL-8 in periodontitis patients were similar to non-periodontitis patients [72,73]. Indeed, both of TNF-α and IL-8 levels in the gingival crevicular fluids of HD patients with periodontitis were reportedly not significantly different compared to patients with gingivitis (p = 0.213 and 0.823, respectively) [53]. However, we should also note that IL-1ra, IL-6, and interferon-γ levels in gingival crevicular fluids were significantly correlated to serum levels, whereas TNF-α and IL-8 were not identified in the serum of periodontitis patients with normal renal function, [74]; however, similar analyses have not been performed in HD patients to date. Thus, the pathological roles of TNF-α and IL-8 in periodontal disease in HD patients are not fully understood. The immune system is regulated by numerous cytokines, growth factors, and immune response-related molecules. However, unfortunately, immune function in the context of periodontal disease in HD patients is only partially understood. We strongly suggest that more detailed studies are necessary to understand the pathological characteristics of periodontal disease in patients undergoing dialysis.

3.4. Correlation with Cardiovascular Diseases, Metabolic Syndromes, and Pneumonia

There is a general agreement that the most important comorbidities and/or causes of death in HD patients are cardiovascular disease and DM [11,37,75]. Therefore, in this section, we reviewed the impact of periodontal disease on cardiovascular diseases in HD patients. In addition, we also reported findings regarding metabolic syndrome and pneumonia because of their frequency and significant contributions to mortality in patients with HD. DM was also discussed in the following section.

3.4.1. Cardiovascular Disease

Kaplan–Meier survival analyses have shown that cardiovascular disease-free survival rates in HD patients with moderate/severe periodontitis (defined as 2 or more teeth with at least 6 mm of inter-proximal attachment loss) were significantly worse ($p = 0.01$) compared to those with no/mild periodontitis [3]. In addition, a multivariate analysis model including age, center, sex, dialysis vintage, smoking status, cause of ESRD, DM, and hypertension demonstrated that moderate/severe periodontitis was an independent predictor of cardiovascular diseases in HD patients (hazard ratio = 5.0, 95% CI; 1.2–19.1, $p = 0.02$) compared to no/mild periodontitis [3]. However, the study also showed that periodontitis does not play a significant role in all-cause mortality among patients with HD (hazard ratio = 1.8 and 95% CI; 0.7–4.5) [3]. In contrast, other investigators showed that periodontal disease was significantly associated with risks of both cardiovascular-related and all-cause mortality [11]. Briefly, Kaplan–Meier survival curves showed that the cumulative survival rates in HD patients with severe periodontitis were significantly worse ($p < 0.001$) than in HD patients with no/mild or moderate periodontitis [11]. In addition, they found that the overall mortality rates in the no/mild ($n = 104$), moderate ($n = 98$), and severe periodontitis ($n = 51$) groups were 24.0%, 41.8%, and 70.6%, respectively, a statistically significant difference ($p < 0.001$) [11]. Interestingly, this study also showed that in a multivariate analysis model including age, serum levels of albumin, hs-CRP, the Charlson Comorbidity index score, education level, and history of smoking, severe periodontitis was an independent risk factor for all-cause mortality (hazard ratio = 1.83, 95% CI; 1.04–3.24, $p < 0.05$), but not cardiovascular-related diseases (hazard ratio = 1.95, 95% CI; 0.90–4.23, $p = 0.09$) [11]. To summarize, while a prior study had demonstrated that periodontitis is closely associated with mortality from cardiovascular disease, but not with all-cause mortality, the latter study showed opposing results.

A contrasting opinion regarding how periodontitis affects the risk for all-cause and cardiovascular mortality in patients on HD has been raised [44]. In short, the risk of all-cause and cardiovascular disease morality in HD patients with moderate-severe periodontitis was lower (hazard ratio = 0.74, CI = 0.61–0.90 and 0.67, 0.51–0.88, respectively) compared to those with none/mild periodontitis [44]. Importantly, these analyses were performed in propensity-matched cohorts.

3.4.2. Metabolic Syndromes and Pneumonia

Poor oral heath was reported to be associated with metabolic syndrome in 312 HD patients [76]. Briefly, HD patients with metabolic syndrome ($n = 145$) had a higher score compared to those without metabolic syndrome ($n = 108$) in terms of PI (mean/SD; 2.23/0.05 vs. 2.03/0.06; $p = 0.01$), GI (1.63/0.07 vs. 1.33/0.08; $p = 0.003$), and PDI (4.35/0.10 vs. 3.84/0.14; $p = 0.002$) [76]. In addition, they found that metabolic syndrome was positively associated with the severity of periodontitis ($p = 0.002$), and multivariate analysis also showed that moderate or severe periodontitis was an independent risk factor for metabolic syndrome in HD patients (odds ratio; 2.74, 95% CI; 1.29–5.79, $p = 0.008$) [76]. Furthermore, other investigators have compared periodontal indices in HD patients with and without metabolic syndrome [77]. The authors found that bone resorption in the metabolic syndrome group (mean/SD: 1.99/0.39 mm) was significantly higher than in the non-metabolic syndrome group (1.45/0.12 mm) [77]. In addition, PPD showed significant differences between the metabolic syndrome and non-metabolic syndrome groups (mean/SD: 2.73/0.47 and 2.17/0.18, respectively; $p < 0.05$).

Conversely, the cumulative incidence of pneumonia mortality in HD patients with periodontal disease was found to be significantly higher than in HD patients without periodontal disease ($p < 0.01$) [41]. Interestingly, another report showed contrasting findings where intensive treatment of periodontal disease led to a reduced risk of acute and sub-acute pneumonia (hazard ratio; 0.77, 95% CI; 0.65–0.78, $p < 0.001$) in patients with HD [78]. Incidentally, this study also demonstrated that periodontal disease treatment in HD patients was associated with a lower risk of endocarditis (hazard ratio; 0.54, 95% CI; 0.35–0.84, $p < 0.01$) and osteomyelitis (hazard ratio; 0.77, 95% CI; 0.62–0.96, $p < 0.05$) [78]. Thus, periodontal disease is speculated to have played an important role in the pathogenesis and mortality due to metabolic syndrome and pneumonia in HD patients.

3.5. Diabetic and Non-Diabetic Nephropathy

Currently, there is a general agreement that DM is a major cause of dialysis. In other words, many patients with dialysis have been receiving treatment for DM for a long time. Conversely, DM is considered to be one of the major causes of periodontal diseases [79,80]. It has been speculated that HD patients with DM have higher risk of periodontal diseases compared to those without DM. Unfortunately, few studies on the prevalence and severity of periodontal disease in HD patients with DM have been performed, and there is no systematic review on this issue to date.

3.5.1. Comparison of the Prevalence

In Japan, a cross-sectional study composed of HD patients with DM ($n = 29$), HD patients with chronic kidney nephropathy (CGN; $n = 69$), and a control group ($n = 106$) was performed. The study showed that mean/SD number of teeth present in HD patients with DM (17.9/9.8) was significantly lower ($p < 0.05$) compared to those with CGN (24.1/6.8) and the control group (25.3/5.8) [81]. In addition, the same study showed that the percentage of sites with bleeding on probing in HD patients with DM (22.2%) was significantly higher ($p < 0.05$) than in those with CGN (15.9%) and in controls (9.3%) [81]. The authors indicated that the reason for this difference in periodontal conditions between HD patients with DM and those with CGN were unclear; however, they speculated that various factors, such as healthy behavior, social, economic, and environmental status, and mental and systemic conditions, might influence the oral status in these patients [81]. Furthermore, the authors found that the SFR and total score of xerostomia in HD patients with DM or those with CGN were significantly different than those of the control group; however, these periodontitis-related parameters were similar between DM and CGN patients [81]. Thus, the oral health status in patients with renal dysfunction was worse than that of individuals with normal renal function, albeit with similarities observed between HD patients with DM or GCN. Interestingly, they showed that smoking status was significantly associated with the number of teeth in HD patients with DM. Smoking is a well-known risk factor for periodontitis and teeth loss, and it is also associated with development of DM. [82,83]. Thus, smoking played an important role, both directly and indirectly, in the oral health of HD patients with DM [81].

In contrast, the prevalence of moderate or severe periodontitis in HD patients with DM (74/76 patients = 97.4%) was reported to be similar to that of those without DM (51/53 ones = 96.2%), and the severity of periodontitis was not significantly associated with DM status ($p = 0.71$) [84]. In addition, this study showed that various periodontal findings, such as the PBI, PPD, CAL, and bleeding on probing, showed no significant differences in HD patients with and without DM ($p = 0.72, 0.40, 0.58,$ and 0.79, respectively) [84]. Thus, the impact of diabetes on the prevalence and/or severity of periodontal disease in HD patients must be clarified by further investigations.

Interestingly, the prevalence of a variety of bacteria differed between HD patients with and without DM (*Capnocytophaga* species $p = 0.02$; *Eubacterium nodatum*, $p = 0.02$; *Parvimonas micra*, $p = 0.03$; *Porphyromonas gingivalis*, $p = 0.02$) [84]. However, the authors could not definitively conclude on the relationships between periodontitis and DM in patients with HD due to several limitations; for example, the plaque index was not assessed, the mean age of patients was different, and the study was performed across multiple centers. However, they concluded that DM has no decisive influence on periodontal conditions in HD patients [84]. Nevertheless, we should consider that their study population included HD patients with well-controlled DM (mean/SD hemoglobin A1c level = 6.3/2.7).

3.5.2. Objective and Subjective Manifestations

The first comparative study of oral health, dental conditions, and periodontal status in HD patients with and without DM was reported in 2005 [85]. Regarding objective manifestations, the study showed that the percentage of HD patients with DM exhibiting uremic odor (12/43 patients; 27.9%) was significantly lower ($p = 0.018$) compared to those without DM (42/85 patients; 49.4%). However, a similar significant difference was not found in tongue coating, mucosa petechia, or ecchymosis [85]. Conversely, other investigators found that all of these objective manifestations, including uremic odor, did not differ significantly between HD patients with ($n = 46$) and without DM ($n = 54$) [86]. Nevertheless, another report showed that uremic odor, tongue coating, and mucosa petechia were significantly different between the two patient groups ($p = 0.044, 0.026,$ and 0.008, respectively) [87].

Another report using a visual analogue scale to assess subjective symptoms, including dry mouth (xerostomia), taste change (dysgeusia), and tongue/mucosa pain, showed that HD patients with DM had significantly higher scores than those without DM ($p = 0.040, 0.004,$ and 0.018, respectively) [85]. This was in contrast to findings indicating that DM status in HD patients was significantly associated with dysgeusia ($p = 0.008$), but not with dry mouth or mucosal pain [87]. Thus, these 2 studies showed that taste change (dysgeusia) in HD patients differed significantly among patients with and without DM; however, another report showed that the frequency of dysgeusia was similar [86]. In addition, no significant relationships with regard to diabetic status or xerostomia have been reported by other studies [81,87]. Thus, there is no general agreement concerning differences in objective and subjective manifestations of HD patients with and without DM.

3.5.3. The Community Periodontal Index and DMFT Index

As mentioned above, the DMFT index has been commonly used to determine the incidence of dental caries, while the community periodontal index (CPI) has been used to assess periodontal condition using a mouth mirror and a probe according to the World Health Organization criteria [88]. The DMFT index consists of 4 parameters (decayed, missing, fillings, and total teeth) and the CPI consists of 6 (healthy periodontium, bleeding on probing, calculus deposition, probing depth of 4 to 5 mm, probing depth of 6 mm or deeper, and 3 or more teeth missing).

We compared the DMFT index of HD patients with and without DM in Table 5. The overall DMFT score in HD patients, which was calculated as the sum of the number of decayed, missing, and filled teeth, was remarkably higher ($p = 0.001$) in DM patients (19.93/81.9) than in non-DM patients (14.26/9.19) [85]. This finding was supported by other investigators [87]. However, the overall DMFT score was not associated with DM status in HD patients (Table 5) [83,85]. Nevertheless, as shown in Table 4, one report showed that the DM status was significantly associated with each index item, while others showed opposing results [84,85,87].

Table 5. Decayed, missing, and filled teeth (DMFT) index in hemodialysis patients with and without diabetes.

Author/Year/Ref	Decay	Missing	Filled	Overall
Chuang/2005/[85]	Not significant	↑ ($p = 0.039$)	Not significant	↑ ($p = 0.001$)
Murali/2012/[86]	–	–	–	Not significant
Swapna/2013/[87]	↑ ($p < 0.001$)	Not significant	↑ ($p < 0.001$)	↑ ($p < 0.001$)
Schmalz/2017/[84]	Not significant	Not significant	Not significant	Not significant

↑ means that variables in the diabetic group were higher compared to the non-diabetic group.

Evaluating the CPI in HP patients, Chuang et al. [85] reported that there was a borderline significant difference in patients with diabetic and non-diabetic nephropathy ($p = 0.055$). Murali et al. [86] also found no significant association between DM status and CPI in HD patients. These results were obtained by using the chi-square test to compare diabetic nephropathy and CPI codes. In contrast, a different study reported that one CPI variable, probing depth of 6 mm or deeper, in the DM patients receiving HD group was significantly higher ($p = 0.015$) than in non-DM patients, whereas other codes, such as calculus deposition and probing depth of 4 to 5 mm, were not [87]. Thus, with the exception of one code (probing depth 6 mm or deeper), a significant difference in CPI scores was not found in previous studies. However, in contrast to this report, another study reported that the percentage of bleeding on probing and sites in HD patients with DM was significantly higher than in non-DM patients (mean/SD%: 13.3/22.2 versus 8.2/15.9; $p < 0.05$) [81]. However, we must note that this result was obtained using the Tukey HSD test, which is a multiple comparison test, to compare among patients on HD for diabetic nephropathy and chronic glomerulonephritis and healthy controls.

3.5.4. Properties of Saliva

Regarding SFRs in patients with HD, unstimulated and stimulated salivary flow, and buffering capacity of stimulated saliva have been reported to have no significant relationship with diabetic status ($p = 0.15, 0.20$, and 1.0, respectively) [83], which was also supported by another study [81]. However, Sung et al. [89] reported that the unstimulated whole SFR in 68 diabetic HD patients was significantly lower ($p = 0.032$) than that in 116 non-diabetic HD patients.

The salivary pH level in DM patients (mean/SD; 7.97/0.67) showed a trend ($p = 0.063$) towards being lower than that of patients without DM (8.22/0.44) [85]. Similarly, another study showed that the frequency of salivary pH >7.0 in the DM patients was lower compared to the non-DM patients (17.0% versus 34.0%, respectively; $p = 0.056$); however, the frequency of salivary pH <7.0 in both patient groups was similar (DM; 36.2% and non-DM; 34.0%; $p = 0.823$) [87]. Chi-square analysis showed that the relationship between diabetic status and salivary pH level was not significant ($p = 0.623$) [87]. In contrast, Schmalz et al. [84] reported an opposing finding, where the mean/SD salivary pH level of HD patients with DM (6.7/0.7) was significantly lower than that of non-DM patients (7.0/0.9; $p < 0.01$) [84].

As shown in Table 6, the changes in the SFR and pH level according to diabetic status are unclear. While the precise reasons underlying this discrepancy are unknown, differences in patients' backgrounds, history of chronic renal failure and HD, duration of DM, and hemoglobin A1c level may be factors. Conversely, an investigation into the relationships between periodontal condition-related parameters and glycemic control in HD patients with DM showed that tongue coating, dry mouth, and tongue/mucosal pain were significantly correlated with hemoglobin A1c levels ($p = 0.001, 0.001$, and 0.004, respectively); however, salivary pH levels were decreased with higher hemoglobin A1c levels (mean/SD pH level in hemoglobin A1c level ≤6%; 8.20/0.36, 6.1%–9%; 8.00/0.58, ≥9.1%; 7.46/1.07), but the differences were not statistically significant ($p = 0.086$) [85]. Therefore, we emphasized the importance of more detailed investigations with a larger study population to arrive at a conclusion.

Table 6. Comparison of properties of saliva in diabetic and non-diabetic patients.

Properties of Saliva	No. of DM/non-DM	Compared to non-Diabetic Patients	Author/Year/Ref
Salivary flow rate	116/68	Lower	Sung/2006/[89]
	29/69	Not significant	Teratani/2013/[81]
	66/93	Not significant	Schmalz/2017/[84]
Salivary pH level	85/43	Not significant	Chung/2005/[85]
	47/50	Not significant	Swapna/2013/[87]
	66/93	Lower	Schmalz/2017/[84]

DM; diabetic mellitus, Ref; Reference.

3.6. Periodontal Indices and Salivary Status with Peritoneal Dialysis

In the above sections, we discussed the changes in periodontal indices and salivary findings in response to HD. However, several reports have shown differences in these parameters between PD and HD patients, and controls (Table 7). For example, Bayraktar et al. [90]. reported that plaque and calculus accumulation in the HD and PD groups were higher than in controls. However, gingival inflammation in PD patients was significantly lower than in HD patients [22,68,90]. Moreover, the SFR in the PD group was significantly higher than that in the HD group, although both groups had significantly lower values than the control group [68]. The reduction in the SFR has been known to increase the risk of caries [91]. In fact, the authors found that the number of filled teeth was higher in the PD group than in the HD group. Differences in the SFR might be associated with better volume status in the PD group and in the relatively more liberal fluid intake because of residual renal function. In fact, the fluid dynamics of the gingiva might influence gingival health in children undergoing PD therapy [92]. We have summarized these results in Table 6. These results seem to show that the pattern of differences in periodontal indices and salivary status between healthy controls and patients with PD was not replicated between HD and PD patients. However, the data was insufficient to draw definitive conclusions.

Table 7. Periodontal parameters in the peritoneal dialysis, hemodialysis, and healthy groups.

Variables	PD Compared in the Healthy Group		PD Compared to HD	
	Difference	Author/Years/Ref	Differences	Author/Years/Ref
GI	NS	Bayrakter/2008, 2009/[68,90]	Lower	Borawski/2007, 2008/[4,90]
PBI	NS	Bayrakter/2008, 2009/[68,90]	Lower	Borawski/2007/[4] Bayrakter/2008/[90]
PI	Higher	Borawski/2007/[4] Bayrakter/2008/[90]	NS	Bayrakter/2008, 2009 /[68,90]
CSI	Higher	Bayrakter/2008/[90]	NS	Bayrakter/2008/[90]
S-pH	Higher	Bayrakter/2009/[68]	Higher	Bayrakter/2009/[68]
SFR	NS	Bayrakter/2009/[68]	Higher	Bayrakter/2009/[68]
PPD	NS	Bayrakter/2008/[90]	NS	Bayrakter/2008/[90]

GI; gingival index, PBI; papillary bleeding index, PI; plaque index, CSI; calculus surface index, S-; salivary-, SFR; salivary flow rate, PPD; probing pocket depth, NS: not significant, Ref; reference.

4. Management of Periodontal Disease

Many investigators have suggested that correct diagnosis and appropriate treatment of periodontal disease are important not only to the improvement of oral infection and inflammation, but also to maintain systemic health in patients receiving dialysis, and that managing oral health can effectively prolong survival [15–17,23,41,61,70]. In fact, brushing the teeth twice daily led to a reduced chance of developing periodontal diseases than brushing once daily, and it was identified as an independent factor [36]. Furthermore, a lower frequency of visits to the dentist has also been reported to be positively associated with higher mortality in HD patients [37]. Conversely, this report also showed that although the mortality of HD patients with chronic periodontitis is worse than of those without, the survival rate of patients treated for chronic periodontitis was not significantly different from that of untreated patients ($p = 0.774$) [37]. Furthermore, Hou et al. emphasized that special efforts for the prevention and management of periodontal disease are important in elderly HD patients because aging is another risk factor for periodontal disease in HD patients [36]. In addition to the prevention of different complex diseases and the prolongation of survival, maintenance of oral health and treatment of periodontal disease are essential for dialysis patients waiting for renal transplantation because patients with active inflammation and/or severe periodontal disease are usually judged as unfit for transplantation.

Thus, many studies support the importance of maintenance of dental health and periodontal treatment in patients with dialysis. However, in the real world, approximately 70% of Japanese HD facilities have no registered dental clinic [93]. Consequently, collaboration with dental facilities was promoted as beneficial for maintenance and management of oral health in HD patients [93], and found support from other investigators [53]. In addition, education on preventive dental care is important to the collaboration with dentists [94]. The prevalence and severity of periodontal disease are reported to vary substantially according to country, rather than being rotted in individual patient characteristics or healthcare [75].

Thus, conscientious efforts are necessary to establish an effective management and/or treatment approach to oral health in patients receiving dialysis treatment. In addition, this system must be modified for different countries in accordance with their specific conditions, including causes of ESRD, complications, and lifestyle habits. However, we believe that such a management approach in collaboration with dentists is well worth implementing because management of oral health and periodontal disease leads to maintenance or improvement in the QoL, reduction of complications, and prolongation of survival in dialysis patients.

5. Conclusions and Future Perspectives

This review showed that periodontal diseases affect the inflammation, immune response, and nutritional status in patients on dialysis. In fact, the severity of periodontal disease was significantly associated with serum levels of CRP, albumin, and a variety of minerals. In addition, several inflammation-related cytokines and molecules, such as IL-6, Il-8, TNF-α, and PTX-3 were influenced by periodontal conditions. As a result, a significant association between periodontal disease and various pathological conditions, including cardiovascular disease, metabolic syndrome, and pneumonia, is observed. Furthermore, we showed how dialysis, especially HD, exacerbates oral conditions via disruption of salivary characteristics, such as pH and flow rate. The deterioration in oral and periodontal tissues subsequently leads to a high frequency and severity of periodontal disease. Importantly, DM plays important roles in these pathological mechanisms. These findings are summarized in Figure 1. Furthermore, based on these facts, we demonstrated that maintenance of oral health and treatment of periodontal disease are important to maintaining QoL, prevention of various pathological conditions, and prolongation of survival in patients with dialysis. Unfortunately, we found that it was difficult to conduct a focused and systematic study into the relationships between periodontal disease and dialysis-related factors. Although numerous studies have been performed, they exhibit significant heterogeneity in patient characteristics, such as age, diabetic nephropathy, duration of chronic kidney disease; and methods of dialysis, such as PD or HD, the specific machine and agents used, timing of sampling, and duration. Data on the pathological roles of periodontal disease in patients with PD in particular is insufficient for a systematic review. However, continuous technological development could enable us to identify new pathogens, determine their interactions, and assess periodontal disease-related parameters in patients on dialysis. In fact, we have developed a research strategy aimed at elucidating the molecular and immune-related mechanisms of periodontal disease in patients on dialysis using novel approaches [95,96]. We emphasized that further studies with larger populations and uniform design are required to determine the pathological significance of periodontal disease and the clinical utility of oral care in patients on dialysis.

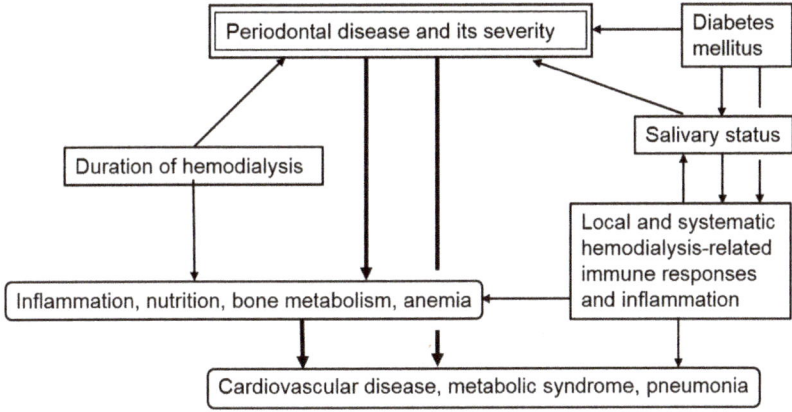

Figure 1. Schema of pathological roles played by periodontal disease in patients on hemodialysis.

Funding: This research was funded in part by a Grant-in-Aid from the Japan Society for the Promotion of Science (to Yasuyoshi Miyata; No. 16K15690).

Acknowledgments: We would like to thank Editage (www.editage.jp) for English language editing.

Conflicts of Interest: The authors declare no conflicts of interest.

References

1. Fenton, S.S.; Schaubel, D.E.; Desmeules, M.; Morrison, H.I.; Mao, Y.; Copleston, P.; Jeffery, J.R.; Kjellstrand, C.M. Hemodialysis versus peritoneal dialysis: A comparison of adjusted mortality rates. *Am. J. Kidney Dis.* **1997**, *30*, 334–342. [CrossRef]
2. Pihlstrom, B.L.; Michalowicz, B.S.; Johnson, N.W. Periodontal diseases. *Lancet* **2005**, *366*, 1809–1820. [CrossRef]
3. Kshirsagar, A.V.; Craig, R.G.; Moss, K.L.; Beck, J.D.; Offenbacher, S.; Kotanko, P.; Klemmer, P.J.; Yoshino, M.; Levin, N.W.; Yip, J.K.; et al. Periodontal disease adversely affects the survival of patients with end-stage renal disease. *Kidney Int.* **2009**, *75*, 746–751. [CrossRef] [PubMed]
4. Borawski, J.; Wilczyńska-Borawska, M.; Stokowska, W.; Myśliwiec, M. The periodontal status of pre-dialysis chronic kidney disease and maintenance dialysis patients. *Nephrol. Dial. Transplant.* **2007**, *22*, 457–464. [CrossRef] [PubMed]
5. Kocyigit, I.; Yucel, H.E.; Cakmak, O.; Dogruel, F.; Durukan, D.B.; Korkar, H.; Unal, A.; Sipahioglu, M.H.; Oymak, O.; Gurgan, C.A.; et al. An ignored cause of inflammation in patients undergoing continuous ambulatory peritoneal dialysis: Periodontal problems. *Int. Urol. Nephrol.* **2014**, *46*, 2021–2028. [CrossRef] [PubMed]
6. Cengiz, M.I.; Bal, S.; Gökçay, S.; Cengiz, K. Does periodontal disease reflect atherosclerosis in continuous ambulatory peritoneal dialysis patients? *J. Periodontol.* **2007**, *78*, 1926–1934. [CrossRef] [PubMed]
7. Thorman, R.; Neovius, M.; Hylander, B. Clinical findings in oral health during progression of chronic kidney disease to end-stage renal disease in a Swedish population. *Scand. J. Urol. Nephrol.* **2009**, *43*, 154–159. [CrossRef]
8. Brito, F.; Almeida, S.; Figueredo, C.M.; Bregman, R.; Suassuna, J.H.; Fischer, R.G. Extent and severity of chronic periodontitis in chronic kidney disease patients. *J. Periodontal. Res.* **2012**, *47*, 426–430. [CrossRef]
9. Kim, Y.J.; Moura, L.M.; Caldas, C.P.; Perozini, C.; Ruivo, G.F.; Pallos, D. Evaluation of periodontal condition and risk in patients with chronic kidney disease on hemodialysis. *Einstein (Sao Paulo)* **2017**, *15*, 173–177. [CrossRef]
10. Cholewa, M.; Madziarska, K.; Radwan-Oczko, M. The association between periodontal conditions, inflammation, nutritional status and calcium-phosphate metabolism disorders in hemodialysis patients. *J. Appl. Oral Sci.* **2018**, *26*, e20170495. [CrossRef]

11. Chen, L.P.; Chiang, C.K.; Peng, Y.S.; Hsu, S.P.; Lin, C.Y.; Lai, C.F.; Hung, K.Y. Relationship between periodontal disease and mortality in patients treated with maintenance hemodialysis. *Am. J. Kidney Dis.* **2011**, *57*, 276–282. [CrossRef]
12. Yazdi, F.K.; Karimi, N.; Rasouli, M.; Roozbeh, J. Effect of nonsurgical periodontal treatment on C-reactive protein levels in maintenance hemodialysis patients. *Ren. Fail.* **2013**, *35*, 711–717. [CrossRef]
13. Rodrigues, V.P.; Libério, S.A.; Lopes, F.F.; Thomaz, E.B.; Guerra, R.N.; Gomes-Filho, I.S.; Pereira, A.L. Periodontal status and serum biomarkers levels in haemodialysis patients. *J. Clin. Periodontol.* **2014**, *41*, 862–868. [CrossRef]
14. Iwasaki, M.; Borgnakke, W.S.; Awano, S.; Yoshida, A.; Hamasaki, T.; Teratani, G.; Kataoka, S.; Kakuta, S.; Soh, I.; Ansai, T.; et al. Periodontitis and health-related quality of life in hemodialysis patients. *Clin. Exp. Dent. Res.* **2016**, *3*, 13–18. [CrossRef]
15. Bayraktar, G.; Kurtulus, I.; Duraduryan, A.; Cintan, S.; Kazancioglu, R.; Yildiz, A.; Bural, C.; Bozfakioglu, S.; Besler, M.; Trablus, S.; et al. Dental and periodontal findings in hemodialysis patients. *Oral Dis.* **2007**, *13*, 393–397. [CrossRef]
16. Cengiz, M.I.; Sümer, P.; Cengiz, S.; Yavuz, U. The effect of the duration of the dialysis in hemodialysis patients on dental and periodontal findings. *Oral Dis.* **2009**, *15*, 336–341. [CrossRef]
17. Altamimi, A.G.; AlBakr, S.A.; Alanazi, T.A.; Alshahrani, F.A.; Chalisserry, E.P.; Anil, S. Prevalence of periodontitis in patients undergoing hemodialysis: A case control study. *Mater. Sociomed.* **2018**, *30*, 58–61. [CrossRef]
18. Boros, P.; Miller, C.M. Hepatocyte growth factor: A multifunctional cytokine. *Lancet* **1995**, *345*, 293–295. [CrossRef]
19. Ohshima, M.; Noguchi, Y.; Ito, M.; Maeno, M.; Otsuka, K. Hepatocyte growth factor secreted by periodontal ligament and gingival fibroblasts is a major chemoattractant for gingival epithelial cells. *J. Periodontal. Res.* **2001**, *36*, 377–383. [CrossRef]
20. Ohshima, M.; Fujikawa, K.; Akutagawa, H.; Kato, T.; Ito, K.; Otsuka, K. Hepatocyte growth factor in saliva: A possible marker for periodontal disease status. *J. Oral Sci.* **2002**, *44*, 35–39. [CrossRef]
21. Ohshima, M.; Sakai, A.; Ito, K.; Otsuka, K. Hepatocyte growth factor (HGF) in periodontal disease: Detection of HGF in gingival crevicular fluid. *J. Periodontal. Res.* **2002**, *37*, 8–14. [CrossRef]
22. Wilczyńska-Borawska, M.; Borawski, J.; Bagińska, J.; Małyszko, J.; Myśliwiec, M. Hepatocyte growth factor in saliva of patients with renal failure and periodontal disease. *Ren. Fail.* **2012**, *34*, 942–951. [CrossRef]
23. Tasdemir, Z.; Özsarı Tasdemir, F.; Gürgan, C.; Eroglu, E.; Gunturk, I.; Kocyigit, I. The effect of periodontal disease treatment in patients with continuous ambulatory peritoneal dialysis. *Int. Urol. Nephrol.* **2018**, *50*, 1519–1528. [CrossRef]
24. Keles, M.; Tozoglu, U.; Uyanik, A.; Eltas, A.; Bayindir, Y.Z.; Cetinkaya, R.; Bilge, O.M. Does peritoneal dialysis affect halitosis in patients with end-stage renal disease? *Perit. Dial. Int.* **2011**, *31*, 168–172.
25. Trimarchi, H.; Dicugno, M.; Muryan, A.; Lombi, F.; Iturbe, L.; Raña, M.S.; Young, P.; Nau, K.; Iriarte, R.; Pomeranz, V.; et al. Pro-calcitonin and inflammation in chronic hemodialysis. *Medicina (B Aires)* **2013**, *73*, 411–416.
26. Guo, M.; Chen, R.; Xiang, F.; Cao, X.; Hu, J.; Lu, Z.; Gong, S.; Chen, X.; Chen, X.; Ding, X.; et al. Decreased percentage of memory B cells is independently associated with increased susceptibility to infection in patients on maintenance hemodialysis. *Int. Urol. Nephrol.* **2018**, *50*, 2081–2090. [CrossRef]
27. Omari, A.M.; Omari, L.S.; Dagash, H.H.; Sweileh, W.M.; Natour, N.; Zyoud, S.H. Assessment of nutritional status in the maintenance of haemodialysis patients: A cross-sectional study from Palestine. *BMC Nephrol.* **2019**, *20*, 92. [CrossRef]
28. Noack, B.; Genco, R.J.; Trevisan, M.; Grossi, S.; Zambon, J.J.; De Nardin, E. Periodontal infections contribute to elevated systemic C-reactive protein level. *J. Periodontol.* **2001**, *72*, 1221–1227. [CrossRef]
29. D'Aiuto, F.; Nibali, L.; Parkar, M.; Suvan, J.; Tonetti, M.S. Short-term effects of intensive periodontal therapy on serum inflammatory markers and cholesterol. *J. Dent. Res.* **2005**, *84*, 269–273. [CrossRef]
30. Kadiroglu, A.K.; Kadiroglu, E.T.; Sit, D.; Dag, A.; Yilmaz, M.E. Periodontitis is an important and occult source of inflammation in hemodialysis patients. *Blood. Purif.* **2006**, *24*, 400–404. [CrossRef]
31. Zhao, D.; Zhang, S.; Chen, X.; Liu, W.; Sun, N.; Guo, Y.; Dong, Y.; Mo, A.; Yuan, Q. Evaluation of periodontitis and bone loss in patients undergoing hemodialysis. *J. Periodontol.* **2014**, *85*, 1515–1520. [CrossRef]

32. Franek, E.; Blaschyk, R.; Kolonko, A.; Mazur-Psonka, L.; Łangowska-Adamczyk, H.; Kokot, F.; Wiecek, A. Chronic periodontitis in hemodialysis patients with chronic kidney disease is associated with elevated serum C-reactive protein concentration and greater intima-media thickness of the carotid artery. *J. Nephrol.* **2006**, *19*, 346–351.
33. Kshirsagar, A.V.; Craig, R.G.; Beck, J.D.; Moss, K.; Offenbacher, S.; Kotanko, P.; Yoshino, M.; Levin, N.W.; Yip, J.K.; Almas, K.; et al. Severe periodontitis is associated with low serum albumin among patients on maintenance hemodialysis therapy. *Clin. J. Am. Soc. Nephrol.* **2007**, *2*, 239–244. [CrossRef]
34. Pallos, D.; Leão, M.V.; Togeiro, F.C.; Alegre, L.; Ricardo, L.H.; Perozini, C.; Ruivo, G.F. Salivary markers in patients with chronic renal failure. *Arch. Oral Biol.* **2015**, *60*, 1784–1788. [CrossRef]
35. Chen, L.P.; Chiang, C.K.; Chan, C.P.; Hung, K.Y.; Huang, C.S. Does periodontitis reflect inflammation and malnutrition status in hemodialysis patients? *Am. J. Kidney Dis.* **2006**, *47*, 815–822. [CrossRef]
36. Hou, Y.; Wang, X.; Zhang, C.X.; Wei, Y.D.; Jiang, L.L.; Zhu, X.Y.; Du, Y.J. Risk factors of periodontal disease in maintenance hemodialysis patients. *Medicina (Baltim.)* **2017**, *96*, e7892. [CrossRef]
37. de Souza, C.M.; Braosi, A.P.; Luczyszyn, S.M.; Olandoski, M.; Kotanko, P.; Craig, R.G.; Trevilatto, P.C.; Pecoits-Filho, R. Association among oral health parameters, periodontitis, and its treatment and mortality in patients undergoing hemodialysis. *J. Periodontol.* **2014**, *85*, e169–178. [CrossRef]
38. Siribamrungwong, M.; Puangpanngam, K. Treatment of periodontal diseases reduces chronic systemic inflammation in maintenance hemodialysis patients. *Ren. Fail.* **2012**, *34*, 171–175. [CrossRef]
39. Rahmati, M.A.; Craig, R.G.; Homel, P.; Kaysen, G.A.; Levin, N.W. Serum markers of periodontal disease status and inflammation in hemodialysis patients. *Am. J. Kidney Dis.* **2002**, *40*, 983–989. [CrossRef]
40. Mandic, A.; Cavar, I.; Skoro, I.; Tomic, I.; Ljubic, K.; Coric, S.; Mikulic, I.; Azinovic, I.; Pravdic, D. Body composition and inflammation in hemodialysis patients. *Apher. Dial.* **2017**, *21*, 556–564. [CrossRef]
41. Iwasaki, M.; Taylor, G.W.; Awano, S.; Yoshida, A.; Kataoka, S.; Ansai, T.; Nakamura, H. Periodontal disease and pneumonia mortality in haemodialysis patients: A 7-year cohort study. *J. Clin. Periodontol.* **2018**, *45*, 38–45. [CrossRef]
42. Choi, S.R.; Lee, Y.K.; Cho, A.J.; Park, H.C.; Han, C.H.; Choi, M.J.; Koo, J.R.; Yoon, J.W.; Noh, J.W. Malnutrition, inflammation, progression of vascular calcification and survival: Inter-relationships in hemodialysis patients. *PLoS ONE* **2019**, *14*, e0216415. [CrossRef]
43. Kanda, E.; Kato, A.; Masakane, I.; Kanno, Y. A new nutritional risk index for predicting mortality in hemodialysis patients: Nationwide cohort study. *PLoS ONE* **2019**, *14*, e0214524. [CrossRef]
44. Ruospo, M.; Palmer, S.C.; Wong, G.; Craig, J.C.; Petruzzi, M.; De Benedittis, M.; Ford, P.; Johnson, D.W.; Tonelli, M.; Natale, P.; et al. Periodontitis and early mortality among adults treated with hemodialysis: A multinational propensity-matched cohort study. *BMC Nephrol.* **2017**, *18*, 166. [CrossRef]
45. Matsuura, S.; Shirai, Y.; Kubo, M.; Nayama, C.; Okitsu, M.; Oiwa, Y.; Yasui, S.; Suzuki, Y.; Murata, T.; Ishikawa, E.; et al. Body fat mass is correlated with serum transthyretin levels in maintenance hemodialysis patients. *J. Med. Invest.* **2017**, *64*, 222–227. [CrossRef]
46. Avramovski, P.; Avramovska, M.; Sotiroski, K.; Sikole, A. Acute-phase proteins as promoters of abdominal aortic calcification in chronic dialysis patients. *Saudi. J. Kidney Dis. Transpl.* **2019**, *30*, 376–386. [CrossRef]
47. Kim, M.; Kim, C.S.; Bae, E.H.; Ma, S.K.; Kim, S.W. Risk factors for peptic ulcer disease in patients with end-stage renal disease receiving dialysis. *Kidney Res. Clin. Pr.* **2019**, *38*, 81–89. [CrossRef]
48. Naghsh, N.; Sabet, N.K.; Vahidi, F.; Mogharehabed, A.; Yaghini, J. Relationship between periodontal disease and serum factors in patients undergoing hemodialysis. *Open Dent. J.* **2017**, *11*, 701–709. [CrossRef]
49. Malhotra, R.; Grover, V.; Kapoor, A.; Kapur, R. Alkaline phosphatase as a periodontal disease marker. *Indian J. Dent. Res.* **2010**, *21*, 531–536. [CrossRef]
50. Tanaka, K.; Miyake, Y.; Okubo, H.; Hanioka, T.; Sasaki, S.; Miyatake, N.; Arakawa, M. Calcium intake is associated with decreased prevalence of periodontal disease in young Japanese women. *Nutr. J.* **2014**, *13*, 109. [CrossRef]
51. Frankenthal, S.; Nakhoul, F.; Machtei, E.E.; Green, J.; Ardekian, L.; Laufer, D.; Peled, M. The effect of secondary hyperparathyroidism and hemodialysis therapy on alveolar bone and periodontium. *J. Clin. Periodontol.* **2002**, *29*, 479–483. [CrossRef]
52. Sousa, L.H.; Linhares, E.V.; Alexandre, J.T.; Lisboa, M.R.; Furlaneto, F.; Freitas, R.; Ribeiro, I.; Val, D.; Marques, M.; Chaves, H.V.; et al. Effects of atorvastatin on periodontitis of rats subjected to glucocorticoid-induced osteoporosis. *J. Periodontol.* **2016**, *87*, 1206–1216. [CrossRef]

53. Dağ, A.; Firat, E.T.; Kadiroğlu, A.K.; Kale, E.; Yilmaz, M.E. Significance of elevated gingival crevicular fluid tumor necrosis factor-alpha and interleukin-8 levels in chronic hemodialysis patients with periodontal disease. *J. Periodontal. Res.* **2010**, *45*, 445–450.
54. Rocha, L.A.; Barreto, D.V.; Barreto, F.C.; Dias, C.B.; Moysés, R.; Silva, M.R.; Moura, L.A.; Draibe, S.A.; Jorgetti, V.; Carvalho, A.B.; et al. Serum ferritin level remains a reliable marker of bone marrow iron stores evaluated by histomorphometry in hemodialysis patients. *Clin. J. Am. Soc. Nephrol.* **2009**, *4*, 105–109. [CrossRef]
55. Kell, D.B.; Pretorius, E. Serum ferritin is an important inflammatory disease marker, as it is mainly a leakage product from damaged cells. *Metallomics* **2014**, *6*, 748–773. [CrossRef]
56. Kalantar-Zadeh, K.; Rodriguez, R.A.; Humphreys, M.H. Association between serum ferritin and measures of inflammation, nutrition and iron in haemodialysis patients. *Nephrol. Dial. Transpl.* **2004**, *19*, 141–149. [CrossRef]
57. Ganu, V.J.; Boima, V.; Adjei, D.N.; Yendork, J.S.; Dey, I.D.; Yorke, E.; Mate-Kole, C.C.; Mate-Kole, M.O. Depression and quality of life in patients on long term hemodialysis at a nationalhospital in Ghana: A cross-sectional study. *Ghana Med. J.* **2018**, *52*, 22–28. [CrossRef]
58. Kondo, T.; Sasa, N.; Yamada, H.; Takagi, T.; Iizuka, J.; Kobayashi, H.; Yoshida, K.; Fukuda, H.; Ishihara, H.; Tanabe, K.; et al. Acquired cystic disease-associated renal cell carcinoma is the most common subtype in long-term dialyzed patients: Central pathology results according to the 2016 WHO classification in a multi-institutional study. *Pathol. Int.* **2018**, *68*, 543–549. [CrossRef]
59. El-Gamasy, M.A. Study of some pulmonary function tests in Egyptian children with end-stage renal disease under regular hemodialysis in correlation with dialysis duration. *Saudi. J. Kidney Dis. Transpl.* **2019**, *30*, 119–128. [CrossRef]
60. Matsumoto, Y.; Mori, Y.; Kageyama, S.; Arihara, K.; Sato, H.; Nagata, K.; Shimada, Y.; Nojima, Y.; Iguchi, K.; Sugiyama, T. Changes in QTc interval in long-term hemodialysis patients. *PLoS ONE* **2019**, *14*, e0209297. [CrossRef]
61. Parkar, S.M.; Ajithkrishnan, C.G. Periodontal status in patients undergoing hemodialysis. *Indian J. Nephrol.* **2012**, *22*, 246–250. [CrossRef]
62. Sekiguchi, R.T.; Pannuti, C.M.; Silva, H.T., Jr.; Medina-Pestana, J.O.; Romito, G.A. Decrease in oral health may be associated with length of time since beginning dialysis. *Spec. Care Dent.* **2012**, *32*, 6–10. [CrossRef]
63. Castillo, A.; Mesa, F.; Liébana, J.; García-Martinez, O.; Ruiz, S.; García-Valdecasas, J.; O'Valle, F. Periodontal and oral microbiological status of an adult population undergoing haemodialysis: A cross-sectional study. *Oral Dis.* **2007**, *13*, 198–205. [CrossRef]
64. Tonetti, M.S.; Freiburghaus, K.; Lang, N.P.; Bickel, M. Detection of interleukin-8 and matrix metalloproteinases transcripts in healthy and diseased gingival biopsies by RNA/PCR. *J. Periodontal. Res.* **1993**, *28*, 511–513. [CrossRef]
65. Afacan, B.; Öztürk, V.Ö.; Paşalı, Ç.; Bozkurt, E.; Köse, T.; Emingil, G. Gingival crevicular fluid and salivary HIF-1α, VEGF, and TNF-α levels in periodontal health and disease. *J. Periodontol.* **2018**, in press. [CrossRef]
66. Sedý, J.; Horká, E.; Foltán, R.; Spacková, J.; Dusková, J. Mechanism of increased mortality in hemodialysed patients with periodontitis. *Med. Hypotheses* **2010**, *74*, 374–376. [CrossRef]
67. Craig, R.G. Interactions between chronic renal disease and periodontal disease. *Oral Dis.* **2008**, *14*, 1–7. [CrossRef]
68. Bayraktar, G.; Kurtulus, I.; Kazancioglu, R.; Bayramgurler, I.; Cintan, S.; Bural, C.; Bozfakioglu, S.; Issever, H.; Yildiz, A. Oral health and inflammation in patients with end-stage renal failure. *Perit. Dial. Int.* **2009**, *29*, 472–479.
69. Malekmakan, L.; Haghpanah, S.; Pakfetrat, M.; Ebrahimic, Z.; Hasanlic, E. Oral health status in Iranian hemodialysis patients. *Indian J. Nephrol.* **2011**, *21*, 235–238.
70. Palmer, S.C.; Ruospo, M.; Wong, G.; Craig, J.C.; Petruzzi, M.; De Benedittis, M.; Ford, P.; Johnson, D.W.; Tonelli, M.; Natale, P.; et al. ORAL-D Study Investigators. Dental health and mortality in people with end-stage kidney disease treated with hemodialysis: A multinational cohort study. *Am. J. Kidney Dis.* **2015**, *66*, 666–676. [CrossRef]
71. Lagdive, S.S.; Marawar, P.P.; Byakod, G.; Lagdive, S.B. Evaluation and comparison of interleukin-8 (IL-8) level in gingival crevicular fluid in health and severity of periodontal disease: A clinico-biochemical study. *Indian J. Dent. Res.* **2013**, *24*, 188–192. [CrossRef]

72. Branco-de-Almeida, L.S.; Cruz-Almeida, Y.; Gonzalez-Marrero, Y.; Huang, H.; Aukhil, I.; Harrison, P.; Wallet, S.M.; Shaddox, L.M. Local and plasma biomarker profiles in localized aggressive periodontitis. *JDR Clin. Trans. Res.* **2017**, *2*, 258–268. [CrossRef]
73. Chatzopoulos, G.S.; Mansky, K.C.; Lunos, S.; Costalonga, M.; Wolff, L.F. Sclerostin and WNT-5a gingival protein levels in chronic periodontitis and health. *J. Periodontal. Res.* **2019**, in press. [CrossRef]
74. Zekeridou, A.; Mombelli, A.; Cancela, J.; Courvoisier, D.; Giannopoulou, C. Systemic inflammatory burden and local inflammation in periodontitis: What is the link between inflammatory biomarkers in serum and gingival crevicular fluid? *Clin. Exp. Dent. Res.* **2019**, *5*, 128–135. [CrossRef]
75. Palmer, S.C.; Ruospo, M.; Wong, G.; Craig, J.C.; Petruzzi, M.; De Benedittis, M.; Ford, P.; Johnson, D.W.; Tonelli, M.; Natale, P.; et al. Patterns of oral disease in adults with chronic kidney disease treated with hemodialysis. *Nephrol. Dial. Transpl.* **2016**, *31*, 1647–1653. [CrossRef]
76. Chen, L.P.; Hsu, S.P.; Peng, Y.S.; Chiang, C.K.; Hung, K.Y. Periodontal disease is associated with metabolic syndrome in hemodialysis patients. *Nephrol. Dial. Transpl.* **2011**, *26*, 4068–4073. [CrossRef]
77. Tavakoli, M.; Izadi, M.; Yaghini, J.; Rastegari, A.; Abed, A.M. A survey on the effects of metabolic syndrome on the periodontal indices of hemodialysis patients. *Dent. Res. J. (Isfahan)* **2016**, *13*, 333–337.
78. Huang, S.T.; Lin, C.L.; Yu, T.M.; Wu, M.J.; Kao, C.H. Intensive periodontal treatment reduces risk of infection-related hospitalization in hemodialysis population: A nationwide population-based cohort study. *Medicina (Baltim.)* **2015**, *94*, e1436. [CrossRef]
79. Casanova, L.; Hughes, F.J.; Preshaw, P.M. Diabetes and periodontal disease: A two-way relationship. *Br. Dent. J.* **2014**, *217*, 433–437. [CrossRef]
80. Gayathri, S.; Elizabeth, K.; Sadasivan, A.; Arunima, P.R.; Jaya Kumar, K. Effect of initial periodontal therapy on serum nitric oxide levels in chronic periodontitis patients with or without type 2 diabetes mellitus. *J. Contemp. Dent. Pract.* **2019**, *20*, 197–203. [CrossRef]
81. Teratani, G.; Awano, S.; Soh, I.; Yoshida, A.; Kinoshita, N.; Hamasaki, T.; Takata, Y.; Sonoki, K.; Nakamura, H.; Ansai, T. Oral health in patients on haemodialysis for diabetic nephropathy and chronic glomerulonephritis. *Clin. Oral Investig.* **2013**, *17*, 483–489. [CrossRef]
82. Chambrone, L.; Chambrone, D.; Lima, L.A.; Chambrone, L.A. Predictors of tooth loss during long-term periodontal maintenance: A systematic review of observational studies. *J. Clin. Periodontol.* **2010**, *37*, 675–684. [CrossRef]
83. Psaltopoulou, T.; Ilias, I.; Alevizaki, M. The role of diet and lifestyle in primary, secondary, and tertiary diabetes prevention: A review of meta-analyses. *Rev. Diabet. Stud.* **2010**, *7*, 26–35. [CrossRef]
84. Schmalz, G.; Schiffers, N.; Schwabe, S.; Vasko, R.; Müller, G.A.; Haak, R.; Mausberg, R.F.; Ziebolz, D. Dental and periodontal health, and microbiological and salivary conditions in patients with or without diabetes undergoing haemodialysis. *Int. Dent. J.* **2017**, *67*, 186–193. [CrossRef]
85. Chuang, S.F.; Sung, J.M.; Kuo, S.C.; Huang, J.J.; Lee, S.Y. Oral and dental manifestations in diabetic and nondiabetic uremic patients receiving hemodialysis. *Oral Surg. Oral Med. Oral Pathol. Oral Radiol. Endod.* **2005**, *99*, 689–695. [CrossRef]
86. Murali, P.; Narasimhan, M.; Periasamy, S.; Harikrishnan, T.C. A comparison of oral and dental manifestations in diabetic and non-diabetic uremic patients receiving hemodialysis. *J. Oral Maxillofac. Pathol.* **2012**, *16*, 374–379. [CrossRef]
87. Swapna, L.A.; Reddy, R.S.; Ramesh, T.; Reddy, R.L.; Vijayalaxmi, N.; Karmakar, P.; Pradeep, K. Oral health status in haemodialysis patients. *J. Clin. Diagn. Res.* **2013**, *7*, 2047–2050. [CrossRef]
88. Pilot, T.; Miyazaki, H. Global results: 15 years of CPITN epidemiology. *Int. Dent. J.* **1994**, *44*, 553–560.
89. Sung, J.M.; Kuo, S.C.; Guo, H.R.; Chuang, S.F.; Lee, S.Y.; Huang, J.J. The role of oral dryness in interdialytic weight gain by diabetic and non-diabetic haemodialysis patients. *Nephrol. Dial. Transpl.* **2006**, *21*, 2521–2528. [CrossRef]
90. Bayraktar, G.; Kurtulus, I.; Kazancioglu, R.; Bayramgurler, I.; Cintan, S.; Bural, C.; Bozfakioglu, S.; Besler, M.; Trablus, S.; Issever, H.; et al. Evaluation of periodontal parameters in patients undergoing peritoneal dialysis or hemodialysis. *Oral Dis.* **2008**, *14*, 185–189. [CrossRef]
91. Vissink, A.; Panders, A.K.; Gravenmade, E.J.; Vermey, A. The causes and consequences of hyposalivation. *Ear Nose Throat J.* **1988**, *67*, 166–168, 173–176.
92. Sakallioğlu, E.E.; Lütfioğlu, M.; Ozkaya, O.; Aliyev, E.; Açikgöz, G.; Firatli, E. Fluid dynamics of gingiva and gingival health in children with end stage renal failure. *Arch. Oral Biol.* **2007**, *52*, 1194–1199. [CrossRef]

93. Yoshioka, M.; Shirayama, Y.; Imoto, I.; Hinode, D.; Yanagisawa, S.; Takeuchi, Y. Current status of collaborative relationships between dialysis facilities and dental facilities in Japan: Results of a nationwide survey. *BMC Nephrol.* **2015**, *16*, 17. [CrossRef]
94. Yoshioka, M.; Shirayama, Y.; Imoto, I.; Hinode, D.; Yanagisawa, S.; Takeuchi, Y.; Bando, T.; Yokota, N. Factors associated with regular dental visits among hemodialysis patients. *World J. Nephrol.* **2016**, *5*, 455–460. [CrossRef]
95. Ohyama, K.; Yoshimi, H.; Aibara, N.; Nakamura, Y.; Miyata, Y.; Sakai, H.; Fujita, F.; Imaizumi, Y.; Chauhan, A.K.; Kishikawa, N.; et al. Immune complexome analysis reveals the specific and frequent presence of immune complex antigens in lung cancer patients: A pilot study. *Int. J. Cancer.* **2017**, *140*, 370–380. [CrossRef]
96. Aibara, N.; Kamohara, C.; Chauhan, A.K.; Kishikawa, N.; Miyata, Y.; Nakashima, M.; Kuroda, N.; Ohyama, K. Selective, sensitive and comprehensive detection of immune complex antigens by immune complexome analysis with papain-digestion and elution. *J. Immunol. Methods* **2018**, *461*, 85–90. [CrossRef]

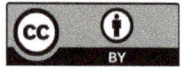

© 2019 by the authors. Licensee MDPI, Basel, Switzerland. This article is an open access article distributed under the terms and conditions of the Creative Commons Attribution (CC BY) license (http://creativecommons.org/licenses/by/4.0/).

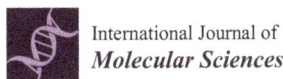

Review

The Possible Causal Link of Periodontitis to Neuropsychiatric Disorders: More Than Psychosocial Mechanisms

Sadayuki Hashioka [1,*], Ken Inoue [2], Tsuyoshi Miyaoka [1], Maiko Hayashida [1], Rei Wake [1], Arata Oh-Nishi [1] and Masatoshi Inagaki [1]

1. Department of Psychiatry, Shimane University, 89-1 Enya-cho, Izumo 693-8501, Japan
2. Health Service Center, Kochi University, 2-5-1 Akebono-cho, Kochi 780-8520, Japan
* Correspondence: hashioka@f2.dion.ne.jp

Received: 22 May 2019; Accepted: 25 July 2019; Published: 30 July 2019

Abstract: Increasing evidence implies a possible causal link between periodontitis and neuropsychiatric disorders, such as Alzheimer's disease (AD) and major depression (MD). A possible mechanism underlying such a link can be explained by neuroinflammation induced by chronic systemic inflammation. This review article focuses on an overview of the biological and epidemiological evidence for a feasible causal link of periodontitis to neuropsychiatric disorders, including AD, MD, Parkinson's disease, and schizophrenia, as well as the neurological event, ischemic stroke. If there is such a link, a broad spectrum of neuropsychiatric disorders associated with neuroinflammation could be preventable and modifiable by simple daily dealings for oral hygiene. However, the notion that periodontitis is a risk factor for neuropsychiatric disorders remains to be effectively substantiated.

Keywords: periodontitis; neuropsychiatric disorders; Alzheimer's disease; Parkinson's disease; major depression; schizophrenia; neuroinflammation; microglia

1. Introduction

Periodontitis is a chronic, oral multi-bacterial infection affecting nearly 50% of the population worldwide and is the most prevalent inflammatory disease in adults [1,2]. Periodontitis is not only an oral localized inflammatory disease, but also elicits low-grade systemic inflammation via both the release of pro-inflammatory cytokines and the invasion of periodontitis bacteria (e.g., *Porphyromonas gingivalis* (*P. gingivalis*)) along with their components (e.g., lipopolysaccharide (LPS) and flagellin) into systemic circulation [3]. Periodontitis thus causes or hastens other chronic systemic inflammatory diseases, including atherosclerosis, cardiovascular diseases, diabetes, and rheumatoid arthritis [4]. In particular, the causal link between periodontitis and infective endocarditis has been known for many decades. Besides inducing systemic inflammation, increasing evidence implies that periodontitis provokes chronic inflammation associated with activation of microglia, the immune cells in the brain, which is referred to as neuroinflammation (reviewed in [5–7]).

The concept of neuroinflammation was originally proposed for neurodegenerative disorders in the 1980s, based on two historical discoveries. The first was the immunohistochemical identification of activated microglia in association with the lesions in Alzheimer's disease (AD) brains [8]. The second was the epidemiologic finding that rheumatoid arthritics, who regularly consume anti-inflammatory agents, were relatively spared from AD [9]. In the ensuing years, activated microglia have also been found in the lesions of Parkinson's disease (PD), multiple sclerosis, and amyotrophic lateral sclerosis [10]. Neuroinflammation has thus become considered as a common prominent feature among a variety of neurodegenerative disorders. Attention on the pathogenetic role of neuroinflammation has, over the past two decades, been expanded to psychiatric disorders. Immunohistochemistry and positron emission tomography studies have revealed microglial activation in the brain of patients with schizophrenia [11–13] and major depression (MD) [14,15], the representative endogenous psychoses. Neuroinflammation could thus be important in many pathological conditions of the brain, including both neurodegenerative disorders and psychiatric disorders (hereinafter referred to as neuropsychiatric disorders in this article).

Based on the aforementioned findings, chronic inflammation can be regarded as a common denominator of periodontitis and neuropsychiatric disorders. Specifically, neuroinflammation may causally link periodontitis to the clinical onset and development of neuropsychiatric disorders. Furthermore, through the biological mechanism of chronic inflammation, periodontitis could causally affect neuropsychiatric disorders, especially MD, because of its psychosocial effects, such as shame, loneliness, impaired quality of life (QOL), and impaired social status [16]. Nonetheless, this review article focuses on the biological and epidemiological evidence for possible causal links of periodontitis to the selected neuropsychiatric disorders, namely AD, MD, PD, and schizophrenia. This article also discusses an association between periodontitis and the neurological event of ischemic stroke.

2. How Does Periodontitis Cause Neuroinflammation?

Neuroinflammation is a key pathogenetic connector between periodontitis and neuropsychiatric disorders. The biological mechanisms by which periodontitis causes neuroinflammation can be presumed to consist of three possibilities, as follows (Figure 1).

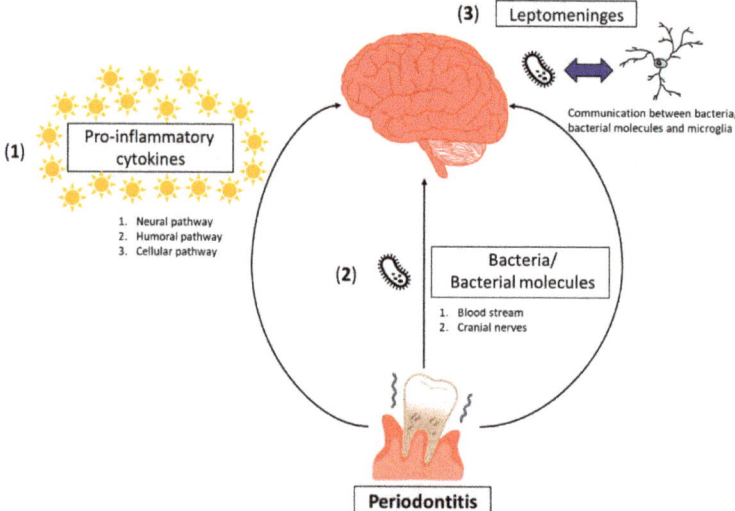

Figure 1. Scheme for presumed mechanisms by which periodontitis causes neuroinflammation. These consist of three possibilities as follows: (**1**) Peripheral pro-inflammatory cytokines associated with periodontitis communicate with the brain via the neural pathway, humoral pathway, and cellular pathway. (**2**) Periodontal bacteria/bacterial molecules can directly invade the brain either through the blood stream or via cranial nerves. (**3**) Communication between periodontal bacteria/bacterial molecules and brain-resident microglia could occur through the leptomeninges.

(**1**) Neuroinflammation can be caused by peripheral pro-inflammatory cytokines generated in systemic inflammation induced by periodontitis without the contact of periodontal bacteria/bacterial molecules with the brain tissue via three pathways, i.e., the neural pathway, the humoral pathway, and the cellular pathway. Through the neural pathway, systemic cytokines directly activate primary afferent nerves, such as the vagus nerve. The signal reaches the primary and secondary projection of the neural pathway, reaching first the nucleus tractus solitaries and subsequently, various hypothalamic brain nuclei [17]. It has been shown that subdiaphragmatic vagotomy blocks the LPS-induced sickness behavior in rats [18], while it does not affect the LPS-induced synthesis of pro-inflammatory cytokines at the periphery. The humoral pathway involves the choroid plexus and circumventricular organs, which lack an intact blood–brain barrier (BBB). These leaky regions may be access points for circulating pro-inflammatory cytokines to enter into the cerebral parenchyma by volume diffusion and elicit downstream signaling events, which are important in altering brain function [19]. The cellular pathway implicates systemic inflammation in association with both activation of endothelial cells (CECs) and an increase in circulating monocytes [19]. Systemic pro-inflammatory cytokines activate CECs, expressing receptors for TNF-α and IL-1β, which in turn, signal to the perivascular macrophages located immediately adjacent to CECs [20]. These perivascular macrophages subsequently communicate with microglia and thus lead to microglial activation. Activated microglia secrete not only pro-inflammatory cytokines but also proteases and chemokines, including monocyte chemoattractant protein (MCP)-1. MCP-1 is supposed to be responsible for the recruitment of monocytes into the motor cortex, hippocampus, and basal ganglia regions, areas of the brain known to be involved in the control of behavior [21].

(2) Periodontal bacteria/bacterial molecules can directly invade the brain either through the blood stream or via cranial nerves. In periodontitis, a periodontal pocket is filled with periodontal bacteria/bacterial molecules that form biofilms. Since periodontal bacteria are capable of invading an intact pocket epithelium, periodontal bacteria/bacterial molecules can gain access to the circulation [22]. It has been shown that LPS deteriorates the BBB and increases its permeability through abnormal activation of matrix metalloproteinase [23]. Circulating periodontal bacteria/bacterial molecules could then penetrate into the brain through the compromised BBB. In fact, *P. gingivalis* DNA has been identified by quantitative polymerase chain reaction (qPCR) in the brain of mice orally infected with *P. gingivalis* [24], and *P. gingivalis*-derived LPS has been detected in the brains of AD patients [25]. Circulating periodontal bacteria/bacterial molecules can also enter the brain through the circumventricular organs and choroid plexuses that lack the contiguous BBB. The cranial nerve may be another entry route for periodontal pathogens into the brain. The olfactory and trigeminal nerves are known to be used by periodontal bacteria to bypass the BBB [26]. The detection of oral *Treponemas* in the trigeminal ganglia supports the idea of neural pathways [27]. Via any of these pathways, infiltration of periodontal bacteria/bacterial molecules into the brain could result in inflammatory activation of microglia, since it has been demonstrated that either *P. gingivalis* infection or LPS of *P. gingivalis* activates microglia in vitro to produce pro-inflammatory cytokines, such as tumor necrosis factor (TNF)-α, interleukin (IL)-1β and IL-6 [28,29].

(3) The leptomeninges could be a site of communication between periodontal bacteria and brain-resident microglia. The leptomeninges covers the brain parenchyma surface and provides a physical boundary at the cerebrospinal fluid (CSF)-blood barrier. Leptomeningeal cells express Toll-like receptors (TLRs) 2 and 4 that are the receptors for *P. gingivalis* LPS. Leptomeningeal cells can be activated by circulating *P. gingivalis* LPS and subsequently produce pro-inflammatory cytokines for the brain [30,31]. The pro-inflammatory cytokines released from leptomeningeal cells activate microglia to evoke neuroinflammation. Accordingly, the leptomeninges could be harmful by transducing peripheral inflammation, including periodontitis, into neuroinflammation.

3. Alzheimer's Disease

AD is currently the best-known neuropsychiatric disease that is associated with periodontitis based on clinical and experimental evidence that is accumulating rapidly. Recent epidemiological studies have pointed out that periodontitis significantly elevates the risk for AD. A prospective pilot study using qPCR identified *P. gingivalis* DNA in the CSF in seven of the 10 clinically diagnosed AD patients who had mild to moderate cognitive impairment [24]. A cross-sectional study reported that plasma TNF-α and antibodies against periodontal bacteria were elevated in AD patients relative to normal controls and were independently associated with AD [32]. Another cross-sectional study demonstrated that the increased serum levels of TNF-α and IL-6 in patients with AD were significantly associated with periodontitis [33]. A case-control study established a significant association between AD and the increased number of deep periodontal pockets [34]. A retrospective matched cohort study on 9291 patients with periodontitis showed that chronic periodontitis exposure for 10 years was associated with a 1.707-fold increase in the risk of developing AD [35]. Another historical cohort study with the larger sample size of 262,349 participants who suffered from chronic periodontitis supports this finding [36]. Prospective cohort studies with relatively small sample sizes demonstrated that serum IgG antibody levels to periodontitis bacteria, such as *P. gingivalis*, *Tannerella forsythia* and *Treponema denticola* (the so-called "red complex"), were significantly increased in baseline serum drawn from subjects who were diagnosed with AD in later years compared to controls [37,38]. Even after the onset of AD, periodontitis may exacerbate cognitive impairment. A six-month observational cohort study tested cognitive function and serum pro-inflammatory markers in 52 patients with mild to moderate AD. The study showed that the presence of periodontitis at baseline was associated with a six-fold increase in the rate of cognitive decline in participants over the six-month follow-up period, and was also associated with a relative increase in the pro-inflammatory state over that period [39]. A meta-analysis based on one cross-sectional study [40] and two case-control studies [41,42], which have not been previously mentioned, and assessed as at a low risk of bias, came to the conclusion that periodontitis is significantly associated with AD (OR 1.69, 95% CI 1.21–2.35) [43]. Furthermore, severe forms of periodontitis show a more intense association with AD (OR 2.98, 95% CI 1.58–5.62) [43]. An interesting study comparing periodontal conditions between countries reported that periodontitis was more prevalent in Germany and that elderly German subjects had significantly more severe periodontal conditions and fewer remaining teeth compared to those in Japan, even after adjustment of the comprehensive risk factor [44]. Accordingly, it would be tempting to examine whether the AD prevalence in Germany is significantly higher than that of Japan by a direct comparison with the adjustment of confounding factors.

Growing evidence based on animal studies also strengthens a possible causal link of periodontitis to AD. Chronic intraperitoneal injection of *P. gingivalis* LPS (1 mg/kg/day, daily for 5 weeks) has been demonstrated to cause learning and memory deficits accompanied with intracellular amyloid β (Aβ) accumulation in neurons and microglial activation (i.e., increased expression of IL-1β and TLR2 restricted to microglia) in the hippocampus in middle-aged mice (12 months old), but not in young mice (2 months old) or in middle-aged cathepsin-B knockout mice [29]. Therefore, cathepsin B, known as an amyloid precursor protein (APP) secretase, may play a critical role in the periodontitis-exacerbated AD and could be a therapeutic target. Even a single intraperitoneal injection of *P. gingivalis* LPS (5 mg/kg) into 8-week old mice has been shown to impair spatial learning and memory with neuroinflammation (i.e., microglial activation, astrocytic activation, and increased expression of TNF-α, IL-1β, and IL-6 in the cortex and/or hippocampus) and activation of the TLR4/nuclear factor-kappa B (NF-κB) signaling pathway (i.e., up-regulation of TLR4, CD14, IL-1 receptor-associated kinase 1, and phospho-p65 in the cortex) [45]. These behavioral and immuno-biochemical findings were considerably abolished by the TLR4 inhibitor TAK242, suggesting that the *P. gingivalis* LPS-induced cognitive dysfunction and neuroinflammation are mediated by the TLR4/NF-κB signaling pathway [45]. Interestingly, this study also tested *E. coli* LPS and reported that either *P. gingivalis* LPS or *E. coli* LPS caused both cognitive impairment and neuroinflammation and there was no significant difference between the effects of the two LPS species [45]. Experimental chronic periodontitis, caused when live *P. gingivalis* (ATCC33277) was given by oral gavage every 48 h over 6 weeks, has been shown to impair learning and memory and elicit neuroinflammation (i.e., increased expression of TNF-α, IL-1β and IL-6 in the brain) in middle-aged mice (12 months old), although not in young individuals (4 weeks old) [46]. Experimental chronic periodontitis, induced by repeated oral application of another live *P. gingivalis* W83 every 48 h over 22 weeks, has been demonstrated to increase extracellular Aβ42 amyloid plaques, ser396 residue of tau protein phosphorylation, neurofibrillary tangle formation, and neuroinflammation (i.e., microglial activation, astrocytic activation, and increased expression of TNF-α, IL-1β and IL-6) in the hippocampus of 6-week old mice [47]. Currently, there is only one study that employed APP-transgenic (Tg) mice and the study implies that periodontitis exacerbates the hallmark pathology and symptoms of AD [48]. Specifically, APP-Tg mice with periodontitis induced by oral infection with *P. gingivalis* ATCC33277, showed greater deposition of Aβ40 and Aβ42 amyloid plaques in both the hippocampus and cortex and increased brain expression of TNF-α and IL-1β, compared with sham-infected APP-Tg mice. Furthermore, cognitive function was significantly impaired in the periodontitis-induced APP-Tg mice relative to sham-infected APP-Tg mice [48].

Postmortem studies have indicated the potentially causal presence of periodontopathic virulence products in AD brains. LPS from *P. gingivalis* was detected in the brain of four out of 10 AD cases by immunofluorescence and Western blot (WB) analyses, whereas *P. gingivalis* LPS was not detected in 10 age-matched non-AD controls. Dominiy et al. (2019) have performed a seminal study, identifying *P. gingivalis* DNA and gingipains, toxic proteases secreted from *P. gingivalis* in AD brains. Immunohistochemical analyses using tissue microarrays showed that gingipain immunoreactivity in AD brains was significantly greater than that in sex- and age-matched non-AD brains, and that gingipain immunoreactivity significantly correlates with tau and ubiquitin loads and AD diagnosis [24]. Using qPCR, the authors identified *P. gingivalis* DNA in the AD brains which were lysine gingipain-positive in WB and immunoprecipitated analyses [24]. In addition to postmortem brain studies, they carried out in vivo studies using wild-type mice and gingipain-knockout mice that were orally infected with *P. gingivalis* W83 every other day for 42 days. Colonization of *P. gingivalis* and Aβ42 levels were increased in the brains of the infected wild-type mice, while the colonization and Aβ42 levels were decreased in the brains of either the infected wild-type mice treated with the gingipain inhibitor COR119 or of the gingipain-knockout mice [24]. Because these findings suggest that gingipain inhibition reduces the *P. gingivali* load and Aβ42 production in the brain, gingipain inhibitors could have therapeutic potential for patients with both AD and periodontitis.

4. Major Depression

MD has also attracted attention and is currently the second elucidated neuropsychiatric disease with respect to its reciprocal association with periodontitis. A recent cross-sectional study on 108 subjects reported that patients with periodontitis showed a significantly higher comorbidity rate of depression (62.5%) compared to periodontally healthy subjects (38.86%), excluding smokers, pregnant women, subjects with systemic pathologies, and subjects taking antidepressants [49]. MD is susceptible to psychosocial factors and periodontitis could increase the risk for developing MD through the psychosocial effects that stem from periodontitis-causing oral troubles, such as halitosis, poor oral hygiene, and edentulousness [16]. Patients with malodorous wounds and poor oral hygiene often experience social isolation, depression, shame, and poor appetite, all of which have a negative impact on their QOL [50]. Also, tooth loss negatively affects the patients' QOL since it worsens not only chewing function, but also body image, self-esteem, and social status [16,51]. Because of all this, many early studies in this field were performed from a psychosocial viewpoint [52,53].

Although several studies have recently focused on the biological relationship between periodontitis and MD, most of them investigated periodontitis as an outcome influenced by MD [54,55]. The effects of antidepressants, which are known to possess anti-inflammatory and immunomodulatory properties [56,57], on chronic periodontitis have been studied in both MD animal models (systematically reviewed in [58]) and in MD patients [59,60]. The majority has established the therapeutic effects of antidepressants on chronic periodontitis. A recent cross-sectional study made by Gomes et al. (2018), who hypothesized that increased root canal LPS accompanying chronic apical periodontitis causes MD, showed that patients with periodontitis and MD had highly increased root canal endotoxin levels relative to patients with periodontitis without MD or normal controls. This study demonstrated a strong positive association between periodontitis or root canal endotoxin levels and the severity of MD, suggesting that the association between periodontitis and MD is attributable, at least in part, to root canal endotoxin levels [61]. In the study, periodontitis-related MD was accompanied with elevated levels of oxidative and nitrosative stress index, including nitric oxide metabolites and hydroperoxides, which are supposed to play a role in the pathogenesis of MD [62]. A recent cohort study composed of a high methodological quality with more than 60,000 participants and a 10-year follow-up period also supports the feasible causal link of periodontitis to MD. The study showed a higher incidence of subsequent depression in the periodontitis group (n = 12,708) than in the non-periodontitis group (n = 50,832) (HR 1.73, 95% CI 1.58–1.89), after adjustment of sex, age and comorbidities [63]. This result suggests that periodontitis is an independent risk factor for subsequent MD regardless of sex, age, and the comorbidities except for diabetes, alcohol abuse, and cancer. On the other hand, in a meta-analysis on four cross-sectional studies [64–67] that were assessed as moderate-high quality of the evidence and considered periodontitis as the outcome and MD as the exposure, the pooled estimate does not show association between periodontitis and MD (OR 0.96, 95% CI 0.84–1.10) [68]. Therefore, more prospective cohort studies that test periodontitis as the independent variable and MD as the outcome, or interventional studies, such as studies that determine the effects of periodontal treatment on MD, are clearly warranted to elucidate the causal relationship between periodontitis and MD.

5. Parkinson's Disease

Compared with AD and MD, any correlation between PD and periodontitis has, traditionally, been less effectively understood. Nevertheless, a few studies have noted an increased prevalence of periodontal disease among individuals with PD relative to age-matched controls [69,70]. PD causes motor disturbance (due to tremor, rigidity, akinesia, and involuntary movement), apathy, and cognitive impairment, all of which appear to make it difficult for patients to maintain daily oral hygiene. Therefore, periodontitis can be considered as a consequence of the poor oral hygiene related to clinical symptoms of PD. Recent epidemiological studies have investigated whether periodontitis increases the risk for developing PD. Chen et al. (2017) conducted a population-based retrospective matched-cohort study and reported that individuals with newly diagnosed periodontitis (n = 5396) had an increased risk of subsequent PD compared to individuals without periodontitis (n = 10,792), regardless of sex, age, comorbidities, and urbanization levels (HR 1.431, 95% CI 1.141–1.794) [71]. The authors also examined the effect of periodontal treatment on developing PD. Their population-based nested case-control study demonstrated that among individuals without periodontitis aged 40–69 (n = 5552), dental scaling over five consecutive years showed a protective effect against PD development, relative to individuals who did not undergo dental scaling (OR 0.204, 95% CI 0.047–0.886) [72]. Moreover, among individuals with periodontitis aged ≥70 (n = 3377), the discontinued scaling (i.e., not five consecutive years) or no treatment were significant risk factors for developing PD [35]. These findings suggest that early and consecutive dental scaling could prevent the development of PD. Although these seminal epidemiological studies imply a feasible causal link of periodontitis to PD and a preventive effect of periodontal treatment on PD development, experimental studies for verifying these concepts are lacking at the present time. Therefore, additional epidemiological studies and experimental studies along this line are required.

6. Schizophrenia

Evidence for a significant relationship between periodontitis and schizophrenia has not yet been accumulated. Only one cross-sectional study with a small sample size has concluded that patients with schizophrenia have a high risk of periodontitis and there is an even higher risk in those who are taking antipsychotics that reduce salivary secretion and cause xerostomia [73]. Intriguingly, human genome/gene analysis on insertion/deletion (D) polymorphism in the angiotensin-converting enzyme (ACE) gene has indicated that the D allele is a protective factor against schizophrenia [74] and chronic periodontitis [75]. Accordingly, the ACE D allele may be a clue to reveal any biological and reciprocal connection between these two diseases.

7. Ischemic Stroke

Epidemiological studies also suggest an association between periodontitis and ischemic stroke. Stroke is the second most common cause of mortality worldwide and approximately 80% of strokes are caused by focal cerebral ischemia [76]. A recent meta-analysis [76] has shown a significant association between periodontitis and ischemic stroke based on three cohort studies [77–79] (pooled RR 2.52, 95% CI 1.77–3.58) and five case-control studies (pooled RR 3.04, 95% CI 1.10–8.43) [80–84]. Chi et al. (2019) examined mice with both experimental periodontitis induced by periodontal injection of LPS and photothrombotic ischemia. The study has demonstrated that chronic periodontitis exacerbates ischemic stroke through increasing the activation of microglia/astrocytes and the expression of nod-like receptor protein 3 inflammasome and IL-1β [85], suggesting that chronic periodontitis is a driving force for neuroinflammation associated with ischemia.

8. Conclusions

The relationship between periodontitis and neuropsychiatric disorders, in particular AD, has recently attracted researchers' attention, and the evidence for their considerable reciprocal association has been accumulated. Specifically, various clinical and experimental studies imply the potentially causal link of periodontitis to neuropsychiatric disorders, and neuroinflammation seems to be a key pathological connector between them. After establishment of such a link, a broad spectrum of neuropsychiatric disorders associated with neuroinflammation may be preventable and modifiable by simple daily dealings for oral hygiene, even though the notion that periodontitis is a risk factor for neuropsychiatric disorders remains to be effectively substantiated.

Author Contributions: S.H. wrote the manuscript. All authors discussed and edited the manuscript. All authors read and approved the final manuscript.

Funding: This study was supported by JSPS KAKENHI Grant Numbers 19K08018 (SH), 17K09194 (KI), 19K08046 (MH).

Acknowledgments: Sincere appreciation is extended to Edith G. McGeer for her invaluable support.

Conflicts of Interest: A.O.-N. has more than 5% shares of RESVO Inc. M.I. received lectures fees from Meiji, Mochida, Takeda, Novartis, Yoshitomi, Pfizer, Eisai, Otsuka, MSD, and Sumitomo Dainippon, personal fees from Technomics and research funds from Novartis, Eisai, Astellas, Pfizer, Daiichi-Sankyo, Takeda, and MSD. The funders had no role in the study design, decision to publish, or preparation of the manuscript.

References

1. Eke, P.I.; Dye, B.A.; Wei, L.; Thornton-Evans, G.O.; Genco, R.J. CDC Periodontal Disease Surveillance Workgroup. Prevalence of periodontitis in adults in the United States: 2009 and 2010. *J. Dent. Res.* **2012**, *91*, 914–920. [CrossRef] [PubMed]
2. Roman-Malo, L.; Bullon, P. Influence of the Periodontal Disease, the Most Prevalent Inflammatory Event, in Peroxisome Proliferator-Activated Receptors Linking Nutrition and Energy Metabolism. *Int. J. Mol. Sci.* **2017**, *18*, 1438. [CrossRef] [PubMed]
3. Gurav, A.N. Alzheimer's disease and periodontitis—An elusive link. *Rev. Assoc. Med. Bras.* **2014**, *60*, 173–180. [CrossRef] [PubMed]
4. Holmstrup, P.; Damgaard, C.; Olsen, I.; Klinge, B.; Flyvbjerg, A.; Nielsen, C.H.; Hansen, P.R. Comorbidity of periodontal disease: Two sides of the same coin? An introduction for the clinician. *J. Oral Microbiol.* **2017**, *9*, 1332710. [CrossRef] [PubMed]
5. Hashioka, S.; Inoue, K.; Hayashida, M.; Wake, R.; Oh-Nishi, A.; Miyaoka, T. Implications of Systemic Inflammation and Periodontitis for Major Depression. *Front. Neurosci.* **2018**, *12*, 483. [CrossRef] [PubMed]
6. Singhrao, S.K.; Olsen, I. Assessing the role of Porphyromonas gingivalis in periodontitis to determine a causative relationship with Alzheimer's disease. *J. Oral Microbiol.* **2019**, *11*, 1563405. [CrossRef] [PubMed]
7. Sochocka, M.; Zwolinska, K.; Leszek, J. The Infectious Etiology of Alzheimer's Disease. *Curr. Neuropharmacol.* **2017**, *15*, 996–1009. [CrossRef] [PubMed]

8. McGeer, P.L.; Itagaki, S.; Tago, H.; McGeer, E.G. Reactive microglia in patients with senile dementia of the Alzheimer type are positive for the histocompatibility glycoprotein HLA-DR. *Neurosci. Lett.* **1987**, *79*, 195–200. [CrossRef]
9. McGeer, P.L.; McGeer, E.; Rogers, J.; Sibley, J. Anti-inflammatory drugs and Alzheimer disease. *Lancet* **1990**, *335*, 1037. [CrossRef]
10. McGeer, P.L.; McGeer, E.G. History of innate immunity in neurodegenerative disorders. *Front. Pharmacol.* **2011**, *2*, 77. [CrossRef]
11. Doorduin, J.; de Vries, E.F.; Willemsen, A.T.; de Groot, J.C.; Dierckx, R.A.; Klein, H.C. Neuroinflammation in schizophrenia-related psychosis: A PET study. *J. Nucl. Med.* **2009**, *50*, 1801–1807. [CrossRef] [PubMed]
12. Fillman, S.G.; Cloonan, N.; Catts, V.S.; Miller, L.C.; Wong, J.; McCrossin, T.; Cairns, M.; Weickert, C.S. Increased inflammatory markers identified in the dorsolateral prefrontal cortex of individuals with schizophrenia. *Mol. Psychiatry* **2013**, *18*, 206–214. [CrossRef] [PubMed]
13. Van Berckel, B.N.; Bossong, M.G.; Boellaard, R.; Kloet, R.; Schuitemaker, A.; Caspers, E.; Luurtsema, G.; Windhorst, A.D.; Cahn, W.; Lammertsma, A.A.; et al. Microglia activation in recent-onset schizophrenia: A quantitative (R)-[11C]PK11195 positron emission tomography study. *Biol. Psychiatry* **2008**, *64*, 820–822. [CrossRef] [PubMed]
14. Su, L.; Faluyi, Y.O.; Hong, Y.T.; Fryer, T.D.; Mak, E.; Gabel, S.; Hayes, L.; Soteriades, S.; Williams, G.B.; Arnold, R.; et al. Neuroinflammatory and morphological changes in late-life depression: The NIMROD study. *Br. J. Psychiatry J. Ment. Sci.* **2016**, *209*, 525–526. [CrossRef] [PubMed]
15. Torres-Platas, S.G.; Cruceanu, C.; Chen, G.G.; Turecki, G.; Mechawar, N. Evidence for increased microglial priming and macrophage recruitment in the dorsal anterior cingulate white matter of depressed suicides. *Brain Behav. Immun.* **2014**, *42*, 50–59. [CrossRef] [PubMed]
16. Dumitrescu, A.L. Depression and Inflammatory Periodontal Disease Considerations-An Interdisciplinary Approach. *Front. Psychol.* **2016**, *7*, 347. [CrossRef] [PubMed]
17. Capuron, L.; Miller, A.H. Immune system to brain signaling: Neuropsychopharmacological implications. *Pharmacol. Ther.* **2011**, *130*, 226–238. [CrossRef]
18. Bluthé, R.M.; Walter, V.; Parnet, P.; Layé, S.; Lestage, J.; Verrier, D.; Poole, S.; Stenning, B.E.; Kelley, K.W.; Dantzer, R. Lipopolysaccharide induces sickness behaviour in rats by a vagal mediated mechanism. *C. R. L'Académie Sci. Ser. III Sci. Vie* **1994**, *317*, 499.
19. D'Mello, C.; Swain, M.G. Immune-to-Brain Communication Pathways in Inflammation-Associated Sickness and Depression. *Curr. Top. Behav. Neurosci.* **2017**, *31*, 73–94. [CrossRef]
20. Perry, V.H. The influence of systemic inflammation on inflammation in the brain: Implications for chronic neurodegenerative disease. *Brain Behav. Immun.* **2004**, *18*, 407–413. [CrossRef]
21. D'Mello, C.; Le, T.; Swain, M.G. Cerebral microglia recruit monocytes into the brain in response to tumor necrosis factoralpha signaling during peripheral organ inflammation. *J. Neurosci.* **2009**, *29*, 2089–2102. [CrossRef] [PubMed]
22. Kamer, A.R.; Craig, R.G.; Dasanayake, A.P.; Brys, M.; Glodzik-Sobanska, L.; de Leon, M.J. Inflammation and Alzheimer's disease: Possible role of periodontal diseases. *Alzheimers Dement.* **2008**, *4*, 242–250. [CrossRef] [PubMed]
23. Frister, A.; Schmidt, C.; Schneble, N.; Brodhun, M.; Gonnert, F.A.; Bauer, M.; Hirsch, E.; Muller, J.P.; Wetzker, R.; Bauer, R. Phosphoinositide 3-kinase gamma affects LPS-induced disturbance of blood-brain barrier via lipid kinase-independent control of cAMP in microglial cells. *Neuromol. Med.* **2014**, *16*, 704–713. [CrossRef] [PubMed]
24. Dominy, S.S.; Lynch, C.; Ermini, F.; Benedyk, M.; Marczyk, A.; Konradi, A.; Nguyen, M.; Haditsch, U.; Raha, D.; Griffin, C.; et al. Porphyromonas gingivalis in Alzheimer's disease brains: Evidence for disease causation and treatment with small-molecule inhibitors. *Sci. Adv.* **2019**, *5*, eaau3333. [CrossRef] [PubMed]
25. Poole, S.; Singhrao, S.K.; Kesavalu, L.; Curtis, M.A.; Crean, S. Determining the presence of periodontopathic virulence factors in short-term postmortem Alzheimer's disease brain tissue. *J. Alzheimers Dis.* **2013**, *36*, 665–677. [CrossRef]
26. Olsen, I.; Singhrao, S.K. Can oral infection be a risk factor for Alzheimer's disease? *J. Oral Microbiol.* **2015**, *7*, 29143. [CrossRef]

27. Riviere, G.R.; Riviere, K.H.; Smith, K.S. Molecular and immunological evidence of oral Treponema in the human brain and their association with Alzheimer's disease. *Oral Microbiol. Immunol.* **2002**, *17*, 113–118. [CrossRef]
28. Liu, Y.; Wu, Z.; Nakanishi, Y.; Ni, J.; Hayashi, Y.; Takayama, F.; Zhou, Y.; Kadowaki, T.; Nakanishi, H. Infection of microglia with Porphyromonas gingivalis promotes cell migration and an inflammatory response through the gingipain-mediated activation of protease-activated receptor-2 in mice. *Sci. Rep.* **2017**, *7*, 11759. [CrossRef]
29. Wu, Z.; Ni, J.; Liu, Y.; Teeling, J.L.; Takayama, F.; Collcutt, A.; Ibbett, P.; Nakanishi, H. Cathepsin B plays a critical role in inducing Alzheimer's disease-like phenotypes following chronic systemic exposure to lipopolysaccharide from Porphyromonas gingivalis in mice. *Brain Behav. Immun.* **2017**, *65*, 350–361. [CrossRef]
30. Liu, Y.; Wu, Z.; Zhang, X.; Ni, J.; Yu, W.; Zhou, Y.; Nakanishi, H. Leptomeningeal cells transduce peripheral macrophages inflammatory signal to microglia in reponse to Porphyromonas gingivalis LPS. *Mediat. Inflamm.* **2013**, *2013*, 407562. [CrossRef]
31. Wu, Z.; Zhang, J.; Nakanishi, H. Leptomeningeal cells activate microglia and astrocytes to induce IL-10 production by releasing pro-inflammatory cytokines during systemic inflammation. *J. Neuroimmunol.* **2005**, *167*, 90–98. [CrossRef] [PubMed]
32. Kamer, A.R.; Craig, R.G.; Pirraglia, E.; Dasanayake, A.P.; Norman, R.G.; Boylan, R.J.; Nehorayoff, A.; Glodzik, L.; Brys, M.; de Leon, M.J. TNF-alpha and antibodies to periodontal bacteria discriminate between Alzheimer's disease patients and normal subjects. *J. Neuroimmunol.* **2009**, *216*, 92–97. [CrossRef] [PubMed]
33. Cestari, J.A.; Fabri, G.M.; Kalil, J.; Nitrini, R.; Jacob-Filho, W.; de Siqueira, J.T.; Siqueira, S.R. Oral Infections and Cytokine Levels in Patients with Alzheimer's Disease and Mild Cognitive Impairment Compared with Controls. *J. Alzheimers Dis.* **2016**, *52*, 1479–1485. [CrossRef] [PubMed]
34. Holmer, J.; Eriksdotter, M.; Schultzberg, M.; Pussinen, P.J.; Buhlin, K. Association between periodontitis and risk of Alzheimer's disease, mild cognitive impairment and subjective cognitive decline: A case-control study. *J. Clin. Periodontol.* **2018**, *45*, 1287–1298. [CrossRef] [PubMed]
35. Chen, C.K.; Wu, Y.T.; Chang, Y.C. Association between chronic periodontitis and the risk of Alzheimer's disease: A retrospective, population-based, matched-cohort study. *Alzheimers Res. Ther.* **2017**, *9*, 56. [CrossRef] [PubMed]
36. Choi, S.; Kim, K.; Chang, J.; Kim, S.M.; Kim, S.J.; Cho, H.J.; Park, S.M. Association of Chronic Periodontitis on Alzheimer's Disease or Vascular Dementia. *J. Am. Geriatr. Soc.* **2019**. [CrossRef] [PubMed]
37. Noble, J.M.; Scarmeas, N.; Celenti, R.S.; Elkind, M.S.; Wright, C.B.; Schupf, N.; Papapanou, P.N. Serum IgG antibody levels to periodontal microbiota are associated with incident Alzheimer disease. *PLoS ONE* **2014**, *9*, e114959. [CrossRef]
38. Sparks Stein, P.; Steffen, M.J.; Smith, C.; Jicha, G.; Ebersole, J.L.; Abner, E.; Dawson, D., 3rd. Serum antibodies to periodontal pathogens are a risk factor for Alzheimer's disease. *Alzheimers Dement. J. Alzheimers Assoc.* **2012**, *8*, 196–203. [CrossRef]
39. Ide, M.; Harris, M.; Stevens, A.; Sussams, R.; Hopkins, V.; Culliford, D.; Fuller, J.; Ibbett, P.; Raybould, R.; Thomas, R.; et al. Periodontitis and Cognitive Decline in Alzheimer's Disease. *PLoS ONE* **2016**, *11*, e0151081. [CrossRef]
40. Syrjala, A.M.; Ylostalo, P.; Ruoppi, P.; Komulainen, K.; Hartikainen, S.; Sulkava, R.; Knuuttila, M. Dementia and oral health among subjects aged 75 years or older. *Gerodontology* **2012**, *29*, 36–42. [CrossRef]
41. De Souza Rolim, T.; Fabri, G.M.; Nitrini, R.; Anghinah, R.; Teixeira, M.J.; de Siqueira, J.T.; Cestari, J.A.; de Siqueira, S.R. Oral infections and orofacial pain in Alzheimer's disease: A case-control study. *J. Alzheimers Dis.* **2014**, *38*, 823–829. [CrossRef] [PubMed]
42. Gil-Montoya, J.A.; Sanchez-Lara, I.; Carnero-Pardo, C.; Fornieles, F.; Montes, J.; Vilchez, R.; Burgos, J.S.; Gonzalez-Moles, M.A.; Barrios, R.; Bravo, M. Is periodontitis a risk factor for cognitive impairment and dementia? A case-control study. *J. Periodontol.* **2015**, *86*, 244–253. [CrossRef] [PubMed]
43. Leira, Y.; Dominguez, C.; Seoane, J.; Seoane-Romero, J.; Pias-Peleteiro, J.M.; Takkouche, B.; Blanco, J.; Aldrey, J.M. Is Periodontal Disease Associated with Alzheimer's Disease? A Systematic Review with Meta-Analysis. *Neuroepidemiology* **2017**, *48*, 21–31. [CrossRef] [PubMed]

44. Hirotomi, T.; Kocher, T.; Yoshihara, A.; Biffar, R.; Micheelis, W.; Hoffmann, T.; Miyazaki, H.; Holtfreter, B. Comparison of periodontal conditions among three elderly populations in Japan and Germany. *J. Clin. Periodontol.* **2014**, *41*, 633–642. [CrossRef] [PubMed]
45. Zhang, J.; Yu, C.; Zhang, X.; Chen, H.; Dong, J.; Lu, W.; Song, Z.; Zhou, W. Porphyromonas gingivalis lipopolysaccharide induces cognitive dysfunction, mediated by neuronal inflammation via activation of the TLR4 signaling pathway in C57BL/6 mice. *J. Neuroinflamm.* **2018**, *15*, 37. [CrossRef] [PubMed]
46. Ding, Y.; Ren, J.; Yu, H.; Yu, W.; Zhou, Y. Porphyromonas gingivalis, a periodontitis causing bacterium, induces memory impairment and age-dependent neuroinflammation in mice. *Immun. Ageing* **2018**, *15*, 6. [CrossRef] [PubMed]
47. Ilievski, V.; Zuchowska, P.K.; Green, S.J.; Toth, P.T.; Ragozzino, M.E.; Le, K.; Aljewari, H.W.; O'Brien-Simpson, N.M.; Reynolds, E.C.; Watanabe, K. Chronic oral application of a periodontal pathogen results in brain inflammation, neurodegeneration and amyloid beta production in wild type mice. *PLoS ONE* **2018**, *13*, e0204941. [CrossRef] [PubMed]
48. Ishida, N.; Ishihara, Y.; Ishida, K.; Tada, H.; Funaki-Kato, Y.; Hagiwara, M.; Ferdous, T.; Abdullah, M.; Mitani, A.; Michikawa, M.; et al. Periodontitis induced by bacterial infection exacerbates features of Alzheimer's disease in transgenic mice. *NPJ Aging Mech. Dis.* **2017**, *3*, 15. [CrossRef] [PubMed]
49. Laforgia, A.; Corsalini, M.; Stefanachi, G.; Pettini, F.; Di Venere, D. Assessment of Psychopatologic Traits in a Group of Patients with Adult Chronic Periodontitis: Study on 108 Cases and Analysis of Compliance during and after Periodontal Treatment. *Int. J. Med. Sci.* **2015**, *12*, 832–839. [CrossRef]
50. Bale, S.; Tebbie, N.; Price, P. A topical metronidazole gel used to treat malodorous wounds. *Br. J. Nurs.* **2004**, *13*, S4–S11. [CrossRef]
51. Saintrain, M.V.; de Souza, E.H. Impact of tooth loss on the quality of life. *Gerodontology* **2012**, *29*, e632–e636. [CrossRef] [PubMed]
52. Monteiro da Silva, A.M.; Oakley, D.A.; Newman, H.N.; Nohl, F.S.; Lloyd, H.M. Psychosocial factors and adult onset rapidly progressive periodontitis. *J. Clin. Periodontol.* **1996**, *23*, 789–794. [CrossRef] [PubMed]
53. Moss, M.E.; Beck, J.D.; Kaplan, B.H.; Offenbacher, S.; Weintraub, J.A.; Koch, G.G.; Genco, R.J.; Machtei, E.E.; Tedesco, L.A. Exploratory case-control analysis of psychosocial factors and adult periodontitis. *J. Periodontol.* **1996**, *67*, 1060–1069. [CrossRef] [PubMed]
54. Breivik, T.; Gundersen, Y.; Murison, R.; Turner, J.D.; Muller, C.P.; Gjermo, P.; Opstad, K. Maternal Deprivation of Lewis Rat Pups Increases the Severity of Experi-mental Periodontitis in Adulthood. *Open Dent. J.* **2015**, *9*, 65–78. [CrossRef] [PubMed]
55. Solis, A.C.O.; Marques, A.H.; Dominguez, W.V.; Prado, E.B.A.; Pannuti, C.M.; Lotufo, R.F.M.; Lotufo-Neto, F. Evaluation of periodontitis in hospital outpatients with major depressive disorder. A focus on gingival and circulating cytokines. *Brain Behav. Immun.* **2016**, *53*, 49–53. [CrossRef]
56. Hashioka, S.; McGeer, P.L.; Monji, A.; Kanba, S. Anti-inflammatory effects of antidepressants: Possibilities for preventives against Alzheimer's disease. *Cent. Nerv. Syst. Agents Med. Chem.* **2009**, *9*, 12–19. [CrossRef]
57. Hashioka, S. Antidepressants and neuroinflammation: Can antidepressants calm glial rage down? *Mini Rev. Med. Chem.* **2011**, *11*, 555–564. [CrossRef]
58. Muniz, F.; Melo, I.M.; Rosing, C.K.; de Andrade, G.M.; Martins, R.S.; Moreira, M.; Carvalho, R.S. Use of antidepressive agents as a possibility in the management of periodontal diseases: A systematic review of experimental studies. *J. Investig. Clin. Dent.* **2018**, *9*. [CrossRef]
59. Bhatia, A.; Sharma, R.K.; Tewari, S.; Khurana, H.; Narula, S.C. Effect of Fluoxetine on Periodontal Status in Patients With Depression: A Cross-Sectional Observational Study. *J. Periodontol.* **2015**, *86*, 927–935. [CrossRef]
60. Bhatia, A.; Sharma, R.K.; Tewari, S.; Narula, S.C.; Khurana, H. Periodontal status in chronic periodontitis depressed patients on desvenlafaxine: An observational study. *J. Indian Soc. Periodontol.* **2018**, *22*, 442–446. [CrossRef]
61. Gomes, C.; Martinho, F.C.; Barbosa, D.S.; Antunes, L.S.; Povoa, H.C.C.; Baltus, T.H.L.; Morelli, N.R.; Vargas, H.O.; Nunes, S.O.V.; Anderson, G.; et al. Increased Root Canal Endotoxin Levels are Associated with Chronic Apical Periodontitis, Increased Oxidative and Nitrosative Stress, Major Depression, Severity of Depression, and a Lowered Quality of Life. *Mol. Neurobiol.* **2018**, *55*, 2814–2827. [CrossRef] [PubMed]
62. Maes, M.; Galecki, P.; Chang, Y.S.; Berk, M. A review on the oxidative and nitrosative stress (O&NS) pathways in major depression and their possible contribution to the (neuro)degenerative processes in that illness. *Prog. Neuro-Psychopharmacol. Biol. Psychiatry* **2011**, *35*, 676–692. [CrossRef]

63. Hsu, C.C.; Hsu, Y.C.; Chen, H.J.; Lin, C.C.; Chang, K.H.; Lee, C.Y.; Chong, L.W.; Kao, C.H. Association of Periodontitis and Subsequent Depression: A Nationwide Population-Based Study. *Medicine* **2015**, *94*, e2347. [CrossRef]
64. Delgado-Angulo, E.K.; Sabbah, W.; Suominen, A.L.; Vehkalahti, M.M.; Knuuttila, M.; Partonen, T.; Nordblad, A.; Sheiham, A.; Watt, R.G.; Tsakos, G. The association of depression and anxiety with dental caries and periodontal disease among Finnish adults. *Community Dent. Oral Epidemiol.* **2015**, *43*, 540–549. [CrossRef] [PubMed]
65. Khambaty, T.; Stewart, J.C. Associations of depressive and anxiety disorders with periodontal disease prevalence in young adults: Analysis of 1999–2004 National Health and Nutrition Examination Survey (NHANES) data. *Ann. Behav. Med.* **2013**, *45*, 393–397. [CrossRef] [PubMed]
66. Park, S.J.; Ko, K.D.; Shin, S.I.; Ha, Y.J.; Kim, G.Y.; Kim, H.A. Association of oral health behaviors and status with depression: Results from the Korean National Health and Nutrition Examination Survey, 2010. *J. Public Health Dent.* **2014**, *74*, 127–138. [CrossRef] [PubMed]
67. Persson, G.R.; Persson, R.E.; MacEntee, C.I.; Wyatt, C.C.; Hollender, L.G.; Kiyak, H.A. Periodontitis and perceived risk for periodontitis in elders with evidence of depression. *J. Clin. Periodontol.* **2003**, *30*, 691–696. [CrossRef]
68. Cademartori, M.G.; Gastal, M.T.; Nascimento, G.G.; Demarco, F.F.; Correa, M.B. Is depression associated with oral health outcomes in adults and elders? A systematic review and meta-analysis. *Clin. Oral Investig.* **2018**, *22*, 2685–2702. [CrossRef]
69. Einarsdóttir, E.R.; Gunnsteinsdóttir, H.; Hallsdóttir, M.H.; Sveinsson, S.; Jónsdóttir, S.R.; Olafsson, V.G.; Bragason, T.H.; Saemundsson, S.R.; Holbrook, W.P. Dental health of patients with Parkinson's disease in Iceland. *Spec. Care Dent.* **2009**, *29*, 123–127. [CrossRef]
70. Schwarz, J.; Heimhilger, E.; Storch, A. Increased periodontal pathology in Parkinson's disease. *J. Neurol.* **2006**, *253*, 608–611. [CrossRef]
71. Chen, C.K.; Huang, J.Y.; Wu, Y.T.; Chang, Y.C. Dental Scaling Decreases the Risk of Parkinson's Disease: A Nationwide Population-Based Nested Case-Control Study. *Int. J. Environ. Res. Public Health* **2018**, *15*, 1587. [CrossRef] [PubMed]
72. Chen, C.K.; Wu, Y.T.; Chang, Y.C. Periodontal inflammatory disease is associated with the risk of Parkinson's disease: A population-based retrospective matched-cohort study. *PeerJ* **2017**, *5*, e3647. [CrossRef] [PubMed]
73. Eltas, A.; Kartalci, S.; Eltas, S.D.; Dundar, S.; Uslu, M.O. An assessment of periodontal health in patients with schizophrenia and taking antipsychotic medication. *Int. J. Dent. Hyg.* **2013**, *11*, 78–83. [CrossRef] [PubMed]
74. Crescenti, A.; Gasso, P.; Mas, S.; Abellana, R.; Deulofeu, R.; Parellada, E.; Bernardo, M.; Lafuente, A. Insertion/deletion polymorphism of the angiotensin-converting enzyme gene is associated with schizophrenia in a Spanish population. *Psychiatry Res.* **2009**, *165*, 175–180. [CrossRef] [PubMed]
75. Gurkan, A.; Emingil, G.; Saygan, B.H.; Atilla, G.; Kose, T.; Baylas, H.; Berdeli, A. Renin-angiotensin gene polymorphisms in relation to severe chronic periodontitis. *J. Clin. Periodontol.* **2009**, *36*, 204–211. [CrossRef] [PubMed]
76. Leira, Y.; Seoane, J.; Blanco, M.; Rodriguez-Yanez, M.; Takkouche, B.; Blanco, J.; Castillo, J. Association between periodontitis and ischemic stroke: A systematic review and meta-analysis. *Eur. J. Epidemiol.* **2017**, *32*, 43–53. [CrossRef] [PubMed]
77. Beck, J.; Garcia, R.; Heiss, G.; Vokonas, P.S.; Offenbacher, S. Periodontal Disease and Cardiovascular Disease. *J. Periodontol.* **1996**, *67*, 1123–1137. [CrossRef] [PubMed]
78. Wu, T.; Trevisan, M.; Genco, R.J.; Dorn, J.P.; Falkner, K.L.; Sempos, C.T. Periodontal disease and risk of cerebrovascular disease: The first national health and nutrition examination survey and its follow-up study. *Arch. Intern. Med.* **2000**, *160*, 2749–2755. [CrossRef]
79. Jimenez, M.; Krall, E.A.; Garcia, R.I.; Vokonas, P.S.; Dietrich, T. Periodontitis and incidence of cerebrovascular disease in men. *Ann. Neurol.* **2009**, *66*, 505–512. [CrossRef]
80. Grau, A.J.; Becher, H.; Ziegler, C.M.; Lichy, C.; Buggle, F.; Kaiser, C.; Lutz, R.; Bultmann, S.; Preusch, M.; Dorfer, C.E. Periodontal disease as a risk factor for ischemic stroke. *Stroke* **2004**, *35*, 496–501. [CrossRef]
81. Dorfer, C.E.; Becher, H.; Ziegler, C.M.; Kaiser, C.; Lutz, R.; Jorss, D.; Lichy, C.; Buggle, F.; Bultmann, S.; Preusch, M.; et al. The association of gingivitis and periodontitis with ischemic stroke. *J. Clin. Periodontol.* **2004**, *31*, 396–401. [CrossRef] [PubMed]

82. Pradeep, A.R.; Hadge, P.; Arjun Raju, P.; Shetty, S.R.; Shareef, K.; Guruprasad, C.N. Periodontitis as a risk factor for cerebrovascular accident: A case-control study in the Indian population. *J. Periodontal. Res.* **2010**, *45*, 223–228. [CrossRef] [PubMed]
83. Sim, S.J.; Kim, H.D.; Moon, J.Y.; Zavras, A.I.; Zdanowicz, J.; Jang, S.J.; Jin, B.H.; Bae, K.H.; Paik, D.I.; Douglass, C.W. Periodontitis and the risk for non-fatal stroke in Korean adults. *J. Periodontol.* **2008**, *79*, 1652–1658. [CrossRef] [PubMed]
84. Lafon, A.; Tala, S.; Ahossi, V.; Perrin, D.; Giroud, M.; Bejot, Y. Association between periodontal disease and non-fatal ischemic stroke: A case-control study. *Acta Odontol. Scand.* **2014**, *72*, 687–693. [CrossRef] [PubMed]
85. Chi, L.; Cheng, X.; He, X.; Sun, J.; Liang, F.; Pei, Z.; Teng, W. Increased cortical infarction and neuroinflammation in ischemic stroke mice with experimental periodontitis. *Neuroreport* **2019**, *30*, 428–433. [CrossRef] [PubMed]

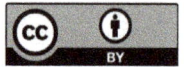 © 2019 by the authors. Licensee MDPI, Basel, Switzerland. This article is an open access article distributed under the terms and conditions of the Creative Commons Attribution (CC BY) license (http://creativecommons.org/licenses/by/4.0/).

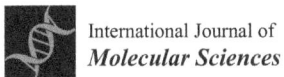

Review

Pathological Characteristics of Periodontal Disease in Patients with Chronic Kidney Disease and Kidney Transplantation

Mineaki Kitamura [1,2], Yasushi Mochizuki [2,3], Yasuyoshi Miyata [3,*], Yoko Obata [1], Kensuke Mitsunari [3], Tomohiro Matsuo [3], Kojiro Ohba, Hiroshi Mukae [4], Atsutoshi Yoshimura [5], Tomoya Nishino [1] and Hideki Sakai [2,3]

1. Department of Nephrology, Nagasaki University Hospital, Nagasaki 852-8501, Japan
2. Division of Blood Purification, Nagasaki University Hospital, Nagasaki 852-8501, Japan
3. Department of Urology, Nagasaki University Graduate School of Biomedical Sciences, Nagasaki 852-8501, Japan
4. Department of Respiratory Medicine, Unit of Basic Medical Sciences, Nagasaki University Graduate School of Biomedical Sciences, Nagasaki 852-8501, Japan
5. Department of Periodontology and Endodontology, Nagasaki University Graduate School of Biomedical Sciences, Nagasaki 852-8501, Japan
* Correspondence: yasu-myt@nagasaki-u.ac.jp; Tel.: +81-95-819-7340; Fax: +81-95-819-7343

Received: 9 June 2019; Accepted: 10 July 2019; Published: 11 July 2019

Abstract: Chronic kidney disease (CKD) is recognized as an irreversible reduction of functional nephrons and leads to an increased risk of various pathological conditions, including cardiovascular disease and neurological disorders, such as coronary artery calcification, hypertension, and stroke. In addition, CKD patients have impaired immunity against bacteria and viruses. Conversely, kidney transplantation (KT) is performed for patients with end-stage renal disease as a renal replacement therapy. Although kidney function is almost normalized by KT, immunosuppressive therapy is essential to maintain kidney allograft function and to prevent rejection. However, these patients are more susceptible to infection due to the immunosuppressive therapy required to maintain kidney allograft function. Thus, both CKD and KT present disadvantages in terms of suppression of immune function. Periodontal disease is defined as a chronic infection and inflammation of oral and periodontal tissues. Periodontal disease is characterized by the destruction of connective tissues of the periodontium and alveolar bone, which may lead to not only local symptoms but also systemic diseases, such as cardiovascular diseases, diabetes, liver disease, chronic obstructive pulmonary disease, and several types of cancer. In addition, the prevalence and severity of periodontal disease are significantly associated with mortality. Many researchers pay special attention to the pathological roles and clinical impact of periodontal disease in patients with CKD or KT. In this review, we provide information regarding important modulators of periodontal disease to better understand the relationship between periodontal disease and CKD and/or KT. Furthermore; we evaluate the impact of periodontal disease on various pathological conditions in patients with CKD and KT. Moreover, pathogens of periodontal disease common to CKD and KT are also discussed. Finally, we examine the importance of periodontal care in these patients. Thus, this review provides a comprehensive overview of the pathological roles and clinical significance of periodontal disease in patients with CKD and KT.

Keywords: periodontal disease; chronic kidney disease; kidney transplantation; immunosuppressive therapy

1. Introduction

Chronic kidney disease (CKD) is defined as either the presence of kidney damage, such as proteinuria and hematuria, or decreased kidney function (estimated glomerular filtration rate (eGFR) < 60 mL/min/1.73 m^2 for >3 months) [1]. CKD is a crucial health issue, as it has a negative impact on prognosis and quality of life (QoL) due to the increasing risk of various pathological conditions including hypertension, diabetes, smoking, aging, autoimmune diseases, systemic inflammation, urinary tract infections, urinary stones, lower urinary tract obstruction, recovery from acute kidney injury, low birth weight, and drug toxicity [2–5]. Conversely, several risk factors of CKD, such as hypertension, diabetes, smoking, and aging have also been identified [1]. Thus, early recognition of CKD and the prevention of CKD progression are highly desirable. Furthermore, growing research has shown that periodontal disease and CKD are positively correlated, although periodontal disease is an important risk factor for CKD as it has the potential to be modified and treated. Several cohort studies have investigated the relationship between CKD and periodontal disease [6–8]. Systematic reviews have also reported that periodontal disease is associated with CKD [9–11]. Moreover, the severity of periodontal disease is correlated with a decline in kidney function [12]. Although periodontal disease is a mixed infection, gram-negative bacilli play a major role. *Porphyromonas gingivalis* is implicated in periodontal disease, and elevated levels of immunoglobulin G (IgG) antibodies against *P. gingivalis* were shown to positively correlate with the onset and progression of CKD [13]. Despite speculations that CKD is closely associated with the occurrence and progression of periodontal disease, detailed pathological characteristics at the molecular level and the clinical significance of periodontal disease in CKD patients are not fully understood and still remain unknown.

Renal replacement therapy is performed to maintain QoL and life in patients with end-stage renal disease (ESRD). As renal replacement therapy, peritoneal dialysis, hemodialysis, and kidney transplantation (KT) are usually selected according to the patient's wishes; his/her clinical condition, the original disease, and/or the presence of transplant organ donor sources. In general, KT has some advantages in the improvement of life expectancy and QoL compared with dialytic therapies [14,15]. In fact, in contrast to peritoneal dialysis and hemodialysis, limitation of amount of drinking water and excessive dietary restriction are necessary the patients received KT when transplanted renal graft achieves normal function [16]. In addition, concentrations of uremic toxins in patients with KT are remarkably lower than those dialysis patients even though technology of dialysis is improving [17]. Such advantages are important to prevent the periodontal disease because oral health is improved by increased drinking of water and normalization of salivary properties [18,19]. Conversely, we also should note that kidney function in KT patients is usually equal to that of CKD patients because there may be still a functional contralateral kidney. Although the differences in renal function are limited between CKD and KT patients, KT should be considered an immunosuppressive status due to the immunosuppressive therapy required in these patients, and this immunoreactivity plays an important role in periodontal disease [20].

In this review, at first, we summarize information regarding the pathogenesis of periodontal disease to provide a better understanding of the specific pathological mechanisms of periodontal disease in CKD and KT patients. Briefly, we pay special attention to common pathological conditions in patients with periodontal diseases and in patients with CKD or KT. Based on this information, we then introduce the impact of periodontal disease on various other diseases and on the pathological status of CKD patients. Moreover, this review also reveals the clinical significance of periodontal disease in patients with KT. Specifically, we discuss the influence of immunosuppressive drugs used to treat oral pathological conditions including gingival overgrowth in patients with KT. Furthermore, we compare the periodontal pathogens implicated in CKD and KT patients. Finally, the impact of periodontal therapy on outcome of kidney function in these patients is discussed, and we comment on the importance of periodic oral care and appropriate periodontal treatment. Thus, this review provides comprehensive and cross-sectional information on the pathological roles of periodontal disease in CKD and KT, while we emphasize that a better understanding of pathogens, pathological roles, and the impact of immunosuppressive therapy is essential to maintain the QoL, avoid complications, and improve survival in these patients.

2. Modulators of Periodontal Disease

It is necessary to exacerbate inflammation in distant tissues for local inflammation of the teeth to injure distant organs. There are several mechanisms through which periodontal bacteria affect multiple organs, such as systemic bacteremia, cytokine release and inflammation, swallowing to the gastrointestinal tract, and direct exposure through alveolar bone destruction. The first two mechanisms are common pathways for multiple organ failure. Bacteremia caused by bacteria invades the blood stream through the periodontitis lesion and an influx of inflammation mediators, such as interleukin (IL)-6 and tumor necrosis factor (TNF)-α, produced in the lesion can be introduced into the systemic circulation. Importantly, the pathological significance of such processes in patients with CKD is different from that of healthy individuals. For example, case fatality rates at 30 and 90 days in ESRD patients with bloodstream infections was 15% and 25%, respectively; however, the rate in control patients was 0% [21]. In addition, a uremic environment due to CKD was reported to modulate the levels of various cytokines and inflammation-related molecules, including toll-like receptor in immune cells, leading to increased inflammation [22]. Furthermore, other investigators have paid special attention to the relationships between CKD and oxidative stress, endothelial dysfunction, and adhesion molecules [23–25]. However, these factors that may be modulated by CKD play important roles in inflammation under various physiological and pathological conditions [23,26–28]. Based on these considerations, we review previous reports describing the pathological significance of bacteremia, cytokines and inflammation-related molecules, oxidative stress, and endothelial dysfunction in periodontal disease.

2.1. Bacteremia

How do periodontal bacteria move via the blood stream and damage multiple organs? First, gingival ulceration in the periodontal pocket enables bacteria to enter the systemic circulation [29]. Recirculating leukocytes engulf and destroy foreign antigens in the immune response; however, some periodontal disease bacteria, such as *P. gingivalis* and *Actinobacillus actinomycetemcomitans*, can survive intracellularly, and may exploit macrophages and/or dendritic cells as vehicles, much like a Trojan horse, which causes silent systemic inflammation [29]. Although it remains unknown as to whether periodontal bacteria proliferate on blood vessel walls, components of periodontitis bacteria have been detected in arteriosclerotic lesions [30]. Thus, bacteremia is an important step in the progression to systematic inflammation in patients with periodontal diseases. In fact, blood bacteria levels were higher in patients with periodontitis than in those with gingivitis ($p < 0.0001$), and its level was positively associated with worse periodontal parameters [31].

2.2. Cytokines and Inflammation-Related Molecules

The biological activity observed in periodontal lesions has suggested that various cytokines are involved in the pathogenesis of periodontal disease [32]. Numerous cytokines are known to be associated with periodontal disease, and cytokines are categorized by their function. Representative inflammatory cytokines include IL-1, IL-6, IL-8, and TNF-α. These inflammatory cytokines enhance vascular permeability, which may enhance bacteremia and stimulate fibroblasts and inflammatory cells, which in turn induce other cytokines. They also enhance the expression of endothelial adhesion molecules, such as intercellular adhesion molecule (ICAM)-1 and vascular cell adhesion molecule (VCAM)-1, E-selectin, and chemokines such as monocyte chemoattractant protein (MCP)-1 and IL-8 [33]. In addition, inflammatory cytokines regulate bone resorption and inhibit bone formation, which are associated with the local expansion of periodontal lesions through alveolar bone loss [32] and systemically with CKD-mineral bone disorder (CKD-MBD). Fibroblast growth factor (FGF)-23, which has been suggested to have a central role in CKD-MBD and in the regulation of serum phosphorus levels, has been associated with higher inflammatory cytokine levels [34]. Moreover, inflammatory cytokines cause an expansion of the mesangial matrix or induce interstitial fibrosis [35]. If bacteremia does not cause direct damage through in situ inflammatory cytokine production in the targeted organ, increased inflammatory cytokines in local periodontal lesions cause systematic inflammation via the blood stream. Other important cytokines are growth factors, such as FGF, platelet-derived growth factor (PDGF), and transforming growth factor-β (TGF-β). Connective tissue growth factor (CTGF), which normally maintains tissue homeostasis, can induce fibrosis during the inflammatory response. Renal fibrosis has a negative impact on renal prognosis, especially in patients with CKD. Considering these findings, cytokines in periodontal diseases increase vascular permeability, enhance the expression of adhesion molecules, and cause up-regulation of TGF-β. These responses may be associated with proteinuria via glomerular permeability, renal thrombosis, and renal fibrosis, respectively, and result in a deterioration of renal function [35,36].

Periodontal disease, which is associated with systemic disorders, is associated with gram-negative organisms such as *P. gingivalis*, rather than gram-positive organisms. Generally, gram-positive cocci and rods are primarily detected in subgingival plaques of healthy people. However, in plaques formed in the gingival pocket of chronic periodontitis patients, gram-negative anaerobic bacilli increase resulting in the transition to bacterial flora, which cause the formation of more complex pathogenic plaques [37]. Lipopolysaccharides (LPS) derived from the periodontal pathogens will be delivered systemically in blood vessels to other organs. An increase in inflammation through Toll-like receptor 2 and/or 4 in the innate immune system will be observed in these organs [29]. The interaction between LPS and toll-like receptors is quite complicated: The toll-like receptor-mediated pathogenic action of LPS in the immune system differs depending on the derived pathogens and the toll-like receptors [38]. For example, LPS derived from *P. gingivalis* has been associated with inducing urinary protein via Toll-like receptor 2 of the renal glomerular vascular endothelial cells and the progression of kidney diseases via Toll-like receptor 4 signaling in a diabetic animal model [39]. Nonetheless, it should be noted that the downstream signaling of Toll-like receptors has crucial roles in inflammation [32].

2.3. Oxidative Stress

Reactive oxygen species (ROS) are an important primary defense factor in periodontal disease [40]. ROS are produced by inflammatory cells such as polymorphonuclear leukocytes and vascular smooth muscle cells, and nicotine adenine dinucleotide phosphate oxidase is a major source of ROS generation. However, although the main target of ROS is nuclear DNA, excessive ROS production will generate lipid peroxide through homeostasis of oxidative balance in tissues, and lipid peroxide in local periodontal lesions is associated with periodontal diseases [41]. Moreover, ROS are associated with oxidative stress and long-lasting systemic oxidative stress, which is thought to cause multi-organ failure [42]. Reactive nitrogen intermediates are also important in oxidative stress. For example, peroxynitrite, which is produced by nitric oxide and superoxide anion causes endothelial damage [43]. There are several oxidative stress markers such as malondialdehyde (MDA), 8-hydroxydeoxyguanosine (8-OHdG), and 4-hydroxy-2-nonenal (4-HNE). It is plausible that oxidative stress has a significant impact on local periodontal lesions, and the effects of oxidative stress on the systemic inflammation have been shown by several research groups. For example, tissue 8-OHdG levels increased in multiple organs, such as the liver, heart, kidneys, and brain in a periodontal inflammation model [41]. Furthermore, in saliva, MDA and 8-OHdG levels are thought to be associated with oxidative periodontal lesions, and 4-HNE levels in the saliva may reflect systemic inflammation [44]. Conversely, there has been a report indicating that nuclear factor erythroid 2-related factor (NrF2), which is a key regulator of antioxidants, plays an important role in protecting against tissue destruction in periodontitis [45]. Thus, the balance between oxidative stress and antioxidants is speculated to be associated with occurrence, severity, and progression of periodontal disease.

2.4. Inflammatory Reaction and Endothelial Dysfunction

One of the most important mechanisms in systemic organ dysfunction in periodontal disease is due to endothelial dysfunction, which is associated with platelet aggregation, foam-cell formation, and development of atheroma [46]. In CKD, proteinuria is one of the most important surrogate markers of kidney prognosis and reflects endothelial dysfunction [34]. As stated above, inflammatory cytokines originating from bacteremia or paracrine from distal periodontal lesions will cause vascular permeability and vascular wall injury [32]. In addition to inflammatory cytokines, endothelial adhesion molecules, such as ICAM-1 and VCAM-1, play an important role in vascular injury via the activation of endothelial cells and smooth muscle cell proliferation [47]. Endothelial injury will cause arterial stenosis, resulting in hypertension [47].

In addition to the above observations, an animal model showed that ridocaine inhibited endothelial dysfunction of the systematic artery in rats with periodontal inflammation and decreased ROS was associated with such a mechanism [48]. Furthermore, investigation in patients with chronic periodontitis demonstrated that endothelial dysfunction of the branchial artery occurred with greater frequency in patients with periodontitis than in those without periodontitis [46]. Interestingly, this study and other investigators showed that together with various cytokines and inflammation-related molecules, oxidative stress regulated the relationship between periodontitis and endothelial dysfunction [49,50].

2.5. Matrix Metalloproteinases and Transglutaminases

When discussing the pathological mechanisms and development of periodontal disease, information regarding gingival remodeling and healing steps is important. In addition, an understanding of the protective system of oral tissues from microbial challenge in periodontal disease is also essential. From this standpoint, there is an interesting study that focused on the pathological roles of matrix metalloproteinase (MMP) and transglutaminases in patients with chronic periodontitis [51]. In short, when MMP-2 and -9 and transglutaminase-1–3 were analyzed in 22 patients with chronic periodontitis and healthy controls, transglutaminase-1 and 3 mRNA levels in chronic periodontitis patients were lower than those in healthy controls [51]. Finally, this study showed that different transglutaminases might regulate gingival remodeling/healing and adaptive processes in patients with chronic periodontitis. Conversely, it has also been reported that transglutaminase-2 may play an important role in vascular calcification in CKD [52]. Thus, the pathological roles of transglutaminases in CKD are not fully understood.

3. Periodontal Disease and Chronic Kidney Disease

3.1. Impact on Periodontal Disease from other Pathological Conditions

As discussed above, there is evidence suggesting that there is a direct relationship between the inflammation of periodontal disease and CKD, and renal function may decline for various reasons. CKD may evolve from any chronic renal disorder etiology, and typically includes diabetes, hypertension, and chronic nephritis [1,4]. In contrast, periodontal diseases can cause dysfunction of various organs, such as the heart, liver, and kidney. Therefore, the reduction in renal function due to the burden of other diseases as a result of periodontal disease should be considered.

3.1.1. Diabetes

The most important complication of periodontal disease is diabetes, and the risk of diabetes mellitus is increased by periodontal disease, suggesting that this association is bidirectional. In fact, the prevalence of diabetes is higher in patients with periodontal disease than in those without periodontitis [53]. Furthermore, the Hisayama study in Japan showed that patients who developed glucose intolerance were more likely to have periodontal disease than the group that did not develop glucose intolerance [54]. Diabetic nephropathy with overt proteinuria occurs as a result of long-term diabetes, but diabetes patients with periodontal disease have a higher risk of cardiovascular disease compared with patients without periodontal disease [55]. Therefore, diabetic nephropathy caused by periodontal disease shortens the clinical course of ESRD [56]. With regard to the molecular mechanisms involved, the inflammatory cytokines IL-1 and IL-6, TNF-α; fibrotic growth factors TGF-β and CTGF; and oxidative stress have all been implicated in the original pathogenesis of diabetic nephropathy [57]. There is a close relationship between diabetes and periodontal disease and glycemic control is crucial, not only for kidney function, but also periodontal disease. Leukocyte function is poorly controlled in diabetic patients and this may worsen and exacerbate periodontal disease [58]. The effects of periodontal disease on diabetic nephropathy vary depended upon the patients' condition. Thus, diabetic patients with periodontal disease should be treated intensively both for glycemic control and periodontal diseases.

3.1.2. Hypertension

Hypertension is one of the most important risk factors of premature cardiovascular disease, including CKD. A systematic review has shown the relationship between periodontal disease and hypertension [59]. As stated above, inflammation in response to bacteremia or inflammatory mediators from periodontal lesions plays a role in hypertension. Possible pathophysiological mechanisms in periodontal disease and high blood pressure are endothelial dysfunction, reduction of nitric oxide bioavailability, oxidative stress, renin-angiotensin-aldosterone system activation, arterial stiffness, and atherosclerosis [47]. Conversely, cross-sectional clinical studies have shown that risk factors for CKD in patients with periodontal disease include diabetes [60,61] and hypertension [60].

3.1.3. Liver Diseases

Periodontal disease is considered to be associated with different forms of liver disease, one of which is nonalcoholic fatty liver disease (s). The correlation between IgG antibody titers against periodontal pathogens has been shown to be increased in non-alcoholic fatty liver disease (NAFLD) patients [62]. Similar to injuries in other organs, the mechanisms involved in periodontal diseases and NAFLD are described as follows: LPS derived from periodontopathic bacteria are transferred to the blood and act directly on the liver, or LPS-derived inflammatory cytokines act indirectly on the liver [63]. NAFLD can affect multiple extrahepatic organs, such as the cardiovascular system, and increases the risk of developing CKD, with insulin resistance being an important mediating factor [64].

3.1.4. Others

In recent years, nutritional status in kidney disease has attracted increasing attention and patients with CKD are facing protein energy wasting (PEW) complications [59]. Since proinflammatory cytokines affect the brain and cause anorexia, persistent inflammation is associated with PEW [65]. CKD is a very complicated disease, and the etiologies of inflammation observed in patients with CKD are multifactorial. Although any form of inflammation can cause PEW, periodontal disease is a potential etiology for persistent inflammation [66]. Periodontal pathogens that are swallowed and reach the intestine cause changes in the intestinal microbiota, resulting in a situation resembling metabolic bacteremia such as that found in obesity. Although the direct effect of periodontal pathogens on the gut microbiota is controversial, oral microbiota could also alter the gut microbiota [67]. Recent studies have revealed that not only diabetes and obesity but also CKD is closely associated with the intestinal flora [68]. Dysbiosis of the gut microbiota is believed to be associated with periodontal disease, and administration of *P. gingivalis* was shown to alter the gut microbiota and affect multiple organs in an animal model [69]. Thus, CKD should be considered a multifactorial disease; it is extremely difficult to identify specific etiological factors, but it should be taken into consideration that periodontal disease indirectly causes renal dysfunction.

A scheme illustrating the complex mechanisms involved in periodontal disease and CKD is shown in Figure 1.

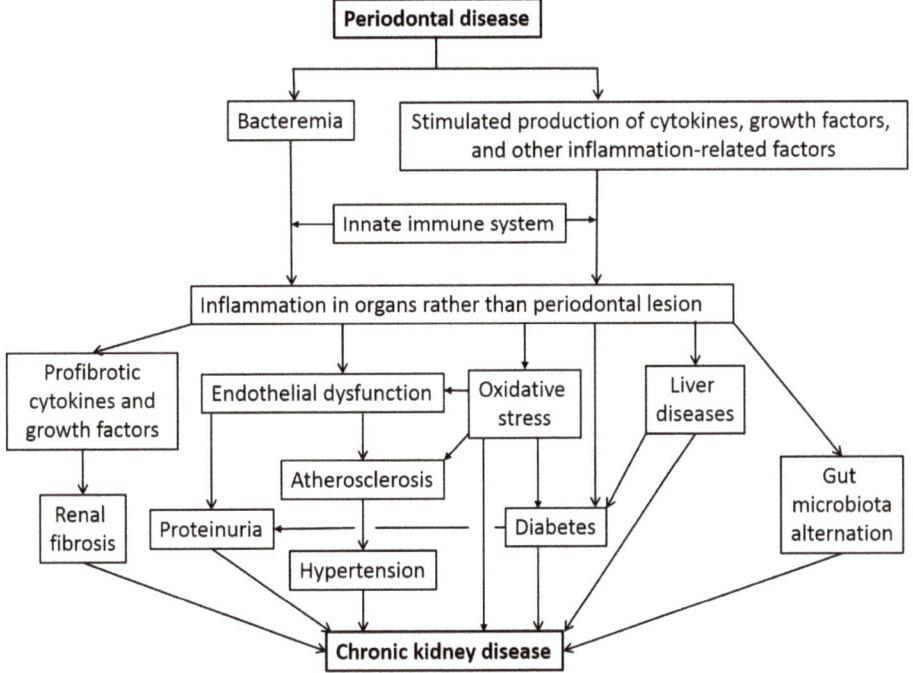

Figure 1. Impact of periodontal disease in the pathogenesis in chronic kidney disease.

3.2. Periodontal Therapy and CKD Patients with Periodontal Disease

There is a bidirectional relationship between periodontal disease and CKD, and between periodontal disease and diabetes [70]. The results of this study still remain unclear, although if CKD proceeds and renal function deteriorates, lymphocyte function and monocyte/macrophage function will be impaired and the immune system will aggregate; consequently, the risk of infection will increase compared to the healthy population [4]. When it comes to CKD-MBD, hyperphosphatemia increases phosphate levels in saliva, which is associated with a higher risk of inflammation of the periodontium. Furthermore, higher levels of phosphorus itself are linked to systemic inflammation [71]. This will enhance the association of periodontal disease and CKD. Although periodontal disease is a crucial risk factor for the onset of kidney disease and progression of renal failure, it is a treatable and modifiable risk factor. eGFR might improve in patients with CKD, however patients with ESRD cannot improve their eGFR.

The treatment of periodontal disease attenuates systemic inflammation and improves surrogate markers of endothelial function [72]. Through the reduction of inflammatory cytokines, renal function was shown to improve after treatment of periodontal disease [73]. A systematic review also showed a favorable effect of periodontal treatment on eGFR [74]. Other reports have indicated that treatment for periodontal disease decreases asymmetric dimethylarginine [75] and 4-hydroxy-2-nonenal, surrogate markers of systemic inflammation [44] and endothelial function [9], respectively.

In a discussion on periodontal therapy in patients with CKD, we must also take into consideration the influence of immunosuppressive agents. In short, a variety of CKD, such as lupus nephritis and IgA nephropathy, is commonly treated with immunosuppressive agents [76,77]. Undoubtedly, the immune response is closely associated with infection control in almost organs and tissues including oral and periodontal tissues. Therefore, in CKD patients treated with immunosuppressive agents, a treatment strategy for periodontal disease must be planned according to its severity, renal function, and response to anti-bacterial agents. In addition, in some patients, decreasing exposure to immunosuppressive agents should also be discussed. Unfortunately, however, there is little information regarding appropriate dosage in these patients. We emphasize the importance of further studies on appropriate dosage and types of immunosuppressive agents to be used in CKD patients with severe periodontal disease, especially in non-responders to anti-bacterial agents.

4. Periodontal Disease and Kidney Transplantation

As mentioned above, KT is one of the major renal replacement approaches to maintain QoL in patients with ESRD, and KT might be the choice of renal replacement therapy to achieve normalized kidney function, which undeniably leads to both social and physical advantages for the patient [14,15]. However, immunosuppressive therapy is essential for maintenance of kidney allograft function to prevent rejection and renal dysfunction, although it may be the cause of several infectious diseases including periodontitis. In addition, there is a general agreement that immunosuppressive conditions sometimes lead to the progression of local infections to general bacteremia. In Japan a total of 1742 KT including 1544 from living donors (LD) and 198 from deceased donors (DD) were performed in the proportion of patients with ABO blood type, incompatible with KT and requiring desensitization for antibody removal before KT, was as large as 27.7% of KT from LD, while the dialysis period before KT was as long as 15.1 years from DD in a Japanese survey [78]. ABO incompatibility and exposure of long-term dialysis therapy lead to susceptibility to immunosuppression, which leads to the risk of developing infectious diseases including periodontal disease. It is important to understand the underlying biological mechanisms of periodontal disease and the immunological status of KT recipients. Moreover, it is important to identify an approach to treat periodontal diseases for the management of KT.

4.1. The Screening of Periodontal Disease Before and After KT

Screening for infectious diseases is important in the preparation of KT. It is well-known that poor oral health is common among CKD patients [79]. KT candidates are considered to have a high prevalence of periodontal disease due to the status of end-stage of renal insufficiency, which is called stage-five CKD. There has been a recent increase in the number of preemptive kidney transplantation (PEKT) procedures, which are defined as transplant before initiation of maintenance dialysis therapy, for the avoidance of complication by dialysis therapy [80]. PEKT is often performed at the progression of renal deterioration in the pre-dialysis stage. Moreover, the progressed renal insufficiency may occasionally fall into a severe immunocompromised state. Oral infections should be treated completely before exposure to immunosuppression for KT candidates, since recent potent immunosuppressive therapy regimens might lead to unexpected onset of infection including periodontitis. Oral health has been reported to be better during the KT period than at the pre-dialysis stage, and it thus is important to treat oral infectious foci at the pre-dialysis stage in order to prevent adverse outcomes after KT [81]. However, lower salivary flow rates and higher numbers of drugs at the KT stage might influence the clinical outcome [81]. Patients with diabetic nephropathy associate with worse periodontal health and higher oral inflammatory conditions at the pre-dialysis stage to the same degree as the pre-transplant stage [82]. Due to the high prevalence of cardiovascular disease and requirements of extracorporeal circulation for hemodialysis, anti-coagulant therapy is used in many KT candidates. The surgical treatment of oral diseases in this condition may lead to active bleeding and cause general bacteremia or fatal sepsis. Preconditioning and necessary treatment are important for the KT recipient before and after exposure to immunosuppressive therapy. Finally, it should be considered that appropriate timing of treatment must be provided to KT recipients depending on the patient's general status, CKD stage, and original cause of renal insufficiency [81,82].

4.2. Periodontal Condition and Clinical Outcome

Several investigators have examined the effects of periodontal conditions in relation to clinical outcome following KT. The studies reported a higher [83,84], similar [85], or lower [86] incidence of periodontitis in transplant recipients than in healthy controls. A limitation to the study results is that these differ depending on the definition of occurrence of periodontitis used. Ioannidou et al. [87] reported that none of the continuous periodontal variables were significantly associated with deterioration of allograft function due to the presence of strict criteria such as HLA-matching or history of acute rejection. A systematic review described the associations between periodontal status and clinical outcomes in KT recipients. A patient's periodontal status might be associated with a larger left ventricular mass, greater carotid thickness, graft rejection, lower graft survival, and higher mortality rate in early KT periods among KT recipients [88]. These studies suggest that periodontal status may affect clinical outcomes of patient survival and graft survival due to the occurrence of cardiovascular disease and abnormal immunological responses with essential immunosuppressive therapy [86–88].

4.3. Influence of Immunosuppressive Drugs

Recently, potent strong immunosuppressive therapy is becoming more commonly used to prevent acute rejection, which has improved outcomes of KT in the modern era [89]. A protocol using everolimus (ERL) is often performed in addition to a standard protocol consisting of mycophenolate mofetil (MMF), tacrolimus (Tac), and corticosteroid (CS), which has allowed further improvements in treatment outcomes of KT [90,91]. However, protocols using multiple agents can lead to a condition of excessive immunosuppression, which may worsen oral status. There are currently different immunosuppressive agents available and it is clinically important to understand differences in each drug relative to the possible occurrence of periodontal disease. Calcineurin inhibitors (CNI) such as Cyclosporin A (CsA) and Tac have played a central role in immunosuppressive therapy of KT since the 1980s. CsA is characterized by a major side effect of gingival overgrowth (GO), which may lead to occasionally worsening of oral health. CsA-induced gingival enlargement has been reported to vary from 7–80% in different transplant centers [92]. Conversely, the use of ERL frequently results in adverse events of stomatitis and compromised status, and so it may be important to properly manage the oral environment during treatment [93]. However, few reports have examined the risk of developing periodontitis and other oral diseases in patients using ERL. Pereira-Lopes et al. compared the oral health status of KT recipients receiving Tac or ERL as immunosuppressants. The study showed that KT recipients receiving the ERL protocol presented reduced periodontal inflammation in comparison with patients receiving Tac [94]. In the study, patients receiving ERL were older and they experienced more limited periodontal inflammation. There might be a bias in the patient selection in the study. ERL is used for CNI minimization or corticosteroid elimination due to protection from CNI nephrotoxicity or various side effects of steroid therapy, which might affect long-term graft survival or patient survival [95–97]. Tac has similar adverse effects as CsA because both drugs share the same pharmacological mechanism of calcineurin inhibition. Several investigators have examined the occurrence of GO with the use of Tac, which has been less frequent than the use of CsA [98,99]. In a clinical study comparing exposure to CsA and Tac, it was reported that GO occurred later in the group using Tac, with the severity of GO in the Tac group being lower than that in the CA group [100]. Another study including a post-hoc analysis revealed that the prevalence of GO was 60.0% for CsA, 28.9% for Tac, and 15.6% for sirolimus, which was used as an mTOR inhibitor for the same purpose of ERL [101]. Tac may be an alternative agent to CsA in attempting to avoid adverse effects of GO [102,103]. Tac seems advantageous with regard to periodontal effects when using CNI as a standard immunosuppression protocol.

4.4. Immunosuppressant-Induced Gingival Overgrowth and Periodontal Condition

Gingival enlargement is commonly observed as a side effect of several different types of drugs, including anticonvulsants, calcium channel blockers, and immunosuppressants [92]. As previously mentioned, GO is common adverse effect of CsA usage, which may lead to the worsening of periodontal conditions in KT recipients. A multitude of factors may affect clinical and histopathological manifestations of immunosuppressant-induced GO. Several investigators have examined the causes of CsA-induced GO, which might associate with periodontal disease. The results of several studies examining specific factors found in the gingival crevicular fluid (GCF) were indicative of CsA-induced GO. Increased LL-37 peptide levels in the GCF is observed at the CsA-induced GO positive site with neutrophil infiltration and extended inflammation. LL-37 is an antimicrobial peptide and an important defense molecule of the host immune response [104]. Gürkan et al. [105] examined the association of many types of cytokine families with CsA-induced GO by the examination of the GCF. TGF-β_1, whose levels are associated with clinical periodontal parameters, might be an exclusive mediator of CsA- or Tac-induced GO. Increased IL-6 and oncostain M under CsA usage have been reported to be involved in regulating the severity of inflammation and presence of GO, but cytokines of the IL-6 family might not be directly involved in the biological mechanisms associated with CsA-induced GO [106]. A study examining transgultaminase (TGM)-2, which had been shown to play a role in fibrosis by extracellular matrix accumulation, showed that TGM-2 might contribute to CsA-induced GO by modifying the GCF and plasma levels of oxidative stress markers [107].

The investigation of molecules contained in the GCF may provide researchers with a variety of insights associated with medication-induced GO. Conversely, several study groups have attempted to elucidate the mechanism of GO by investigating gene polymorphisms. IL-10 gene polymorphism might be associated with CsA-induced GO in KT recipients. A special genotype and allele might indicate an association with susceptibility to GO [108]. Alpha-2 integrin gene polymorphisms were not associated with CsA-induced GO but were associated with CsA-independent GO in KT recipients [109]. Interestingly, the length of the CAG repeat of the androgen receptor gene might link to CsA-induced GO via the analysis of polymorphisms [110]. Thus, many studies have been attempted to elucidate the mechanisms involved in drug-induced GO [104–110], but the biological mechanism of the gingival tissue response involved in immunosuppressant-induced GO is still not fully understood. Since gingival enlargement is directly associated with QoL, it is necessary to elucidate the causes of drug-induced GO by further scientific research and the challenge is to modify present immunosuppressive therapy regimens to avoid GO.

4.5. Inflammatory Markers of Periodontitis in KT

Inflammation may be associated with the deterioration of solid-organ function in transplantation recipients. Systemic inflammation occasionally originates from periodontal inflammation. There is clinical evidence that periodontal inflammation is linked to the occurrence of different systemic diseases including ESRD [111]. Moreover, the chronic inflammation of kidney allograft is often modulated by alloimmune-dependent mechanisms. The main cause of inflammation in solid-organ transplantation is dependent on human leukocyte antigen (HLA) mismatches or panel reactive antibody (PRA) scores, which may lead to acute humoral rejection [112,113]. Several inflammatory markers such as IL-6 and C-reactive protein (CRP) may be predictors of renal allograft survival associated with alloimmune-dependent acute rejection [114,115]. Moreover, specific cells associated with periodontal disease may produce significantly higher levels of IL-6, and serum CRP was reported to be elevated in patients with periodontal inflammation [116]. Shaqman et al. [117] compared periodontal disease and systemic inflammatory status of transplant recipients and age-matched controls, which led to the conclusion of the absence of any significant predictors of systemic inflammation in the population. In another study Blach et al. [118] examined several inflammatory markers such as TNF-α, IL-6, and high-sensitive CRP (hs-CRP) in KT recipients. The study demonstrated that severe chronic periodontitis was associated with increased serum hs-CRP, but not with any significant elevation of TNF-α or CRP. Elevated hs-CRP levels appeared to influence mortality after KT [118]; thus, it is important to monitor the levels of inflammatory markers such as hs-CRP, which may lead to the early detection and early treatment of periodontal disease. Furthermore, it would be more useful if an inflammatory marker specific to KT recipients undergoing immunosuppressive therapy were identified in real world studies.

5. Periodontal Pathogens in Chronic Kidney Disease and Kidney Transplantation

Several investigators have reported an increased frequency of periodontal pathogens in CKD and KT patients. There is general agreement that periodontal disease occurred by mixed infection, but not by a single pathogen alone [119,120]. With regard to CKD, Bastos et al. [121] reported that the frequencies of *P. gingivalis* and *Candida albicans* in pre-dialysis CKD patients showed a higher trend than the control group (94.7 versus 72.2% and 52.0% versus 26.3%, respectively); however, such difference did not reach statistical significance ($p = 0.078$ and $p = 0.079$, respectively). Conversely, the frequencies of *P. gingivalis* and *Treponema denticola* (*T. denticola*) were significantly associated with clinical detectable levels ($p = 0.008$ and $p = 0.013$, respectively) in CKD patients with periodontitis [121]. Conversely, other investigators have shown that *T. denticola*, *Tanerella forsythia* (*T. forsythia*), and *Parvimonas micra* (*P. micra*) were significantly associated with periodontal disease in patients with CKD [122]. In addition, the authors also found that *T. forsythia* was independently associated with periodontal disease in a multivariate analysis model including other significant pathogens, age, and estimated glomerular filtration rate ($p = 0.008$) [122].

Regarding KT patients, the frequency of *Streptococcus constellatus* in plaque samples form subjects with alveolar bone loss (36.4%) was significantly higher ($p = 0.019$) than that in samples without alveolar bone loss (3.7%) [83]. Conversely, a report also indicated that total counts of micro-organisms were increased between day 0 and day 90 after renal transplantation and between day 30 and day 90 after surgery [123]. In addition, the same study also showed that the frequency of β-hemolytic Streptococcus on day 90 after surgery (28.6%) was significantly lower ($p = 0.031$) than that on day 30 (44.4%) in KT patients with GO, but not in patients without GO [123]. Thus, in KT patients, quantitative and qualitative changes of microorganisms in the subgingival plaque might occur 90 days after surgery, and GO had an effect on expression of these microorganisms [117]. Unfortunately, there is limited information on the pathological significance of pathogens in patients with KT.

Conversely, a recent study evaluated the relationships between immunosuppressive agents and periodontal pathogenic bacteria in patients following solid organ transplantation [124]. Although it should be noted that the study population included three different types of organs (kidney, liver, and lung), the study demonstrated that changes in the levels of periodontal pathogenic bacteria dependent on immunosuppressive agents. In short, the prevalence of *P. micra*, was associated with immunosuppression exclusively with glucocorticoids; however, *P. gingivalis* was associated with combined immunosuppression of glucocorticoids, MMF, and Tac [124]. A summary is shown in Table 1.

Table 1. Pathological significance and levels of pathogens according to kidney status.

Pathogens	Status	Pathological Significance and Level of Pathogens	Ref.
β-hemolytic Streptococcus	KT	Associated with gingival overgrowth after transplantation	[123]
Capnocytophaga spec	KT	Lower compared to HD	[120]
Enterococcus faecalis	CKD	Higher compared to control	[125]
Fusobacterium nucleatum	KT	Lower in immunosuppression with glucocorticoid and mycophenolate	[124]
	CRF	Correlation with periodontal disease in multi-variate analysis model	[122]
Parvimonas micra	KT	Lower compared to HD	[122]
	SOT	Higher in immunosuppression with glucocorticoid	[124]
Porphyromonas gingivalis	CRF	Positively associated with clinical attachment level	[122]
	SOT	Lower immunosuppression with glucocorticoid, mycophenolate, and tacrolimus	[124]
Prevotella nigrescens	CRF	Higher compared to control	[125]
Streptococcus constellatus	KT	Lower in subjects with peritoneal destruction	[83]
Tanerella forsythia	CKD	Correlation with periodontal disease in a multi-variate analysis model	[122]
	SOT	Lower in immunosuppression with glucocorticoid and mycophenolate	[124]
Treponema denticola	CRF	Positively associated with clinical attachment level	[121]
	CKD	Associated with periodontal disease	[122]

CKD—chronic kidney disease, KT—kidney transplantation, SOT—solid organ transplantation, and ref—reference.

6. Care of Periodontal Conditions in Chronic Kidney Disease and Kidney Transplantation

Many investigators pay special attention to the prevalence and severity of periodontal disease. In addition, the importance of periodontal treatment has been reported in CKD and KT patients because they may exhibit periodontal conditions worse than that of the healthy general population [124,125]. Currently, several pilot studies support this opinion in these patient groups [75,126]. Unfortunately, CRF or KT patients do not have much interest in screening and/or treatment of periodontal disease. Although we have no data in CRF and KT, there is a report that approximately 70% of hemodialysis facilities have no associated dental clinic [127]. There is an opinion that immunosuppressive therapy is not associated with the necessity of dental and periodontal treatment in patients with transplantation [124]. However, there is no general consensus for KT patients. Conversely, other investigators have suggested the importance of appropriate oral health in KT patients because oral hygiene status was closely associated with the development and degree of GO [128]. Finally, we also emphasize that periodic oral care and appropriate periodontal treatment with dentists are important to maintain QoL, inhibit the complications, and prolong the survival periods in CKD and KT patients. In recent years, the usefulness of various treatment strategies for improvement of oral health has been analyzed [129,130]. In addition, there is the opinion that clinical conditions, such as lipidemia in obesity, affect preventive and treatment strategies of chronic periodontitis [131]. Based on these facts, further detailed studies with larger study populations, longer observation periods, and analyses including broader periodontal disease-related factors are necessary to be able to reach definitive conclusions.

7. Conclusions

In this review, we introduced the pathological significance of periodontal diseases in patients with CKD. Specifically, we showed the increased risks of various pathological conditions, such as diabetes, hypertension, atherosclerosis, liver diseases, and gut microbiota alternation in these patients. Furthermore, in addition to the pathological roles of periodontal diseases in KT patients, we focused on the influence of immunosuppressive drugs on oral health, such as periodontitis, periodontal inflammation, and gingival enlargement. Moreover, the pathological significance and levels of pathogens were compared between patients with CKD and those with KT. Finally, we emphasized the importance of care of oral and periodontal condition to maintain the QoL, prevent complications, and improve survival in patients with CKD and KT. Conversely, a discussion regarding comprehensive preventive strategies of oral health, information on genetic polymorphisms and DNA methylation of oral diseases-related molecules is essential [132]. Based on such information, we suggest that further detailed prospective studies with larger populations and analyses at the molecular level should be performed to clarify the importance of oral health in these patients.

Funding: This research was supported by JSPS KAKENHI Grant Number 16K15690 (to Yasuyoshi Miyata).

Acknowledgments: We would like to thank Editage (www.editage.jp) for English language editing.

Conflicts of Interest: The authors declare no conflicts of interest.

References

1. National Kidney Foundation. K/DOQI clinical practice guidelines for chronic kidney disease: Evaluation, classification, and stratification. *Am. J. Kidney Dis.* **2002**, *39* (Suppl. 1), S1–S266.
2. Ishigami, J.; Grams, M.E.; Chang, A.R.; Carrero, J.J.; Coresh, J.; Matsushita, K. CKD and Risk for Hospitalization with Infection: The Atherosclerosis Risk in Communities (ARIC) Study. *Am. J. Kidney Dis.* **2017**, *69*, 752–761. [CrossRef] [PubMed]
3. Chen, D.P.; Davis, B.R.; Simpson, L.M.; Cushman, W.C.; Cutler, J.A.; Dobre, M.; Ford, C.E.; Louis, G.T.; Muntner, P.; Oparil, S.; et al. Association between chronic kidney disease and cancer mortality: A report from the ALLHAT. *Clin. Nephrol.* **2017**, *87*, 11–20. [CrossRef] [PubMed]
4. Webster, A.C.; Nagler, E.V.; Morton, R.L.; Masson, P. Chronic Kidney Disease. *Lancet* **2017**, *389*, 1238–1252. [CrossRef]

5. Jabbari, B.; Vaziri, N.D. The nature, consequences, and management of neurological disorders in chronic kidney disease. *Hemodial. Int.* **2018**, *22*, 150–160. [CrossRef] [PubMed]
6. Grubbs, V.; Vittinghoff, E.; Taylor, G.; Kritz-Silverstein, D.; Powe, N.; Bibbins-Domingo, K.; Ishani, A.; Cummings, S.R. Osteoporotic Fractures in Men (MrOS) Study Research Group. The association of periodontal disease with kidney function decline: A longitudinal retrospective analysis of the MrOS dental study. *Nephrol. Dial. Transplant.* **2016**, *31*, 466–472. [CrossRef]
7. Ricardo, A.C.; Athavale, A.; Chen, J.; Hampole, H.; Garside, D.; Marucha, P.; Lash, J.P. Periodontal disease, chronic kidney disease and mortality: Results from the third National Health and Nutrition Examination Survey. *BMC Nephrol.* **2015**, *16*, 97. [CrossRef]
8. Sharma, P.; Dietrich, T.; Ferro, C.J.; Cockwell, P.; Chapple, I.L. Association between periodontitis and mortality in stages 3-5 chronic kidney disease: NHANES III and linked mortality study. *J. Clin. Periodontol.* **2016**, *43*, 104–113. [CrossRef] [PubMed]
9. Deschamps-Lenhardt, S.; Martin-Cabezas, R.; Hannedouche, T.; Huck, O. Association between periodontitis and chronic kidney disease: Systematic review and meta-analysis. *Oral Dis.* **2019**, *25*, 385–402. [CrossRef]
10. Kapellas, K.; Singh, A.; Bertotti, M.; Nascimento, G.G.; Jamieson, L.M. Perio-CKD collaboration. Periodontal and chronic kidney disease association: A systematic review and meta-analysis. *Nephrology* **2019**, *24*, 202–212. [CrossRef]
11. Zhang, J.; Jiang, H.; Sun, M.; Chen, J. Association between periodontal disease and mortality in people with CKD: A meta-analysis of cohort studies. *BMC Nephrol.* **2017**, *18*, 269. [CrossRef] [PubMed]
12. Grubbs, V.; Vittinghoff, E.; Beck, J.D.; Kshirsagar, A.V.; Wang, W.; Griswold, M.E.; Powe, N.R.; Correa, A.; Young, B. Association Between Periodontal Disease and Kidney Function Decline in African Americans: The Jackson Heart Study. *J. Periodontol.* **2015**, *86*, 1126–1132. [CrossRef] [PubMed]
13. Kshirsagar, A.V.; Offenbacher, S.; Moss, K.L.; Barros, S.P.; Beck, J.D. Antibodies to periodontal organisms are associated with decreased kidney function. The Dental Atherosclerosis Risk in Communities study. *Blood Purif.* **2007**, *25*, 125–132. [CrossRef] [PubMed]
14. Wang, J.H.; Skeans, M.A.; Israni, A.K. Current Status of Kidney Transplant Outcomes: Dying to Survive. *Adv. Chronic Kidney Dis.* **2016**, *23*, 281–286. [CrossRef] [PubMed]
15. Ju, A.; Chow, B.Y.; Ralph, A.F.; Howell, M.; Josephson, M.A.; Ahn, C.; Butt, Z.; Dobbels, F.; Fowler, K.; Jowsey-Gregoire, S.; et al. Patient-reported outcome measures for life participation in kidney transplantation: A systematic review. *Am. J. Transplant.* **2019**, in press. [CrossRef]
16. Nagaoka, Y.; Onda, R.; Sakamoto, K.; Izawa, Y.; Kono, H.; Nakagawa, K.; Shinoda, K.; Morita, S.; Kanno, Y. Dietary intake in Japanese patients with kidney transplantation. *Clin. Exp. Nephrol.* **2016**, *20*, 972–981. [CrossRef]
17. Liabeuf, S.; Cheddani, L.; Massy, Z.A. Uremic Toxins and Clinical Outcomes: The Impact of Kidney Transplantation. *Toxins* **2018**, *10*, 229. [CrossRef]
18. Björnsson, M.J.; Velschow, S.; Stoltze, K.; Havemose-Poulsen, A.; Schou, S.; Holmstrup, P. The influence of diet consistence, drinking water and bedding on periodontal disease in Sprague-Dawley rats. *J. Periodontal Res.* **2003**, *38*, 543–550. [CrossRef]
19. Podzimek, S.; Vondrackova, L.; Duskova, J.; Janatova, T.; Broukal, Z. Salivary Markers for Periodontal and General Diseases. *Dis. Markers* **2016**, *2016*. [CrossRef]
20. Park, C.S.; Lee, J.Y.; Kim, S.J.; Choi, J.I. Identification of immunological parameters associated with the alveolar bone level in periodontal patients. *J. Periodontal Implant Sci.* **2010**, *40*, 61–68. [CrossRef]
21. Dagasso, G.; Conley, J.; Parfitt, E.; Pasquill, K.; Steele, L.; Laupland, K. Risk factors associated with bloodstream infections in end-stage renal disease patients: A population-based study. *Infect. Dis.* **2018**, *50*, 831–836. [CrossRef] [PubMed]
22. Grabulosa, C.C.; Manfredi, S.R.; Canziani, M.E.; Quinto, B.M.R.; Barbosa, R.B.; Rebello, J.F.; Batista, M.C.; Cendoroglo, M.; Dalboni, M.A. Chronic kidney disease induces inflammation by increasing Toll-like receptor-4, cytokine and cathelicidin expression in neutrophils and monocytes. *Exp. Cell Res.* **2018**, *365*, 157–162. [CrossRef] [PubMed]
23. Feng, Y.M.; Thijs, L.; Zhang, Z.Y.; Yang, W.Y.; Huang, Q.F.; Wei, F.F.; Kuznetsova, T.; Jennings, A.M.; Delles, C.; Lennox, R.; et al. Glomerular function in relation to circulating adhesion molecules and inflammation markers in a general population. *Nephrol. Dial. Transplant.* **2018**, *33*, 426–435. [CrossRef] [PubMed]

24. Krata, N.; Zagożdżon, R.; Foroncewicz, B.; Mucha, K. Oxidative Stress in Kidney Diseases: The Cause or the Consequence? *Arch. Immunol. Ther. Exp.* **2018**, *66*, 211–220. [CrossRef] [PubMed]
25. Khukhlina, O.S.; Antoniv, A.A.; Mandryk, O.Y.; Smandych, V.S.; Matushchak, M.R. The role of endothelial dysfunction in the progression mechanisms of non-alcoholic steatohepatitis in patients with obesity and chronic kidney disease. *Wiad. Lek.* **2019**, *72*, 523–526. [PubMed]
26. Yang, X.; Chang, Y.; Wei, W. Endothelial Dysfunction and Inflammation: Immunity in Rheumatoid Arthritis. *Mediat. Inflamm.* **2016**, *2016*, 6813016. [CrossRef]
27. Molteni, M.; Gemma, S.; Rossetti, C. The Role of Toll-Like Receptor 4 in Infectious and Noninfectious Inflammation. *Mediat. Inflamm.* **2016**, *2016*, 6978936. [CrossRef] [PubMed]
28. Nasef, N.A.; Mehta, S.; Ferguson, L.R. Susceptibility to chronic inflammation: An update. *Arch. Toxicol.* **2017**, *91*, 1131–1141. [CrossRef]
29. Hajishengallis, G. Periodontitis: From microbial immune subversion to systemic inflammation. *Nat. Rev. Immunol.* **2015**, *15*, 30–44. [CrossRef]
30. Tsuchida, S.; Satoh, M.; Takiwaki, M.; Nomura, F. Ubiquitination in Periodontal Disease: A Review. *Int. J. Mol. Sci.* **2017**, *18*, 1476. [CrossRef]
31. Balejo, R.D.P.; Cortelli, J.R.; Costa, F.O.; Cyrino, R.M.; Aquino, D.R.; Cogo-Müller, K.; Miranda, T.B.; Moura, S.P.; Cortelli, S.C. Effects of chlorhexidine preprocedural rinse on bacteremia in periodontal patients: A randomized clinical trial. *J. Appl. Oral Sci.* **2017**, *25*, 586–595. [CrossRef]
32. Okada, H.; Murakami, S. Cytokine expression in periodontal health and disease. *Crit. Rev. Oral Biol. Med.* **1998**, *9*, 248–266. [CrossRef] [PubMed]
33. Gimbrone, M.A., Jr.; García-Cardeña, G. Endothelial Cell Dysfunction and the Pathobiology of Atherosclerosis. *Circ. Res.* **2016**, *118*, 620–636. [CrossRef] [PubMed]
34. Munoz Mendoza, J.; Isakova, T.; Ricardo, A.C.; Xie, H.; Navaneethan, S.D.; Anderson, A.H.; Bazzano, L.A.; Xie, D.; Kretzler, M.; Nessel, L.; et al. Fibroblast growth factor 23 and Inflammation in CKD. *Clin. J. Am. Soc. Nephrol.* **2012**, *7*, 1155–1162. [CrossRef] [PubMed]
35. Gewin, L.; Zent, R.; Pozzi, A. Progression of chronic kidney disease: Too much cellular talk causes damage. *Kidney Int.* **2017**, *91*, 552–560. [CrossRef] [PubMed]
36. Paisley, K.E.; Beaman, M.; Tooke, J.E.; Mohamed-Ali, V.; Lowe, G.D.; Shore, A.C. Endothelial dysfunction and inflammation in asymptomatic proteinuria. *Kidney Int.* **2003**, *63*, 624–633. [CrossRef] [PubMed]
37. Larsen, T.; Fiehn, N.E. Dental biofilm infections—An update. *APMIS* **2017**, *125*, 376–384. [CrossRef]
38. Pulendran, B.; Kumar, P.; Cutler, C.W.; Mohamadzadeh, M.; Van Dyke, T.; Banchereau, J. Lipopolysaccharides from distinct pathogens induce different classes of immune responses in vivo. *J. Immunol.* **2001**, *167*, 5067–5076. [CrossRef]
39. Kajiwara, K.; Takata, S.; To, T.T.; Takara, K.; Hatakeyama, Y.; Tamaoki, S.; Darveau, R.P.; Ishikawa, H.; Sawa, Y. The promotion of nephropathy by Porphyromonas gingivalis lipopolysaccharide via toll-like receptors. *Diabetol. Metab. Syndr.* **2017**, *9*, 73. [CrossRef]
40. Kanzaki, H.; Wada, S.; Narimiya, T.; Yamaguchi, Y.; Katsumata, Y.; Itohiya, K.; Fukaya, S.; Miyamoto, Y.; Nakamura, Y. Pathways that Regulate ROS Scavenging Enzymes, and Their Role in Defense Against Tissue Destruction in Periodontitis. *Front. Physiol.* **2017**, *8*, 51. [CrossRef]
41. Tomofuji, T.; Ekuni, D.; Irie, K.; Azuma, T.; Tamaki, N.; Maruyama, T.; Yamamoto, T.; Watanabe, T.; Morita, M. Relationships between periodontal inflammation, lipid peroxide and oxidative damage of multiple organs in rats. *Biomed. Res.* **2011**, *32*, 343–349. [CrossRef] [PubMed]
42. D'Aiuto, F.; Nibali, L.; Parkar, M.; Patel, K.; Suvan, J.; Donos, N. Oxidative stress, systemic inflammation, and severe periodontitis. *J. Dent. Res.* **2010**, *89*, 1241–1246. [CrossRef]
43. Jha, N.; Ryu, J.J.; Choi, E.H.; Kaushik, N.K. Generation and Role of Reactive Oxygen and Nitrogen Species Induced by Plasma, Lasers, Chemical Agents, and Other Systems in Dentistry. *Oxid. Med. Cell. Longev.* **2017**, *2017*, 7542540. [CrossRef] [PubMed]
44. Önder, C.; Kurgan, Ş.; Altıngöz, S.M.; Bağış, N.; Uyanık, M.; Serdar, M.A.; Kantarcı, A.; Günhan, M. Impact of non-surgical periodontal therapy on saliva and serum levels of markers of oxidative stress. *Clin. Oral Investig.* **2017**, *21*, 1961–1969. [CrossRef] [PubMed]
45. Chiu, A.V.; Saigh, M.A.; McCulloch, C.A.; Glogauer, M. The Role of NrF2 in the Regulation of Periodontal Health and Disease. *J. Dent. Res.* **2017**, *96*, 975–983. [CrossRef] [PubMed]

46. Bartova, J.; Sommerova, P.; Lyuya-Mi, Y.; Mysak, J.; Prochazkova, J.; Duskova, J.; Janatova, T.; Podzimek, S. Periodontitis as a risk factor of atherosclerosis. *J. Immunol. Res.* **2014**, *2014*, 636893. [CrossRef] [PubMed]
47. Macedo Paizan, M.L.; Vilela-Martin, J.F. Is there an association between periodontitis and hypertension? *Curr. Cardiol. Rev.* **2014**, *10*, 355–361. [CrossRef]
48. Saito, T.; Yamamoto, Y.; Feng, G.G.; Kazaoka, Y.; Fujiwara, Y.; Kinoshita, H. Lidocaine Prevents Oxidative Stress-Induced Endothelial Dysfunction of the Systemic Artery in Rats with Intermittent Periodontal Inflammation. *Anesth. Analg.* **2017**, *124*, 2054–2062. [CrossRef]
49. Moura, M.F.; Navarro, T.P.; Silva, T.A.; Cota, L.O.M.; Soares Dutra Oliveira, A.M.; Costa, F.O. Periodontitis and Endothelial Dysfunction: Periodontal Clinical Parameters and Levels of Salivary Markers Interleukin-1β, Tumor Necrosis Factor-α, Matrix Metalloproteinase-2, Tissue Inhibitor of Metalloproteinases-2 Complex, and Nitric Oxide. *J. Periodontol.* **2017**, *88*, 778–787. [CrossRef]
50. Scicchitano, P.; Cortese, F.; Gesualdo, M.; De Palo, M.; Massari, F.; Giordano, P.; Ciccone, M.M. The role of endothelial dysfunction and oxidative stress in cerebrovascular diseases. *Free Radic. Res.* **2019**, *20*, 1–471. [CrossRef]
51. Currò, M.; Matarese, G.; Isola, G.; Caccamo, D.; Ventura, V.P.; Cornelius, C.; Lentini, M.; Cordasco, G.; Ientile, R. Differential expression of transglutaminase genes in patients with chronic periodontitis. *Oral Dis.* **2014**, *20*, 616–623. [CrossRef]
52. Chen, N.X.; O'Neill, K.; Chen, X.; Kiattisunthorn, K.; Gattone, V.H.; Moe, S.M. Transglutaminase 2 accelerates vascular calcification in chronic kidney disease. *Am. J. Nephrol.* **2013**, *37*, 191–198. [CrossRef] [PubMed]
53. Ziukaite, L.; Slot, D.E.; Van der Weijden, F.A. Prevalence of diabetes mellitus in people clinically diagnosed with periodontitis: A systematic review and meta-analysis of epidemiologic studies. *J. Clin. Periodontol.* **2018**, *45*, 650–662. [CrossRef] [PubMed]
54. Saito, T.; Shimazaki, Y.; Kiyohara, Y.; Kato, I.; Kubo, M.; Iida, M.; Koga, T. The severity of periodontal disease is associated with the development of glucose intolerance in non-diabetics: The Hisayama study. *J. Dent. Res.* **2004**, *83*, 485–490. [CrossRef] [PubMed]
55. Liccardo, D.; Cannavo, A.; Spagnuolo, G.; Ferrara, N.; Cittadini, A.; Rengo, C.; Rengo, G. Periodontal Disease: A Risk Factor for Diabetes and Cardiovascular Disease. *Int. J. Mol. Sci.* **2019**, *20*, 1414. [CrossRef] [PubMed]
56. Shultis, W.A.; Weil, E.J.; Looker, H.C.; Curtis, J.M.; Shlossman, M.; Genco, R.J.; Knowler, W.C.; Nelson, R.G. Effect of periodontitis on overt nephropathy and end-stage renal disease in type 2 diabetes. *Diabetes Care* **2007**, *30*, 306–311. [CrossRef] [PubMed]
57. Elmarakby, A.A.; Sullivan, J.C. Relationship between oxidative stress and inflammatory cytokines in diabetic nephropathy. *Cardiovasc. Ther.* **2012**, *30*, 49–59. [CrossRef] [PubMed]
58. Mauri-Obradors, E.; Estrugo-Devesa, A.; Jané-Salas, E.; Viñas, M.; López-López, J. Oral manifestations of Diabetes Mellitus. A systematic review. *Med. Oral Patol. Oral Cir. Bucal* **2017**, *22*, e586–e594. [CrossRef] [PubMed]
59. Martin-Cabezas, R.; Seelam, N.; Petit, C.; Agossa, K.; Gaertner, S.; Tenenbaum, H.; Davideau, J.L.; Huck, O. Association between periodontitis and arterial hypertension: A systematic review and meta-analysis. *Am. Heart J.* **2016**, *180*, 98–112. [CrossRef]
60. Han, S.S.; Shin, N.; Lee, S.M.; Lee, H.; Kim, D.K.; Kim, Y.S. Correlation between periodontitis and chronic kidney disease in Korean adults. *Kidney Res. Clin. Pract.* **2013**, *32*, 164–170. [CrossRef]
61. Liu, K.; Liu, Q.; Chen, W.; Liang, M.; Luo, W.; Wu, X.; Ruan, Y.; Wang, J.; Xu, R.; Zhan, X.; et al. Prevalence and risk factors of CKD in Chinese patients with periodontal disease. *PLoS ONE* **2013**, *8*, e70767. [CrossRef] [PubMed]
62. Komazaki, R.; Katagiri, S.; Takahashi, H.; Maekawa, S.; Shiba, T.; Takeuchi, Y.; Kitajima, Y.; Ohtsu, A.; Udagawa, S.; Sasaki, N.; et al. Periodontal pathogenic bacteria, Aggregatibacter actinomycetemcomitans affect non-alcoholic fatty liver disease by altering gut microbiota and glucose metabolism. *Sci. Rep.* **2017**, *7*, 13950. [CrossRef] [PubMed]
63. Tomofuji, T.; Ekuni, D.; Yamanaka, R.; Kusano, H.; Azuma, T.; Sanbe, T.; Tamaki, N.; Yamamoto, T.; Watanabe, T.; Miyauchi, M.; et al. Chronic administration of lipopolysaccharide and proteases induces periodontal inflammation and hepatic steatosis in rats. *J. Periodontol.* **2007**, *78*, 1999–2006. [CrossRef] [PubMed]
64. Targher, G.; Byrne, C.D. Non-alcoholic fatty liver disease: An emerging driving force in chronic kidney disease. *Nat. Rev. Nephrol.* **2017**, *13*, 297–310. [CrossRef] [PubMed]

65. Lodebo, B.T.; Shah, A.; Kopple, J.D. Is it Important to Prevent and Treat Protein-Energy Wasting in Chronic Kidney Disease and Chronic Dialysis Patients? *J. Ren. Nutr.* **2018**, *28*, 369–379. [CrossRef]
66. Machowska, A.; Carrero, J.J.; Lindholm, B.; Stenvinkel, P. Therapeutics targeting persistent inflammation in chronic kidney disease. *Transl. Res.* **2016**, *167*, 204–213. [CrossRef]
67. Atarashi, K.; Suda, W.; Luo, C.; Kawaguchi, T.; Motoo, I.; Narushima, S.; Kiguchi, Y.; Yasuma, K.; Watanabe, E.; Tanoue, T.; et al. Ectopic colonization of oral bacteria in the intestine drives T(H)1 cell induction and inflammation. *Science* **2017**, *358*, 359–365. [CrossRef]
68. Tang, W.H.; Kitai, T.; Hazen, S.L. Gut Microbiota in Cardiovascular Health and Disease. *Circ. Res.* **2017**, *120*, 1183–1196. [CrossRef]
69. Nakajima, M.; Arimatsu, K.; Kato, T.; Matsuda, Y.; Minagawa, T.; Takahashi, N.; Ohno, H.; Yamazaki, K. Oral Administration of P. gingivalis Induces Dysbiosis of Gut Microbiota and Impaired Barrier Function Leading to Dissemination of Enterobacteria to the Liver. *PLoS ONE* **2015**, *10*, e0134234. [CrossRef]
70. Fisher, M.A.; Taylor, G.W.; West, B.T.; McCarthy, E.T. Bidirectional relationship between chronic kidney and periodontal disease: A study using structural equation modeling. *Kidney Int.* **2011**, *79*, 347–355. [CrossRef]
71. Brown, R.B. Dysregulated Phosphate Metabolism, Periodontal Disease, and Cancer: Possible Global Health Implications. *Dent. J.* **2019**, *7*, 18. [CrossRef] [PubMed]
72. Tonetti, M.S.; D'Aiuto, F.; Nibali, L.; Donald, A.; Storry, C.; Parkar, M.; Suvan, J.; Hingorani, A.D.; Vallance, P.; Deanfield, J. Treatment of periodontitis and endothelial function. *N. Engl. J. Med.* **2007**, *356*, 911–920. [CrossRef] [PubMed]
73. Fang, F.; Wu, B.; Qu, Q.; Gao, J.; Yan, W.; Huang, X.; Ma, D.; Yue, J.; Chen, T.; Liu, F.; et al. The clinical response and systemic effects of non-surgical periodontal therapy in end-stage renal disease patients: A 6-month randomized controlled clinical trial. *J. Clin. Periodontol.* **2015**, *42*, 537–546. [CrossRef] [PubMed]
74. Chambrone, L.; Foz, A.M.; Guglielmetti, M.R.; Pannuti, C.M.; Artese, H.P.; Feres, M.; Romito, G.A. Periodontitis and chronic kidney disease: A systematic review of the association of diseases and the effect of periodontal treatment on estimated glomerular filtration rate. *J. Clin. Periodontol.* **2013**, *40*, 443–456. [CrossRef] [PubMed]
75. Almeida, S.; Figueredo, C.M.; Lemos, C.; Bregman, R.; Fischer, R.G. Periodontal treatment in patients with chronic kidney disease: A pilot study. *J. Periodontal Res.* **2017**, *52*, 262–267. [CrossRef] [PubMed]
76. Park, D.J.; Kang, J.H.; Lee, J.W.; Lee, K.E.; Kim, T.J.; Park, Y.W.; Lee, J.S.; Choi, Y.D.; Lee, S.S. Risk factors to predict the development of chronic kidney disease in patients with lupus nephritis. *Lupus* **2017**, *26*, 1139–1148. [CrossRef] [PubMed]
77. Tomino, Y. How to treat patients with chronic kidney disease: With special focus on IgA nephropathy. *Nephrology* **2018**, *23*, 76–79. [CrossRef] [PubMed]
78. Japanese Society for Clinical Renal Transplantation; The Japan Society for Transplantation. Annual progress report from the Japanese renal transplant registry: Number of renal transplantations in 2017 and a follow-up survey. *Ishoku* **2018**, *53*, 89–108.
79. Ruospo, M.; Palmer, S.C.; Craig, J.C.; Gentile, G.; Johnson, D.W.; Ford, P.J.; Tonelli, M.; Petruzzi, M.; De Benedittis, M.; Strippoli, G.F. Prevalence and severity of oral disease in adults with chronic kidney disease: A systematic review of observational studies. *Nephrol. Dial. Transplant.* **2014**, *29*, 364–375. [CrossRef]
80. Okumi, M.; Sato, Y.; Unagami, K.; Hirai, T.; Ishida, H.; Tanabe, K.; Japan Academic Consortium of Kidney Transplantation (JACK). Preemptive kidney transplantation: A propensity score matched cohort study. *Clin. Exp. Nephrol.* **2017**, *21*, 1105–1112. [CrossRef]
81. Nylund, K.M.; Meurman, J.H.; Heikkinen, A.M.; Furuholm, J.O.; Ortiz, F.; Ruokonen, H.M. Oral health in patients with renal disease: A longitudinal study from predialysis to kidney transplantation. *Clin. Oral. Investig.* **2018**, *22*, 339–347. [CrossRef] [PubMed]
82. Nylund, K.; Meurman, J.H.; Heikkinen, A.M.; Honkanen, E.; Vesterinen, M.; Ruokonen, H. Oral health in predialysis patients with emphasis on periodontal disease. *Quintessence Int.* **2015**, *46*, 899–907. [PubMed]
83. Leung, W.K.; Yau, J.Y.; Jin, L.J.; Chan, A.W.; Chu, F.C.; Tsang, C.S.; Chan, T.M. Subgingival microbiota of renal transplant recipients. *Oral Microbiol. Immunol.* **2003**, *18*, 37–44. [CrossRef] [PubMed]
84. Lessem, J.; Drisko, C.; Greenwell, H.; Persson, R.; Newman, H.; Smart, G.; Hopkins, L.; Parameshwar, J.; Fishbein, D.; Partridge, C.; et al. Are cardiac transplant patients more likely to have periodontitis? A case record study. *J. Int. Acad. Periodontol.* **2002**, *4*, 95–100. [PubMed]

85. Oshrain, H.I.; Telsey, B.; Mandel, I.D. A longitudinal study of periodontal disease in patients with reduced immunocapacity. *J. Periodontol.* **1983**, *54*, 151–154. [CrossRef] [PubMed]
86. Rahman, M.M.; Caglayan, F.; Rahman, B. Periodontal health parameters in patients with chronic renal failure and renal transplants receiving immunosuppressive therapy. *J. Nihon Univ. Sch. Dent.* **1992**, *34*, 265–272.
87. Ioannidou, E.; Shaqman, M.; Burleson, J.; Dongari-Bagtzoglou, A. Periodontitis case definition affects the association with renal function in kidney transplant recipients. *Oral Dis.* **2010**, *16*, 636–642. [CrossRef] [PubMed]
88. Nunes-Dos-Santos, D.L.; Gomes, S.V.; Rodrigues, V.P.; Pereira, A.L.A. Periodontal status and clinical outcomes in kidney transplant recipients: A systematic review. *Oral Dis.* **2019**, in press. [CrossRef]
89. Bamoulid, J.; Staeck, O.; Halleck, F.; Khadzhynov, D.; Brakemeier, S.; Dürr, M.; Budde, K. The need for minimization strategies: Current problems of immunosuppression. *Transpl. Int.* **2015**, *28*, 891–900. [CrossRef]
90. Karam, S.; Wali, R.K. Current State of Immunosuppression: Past, Present, and Future. *Crit. Rev. Eukaryot. Gene Expr.* **2015**, *25*, 113–134. [CrossRef]
91. Ventura-Aguiar, P.; Campistol, J.M.; Diekmann, F. Safety of mTOR inhibitors in adult solid organ transplantation. *Expert Opin. Drug Saf.* **2016**, *15*, 303–319. [CrossRef] [PubMed]
92. Dongari-Bagtzoglou, A. Research, Science and Therapy Committee, American Academy of Periodontology. Drug-associated gingival enlargement. *J. Periodontol.* **2004**, *75*, 1424–1431.
93. Ji, Y.D.; Aboalela, A.; Villa, A. Everolimus-associated stomatitis in a patient who had renal transplant. *BMJ Case Rep.* **2016**, *2016*, 2016217513. [CrossRef] [PubMed]
94. Pereira-Lopes, O.; Sampaio-Maia, B.; Sampaio, S.; Vieira-Marques, P.; Monteiro-da-Silva, F.; Braga, A.C.; Felino, A.; Pestana, M. Periodontal inflammation in renal transplant recipients receiving everolimus or tacrolimus—Preliminary results. *Oral Dis.* **2013**, *19*, 666–672. [CrossRef] [PubMed]
95. Diekmann, F. Immunosuppressive minimization with mTOR inhibitors and belatacept. *Transpl. Int.* **2015**, *28*, 921–927. [CrossRef] [PubMed]
96. Sommerer, C.; Budde, K.; Zeier, M.; Wüthrich, R.P.; Reinke, P.; Eisenberger, U.; Mühlfeld, A.; Arns, W.; Stahl, R.; Heller, K.; et al. Early conversion from cyclosporine to everolimus following living-donor kidney transplantation: Outcomes at 5 years posttransplant in the randomized ZEUS trial. *Clin. Nephrol.* **2016**, *85*, 215–225. [CrossRef] [PubMed]
97. Sommerer, C.; Duerr, M.; Witzke, O.; Lehner, F.; Arns, W.; Kliem, V.; Ackermann, D.; Guba, M.; Jacobi, J.; Hauser, I.A.; et al. Five-year outcomes in kidney transplant patients randomized to everolimus with cyclosporine withdrawal or low-exposure cyclosporine versus standard therapy. *Am. J. Transplant.* **2018**, *18*, 2965–2976. [CrossRef] [PubMed]
98. Ellis, J.S.; Seymour, R.A.; Taylor, J.J.; Thomason, J.M. Prevalence of gingival overgrowth in transplant patients immunosuppressed with tacrolimus. *J. Clin. Periodontol.* **2004**, *31*, 126–131. [CrossRef] [PubMed]
99. Sekiguchi, R.T.; Paixão, C.G.; Saraiva, L.; Romito, G.A.; Pannuti, C.M.; Lotufo, R.F. Incidence of tacrolimus-induced gingival overgrowth in the absence of calcium channel blockers: A short-term study. *J. Clin. Periodontol.* **2007**, *34*, 545–550. [CrossRef] [PubMed]
100. Paixão, C.G.; Sekiguchi, R.T.; Saraiva, L.; Pannuti, C.M.; Silva, H.T.; Medina-Pestana, J.; Romito, G.A. Gingival overgrowth among patients medicated with cyclosporin A and tacrolimus undergoing renal transplantation: A prospective study. *J. Periodontol.* **2011**, *82*, 251–258. [CrossRef] [PubMed]
101. Cota, L.O.; Aquino, D.R.; Franco, G.C.; Cortelli, J.R.; Cortelli, S.C.; Costa, F.O. Gingival overgrowth in subjects under immunosuppressive regimens based on cyclosporine, tacrolimus, or sirolimus. *J. Clin. Periodontol.* **2010**, *37*, 894–902. [CrossRef] [PubMed]
102. Greenberg, K.V.; Armitage, G.C.; Shiboski, C.H. Gingival enlargement among renal transplant recipients in the era of new-generation immunosuppressants. *J. Periodontol.* **2008**, *79*, 453–460. [CrossRef] [PubMed]
103. Párraga-Linares, L.; Almendros-Marqués, N.; Berini-Aytés, L.; Gay-Escoda, C. Effectiveness of substituting cyclosporin A with tacrolimus in reducing gingival overgrowth in renal transplant patients. *Med. Oral Patol. Oral Cir. Bucal* **2009**, *14*, e429–e433.
104. Türkoğlu, O.; Gürkan, A.; Emingil, G.; Afacan, B.; Töz, H.; Kütükçüler, N.; Atilla, G. Are antimicrobial peptides related to cyclosporine A-induced gingival overgrowth? *Arch. Oral Biol.* **2015**, *60*, 508–515. [CrossRef] [PubMed]

105. Gürkan, A.; Afacan, B.; Emingil, G.; Töz, H.; Başkesen, A.; Atilla, G. Gingival crevicular fluid transforming growth factor-beta1 in cyclosporine and tacrolimus treated renal transplant patients without gingival overgrowth. *Arch. Oral Biol.* **2008**, *53*, 723–728. [CrossRef]
106. Gürkan, A.; Becerik, S.; Öztürk, V.Ö.; Atmaca, H.; Atilla, G.; Emingil, G. Interleukin-6 Family of Cytokines in Crevicular Fluid of Renal Transplant Recipients with and Without Cyclosporine A-Induced Gingival Overgrowth. *J. Periodontol.* **2015**, *86*, 1069–1077. [CrossRef] [PubMed]
107. Becerik, S.; Celec, P.; Gürkan, A.; Öztürk, V.Ö.; Kamodyova, N.; Atilla, G.; Emingil, G. Gingival Crevicular Fluid and Plasma Levels of Transglutaminase-2 and Oxidative Stress Markers in Cyclosporin A-Induced Gingival Overgrowth. *J. Periodontol.* **2016**, *87*, 1508–1516. [CrossRef]
108. Luo, Y.; Gong, Y.; Yu, Y. Interleukin-10 gene promoter polymorphisms are associated with cyclosporin A-induced gingival overgrowth in renal transplant patients. *Arch. Oral Biol.* **2013**, *58*, 1199–1207. [CrossRef]
109. Gürkan, A.; Emingil, G.; Afacan, B.; Berdeli, A.; Atilla, G. Alpha 2 integrin gene (ITGA2) polymorphism in renal transplant recipients with and without drug inducedgingival overgrowth. *Arch. Oral Biol.* **2014**, *59*, 283–288. [CrossRef]
110. Al Sayed, A.A.; Al Sulaiman, M.H.; Mishriky, A.; Anil, S. The role of androgen receptor gene in cyclosporine induced gingival overgrowth. *J. Periodontal Res.* **2014**, *49*, 609–614. [CrossRef]
111. Kshirsagar, A.V.; Craig, R.G.; Moss, K.L.; Beck, J.D.; Offenbacher, S.; Kotanko, P.; Klemmer, P.J.; Yoshino, M.; Levin, N.W.; Yip, J.K.; et al. Periodontal disease adversely affects the survival of patients with end-stage renal disease. *Kidney Int.* **2009**, *75*, 746–751. [CrossRef] [PubMed]
112. Ramzy, D.; Rao, V.; Brahm, J.; Miriuka, S.; Delgado, D.; Ross, H.J. Cardiac allograft vasculopathy: A review. *Can. J. Surg.* **2005**, *48*, 319–327. [PubMed]
113. Yates, P.J.; Nicholson, M.L. The aetiology and pathogenesis of chronic allograft nephropathy. *Transpl. Immunol.* **2006**, *16*, 148–157. [CrossRef] [PubMed]
114. Hartono, C.; Dadhania, D.; Suthanthiran, M. Noninvasive diagnosis of acute rejection of solid organ transplants. *Front. Biosci.* **2004**, *9*, 145–153. [CrossRef] [PubMed]
115. van Ree, R.M.; Oterdoom, L.H.; de Vries, A.P.; Gansevoort, R.T.; van der Heide, J.J.; van Son, W.J.; Ploeg, R.J.; de Jong, P.E.; Gans, R.O.; Bakker, S.J. Elevated levels of C-reactive protein independently predict accelerated deterioration of graft function in renal transplant recipients. *Nephrol. Dial. Transplant.* **2007**, *22*, 246–253. [CrossRef] [PubMed]
116. Paraskevas, S.; Huizinga, J.D.; Loos, B.G. A systematic review and meta-analyses on C-reactive protein in relation to periodontitis. *J. Clin. Periodontol.* **2008**, *35*, 277–290. [CrossRef] [PubMed]
117. Shaqman, M.; Ioannidou, E.; Burleson, J.; Hull, D.; Dongari-Bagtzoglou, A. Periodontitis and inflammatory markers in transplant recipients. *J. Periodontol.* **2010**, *81*, 666–672. [CrossRef]
118. Blach, A.; Franek, E.; Witula, A.; Kolonko, A.; Chudek, J.; Drugacz, J.; Wiecek, A. The influence of chronic periodontitis on serum TNF-alpha, IL-6 and hs-CRP concentrations, and function of graft and survival of kidney transplant recipients. *Clin. Transplant.* **2009**, *23*, 213–219. [CrossRef]
119. Alves, L.A.; Souza, R.C.; da Silva, T.M.; Watanabe, A.; Dias, M.; Mendes, M.A.; Ciamponi, A.L. Identification of microorganisms in biofluids of individuals with periodontitis and chronic kidney disease using matrix-assisted laser desorption/ionization time-of-flight mass spectrometry. *Rapid Commun. Mass Spectrom.* **2016**, *30*, 1228–1232. [CrossRef]
120. Schmalz, G.; Kauffels, A.; Kollmar, O.; Slotta, J.E.; Vasko, R.; Müller, G.A.; Haak, R.; Ziebolz, D. Oral behavior, dental, periodontal and microbiological findings in patients undergoing hemodialysis and after kidney transplantation. *BMC Oral Health* **2016**, *16*, 72. [CrossRef]
121. Bastos, J.A.; Diniz, C.G.; Bastos, M.G.; Vilela, E.M.; Silva, V.L.; Chaoubah, A.; Souza-Costa, D.C.; Andrade, L.C. Identification of periodontal pathogens and severity of periodontitis in patients with and without chronic kidney disease. *Arch. Oral Biol.* **2011**, *56*, 804–811. [CrossRef] [PubMed]
122. Ismail, F.B.; Ismail, G.; Dumitriu, A.S.; Baston, C.; Berbecar, V.; Jurubita, R.; Andronesi, A.; Dumitriu, H.T.; Sinescu, I. Identification of subgingival periodontal pathogens and association with the severity of periodontitis in patients with chronic kidney diseases: A cross-sectional study. *Biomed. Res. Int.* **2015**, *2015*, 370314. [CrossRef] [PubMed]
123. Saraiva, L.; Lotufo, R.F.; Pustiglioni, A.N.; Silva, H.T., Jr.; Imbronito, A.V. Evaluation of subgingival bacterial plaque changes and effects on periodontal tissues in patients with renal transplants under immunosuppressive therapy. *Oral Surg. Oral Med. Oral Pathol. Oral Radiol. Endodontol.* **2006**, *101*, 457–462. [CrossRef] [PubMed]

124. Schmalz, G.; Berisha, L.; Wendorff, H.; Widmer, F.; Marcinkowski, A.; Teschler, H.; Sommerwerck, U.; Haak, R.; Kollmar, O.; Ziebolz, D. Association of time under immunosuppression and different immunosuppressive medication on periodontal parameters and selected bacteria of patients after solid organ transplantation. *Med. Oral Patol. Oral Cir. Bucal* **2018**, *23*, e326–e334. [CrossRef] [PubMed]
125. Artese, H.P.; de Sousa, C.O.; Torres, M.C.; Silva-Boghossian, C.M.; Colombo, A.P. Effect of non-surgical periodontal treatment on the subgingival microbiota of patients with chronic kidney disease. *Braz. Oral Res.* **2012**, *26*, 366–372. [CrossRef]
126. Grubbs, V.; Garcia, F.; Jue, B.L.; Vittinghoff, E.; Ryder, M.; Lovett, D.; Carrillo, J.; Offenbacher, S.; Ganz, P.; Bibbins-Domingo, K.; et al. The Kidney and Periodontal Disease (KAPD) study: A pilot randomized controlled trial testing the effect of non-surgical periodontal therapy on chronic kidney disease. *Contemp. Clin. Trials* **2017**, *53*, 143–150. [CrossRef]
127. Yoshioka, M.; Shirayama, Y.; Imoto, I.; Hinode, D.; Yanagisawa, S.; Takeuchi, Y. Current status of collaborative relationships between dialysis facilities and dental facilities in Japan: Results of a nationwide survey. *BMC Nephrol.* **2015**, *16*, 17. [CrossRef]
128. Pejcic, A.; Djordjevic, V.; Kojovic, D.; Zivkovic, V.; Minic, I.; Mirkovic, D.; Stojanovic, M. Effect of periodontal treatment in renal transplant recipients. *Med. Princ. Pract.* **2014**, *23*, 149–153. [CrossRef]
129. Isola, G.; Matarese, M.; Ramaglia, L.; Iorio-Siciliano, V.; Cordasco, G.; Matarese, G. Efficacy of a drug composed of herbal extracts on postoperative discomfort after surgical removal of impacted mandibular third molar: A randomized, triple-blind, controlled clinical trial. *Clin. Oral Investig.* **2019**, *23*, 2443–2453. [CrossRef]
130. Matarese, G.; Ramaglia, L.; Fiorillo, L.; Cervino, G.; Lauritano, F.; Isola, G. Implantology and Periodontal Disease: The Panacea to Problem Solving? *Open Dent. J.* **2017**, *11*, 460–465. [CrossRef]
131. Cury, E.Z.; Santos, V.R.; Maciel, S.D.S.; Gonçalves, T.E.D.; Zimmermann, G.S.; Mota, R.M.S.; Figueiredo, L.C.; Duarte, P.M. Lipid parameters in obese and normal weight patients with or without chronic periodontitis. *Clin. Oral Investig.* **2018**, *22*, 161–167. [CrossRef] [PubMed]
132. Ferlazzo, N.; Currò, M.; Zinellu, A.; Caccamo, D.; Isola, G.; Ventura, V.; Carru, C.; Matarese, G.; Ientile, R. Influence of MTHFR Genetic Background on p16 and MGMT Methylation in Oral Squamous Cell Cancer. *Int. J. Mol. Sci.* **2017**, *18*, 724. [CrossRef] [PubMed]

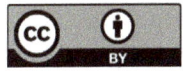

© 2019 by the authors. Licensee MDPI, Basel, Switzerland. This article is an open access article distributed under the terms and conditions of the Creative Commons Attribution (CC BY) license (http://creativecommons.org/licenses/by/4.0/).

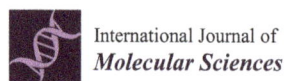

Review

Th17 Cells and the IL-23/IL-17 Axis in the Pathogenesis of Periodontitis and Immune-Mediated Inflammatory Diseases

Kübra Bunte and Thomas Beikler *

Department of Periodontics, Preventive and Restorative Dentistry,
University Medical Centre Hamburg-Eppendorf, 20246 Hamburg, Germany
* Correspondence: t.beikler@uke.de; Tel.: +49-(0)-40-7410-52282; Fax: +49-(0)-40-7410-55168

Received: 23 May 2019; Accepted: 8 July 2019; Published: 10 July 2019

Abstract: Innate immunity represents the semi-specific first line of defense and provides the initial host response to tissue injury, trauma, and pathogens. Innate immunity activates the adaptive immunity, and both act highly regulated together to establish and maintain tissue homeostasis. Any dysregulation of this interaction can result in chronic inflammation and autoimmunity and is thought to be a major underlying cause in the initiation and progression of highly prevalent immune-mediated inflammatory diseases (IMIDs) such as psoriasis, rheumatoid arthritis, inflammatory bowel diseases among others, and periodontitis. Th1 and Th2 cells of the adaptive immune system are the major players in the pathogenesis of IMIDs. In addition, Th17 cells, their key cytokine IL-17, and IL-23 seem to play pivotal roles. This review aims to provide an overview of the current knowledge about the differentiation of Th17 cells and the role of the IL-17/IL-23 axis in the pathogenesis of IMIDs. Moreover, it aims to review the association of these IMIDs with periodontitis and briefly discusses the therapeutic potential of agents that modulate the IL-17/IL-23 axis.

Keywords: periodontitis; psoriasis; rheumatoid arthritis; Crohn's disease; ulcerative colitis; systemic lupus erythematosus; Sjögren syndrome; type 1 diabetes mellitus; cytokines; Th17 cells; interleukin-17; interleukin-23

1. Introduction

Innate immunity represents the semi-specific first line of defense for all primitive and complex multicellular organisms and provides the initial acute inflammatory reaction to tissue injury, trauma, or pathogens [1]. Innate immunity is a rather unspecific and immediate reaction that recruits immune cells to the injury or infection site through various cytokines (e.g., prostaglandins, tumor necrosis factor (TNF), interleukin (IL)-1β, and others). Moreover, it promotes phagocytosis, and activates the complement and adaptive immune system [2]. In contrast to the innate immune system, the activation of the adaptive immune system results in an antigen specific host response that is mediated by T and B cells. It usually requires more time than the innate immune system to react since it turns progenitor cells into regulatory and effector cells with distinct functions, such as (i) self and non-self-antigen recognition, (ii) enhanced elimination of pathogens or infected cells, and (iii) development of immune memory [3].

The innate and adaptive immunity interaction represents a complex system. They are equally required to establish and maintain health and tissue homeostasis and both comprise cellular and humoral immunity components. Humoral immunity refers to antigen-specific antibody production to neutralize toxins and pathogens, mediation of allergic reactions and autoimmunity, generation of immune memory cells, and stimulation of cytokine secretion; whereas, cellular immunity eradicates pathogens by macrophages or natural killer cells, eliminates intracellular bacteria via induction of cytotoxic T-cell-mediated apoptosis, and stimulates tissue cells, such as fibroblasts, to secrete cytokines that further modulate innate and adaptive immune system responses [4]. The inflammation triggered by pathogens, tissue injury, or trauma is typically self-limiting and results in tissue repair and reestablishment of tissue homeostasis following elimination of the cause. However, an alteration of the regular immune response may result in persistence of the acute inflammation, its transition into chronic inflammation, and could even induce autoimmune reactions in susceptible individuals. This altered inflammatory response is believed to be a major underlying cause in the initiation and progression of disorders, such as immune-mediated inflammatory diseases (IMIDs) [5].

IMIDs are the definition of a group of seemingly unrelated diseases that share common inflammatory pathways and are triggered by or result in the dysregulation of innate and adaptive immune system functions [6]. The definitive etiology is still unclear; however, genetic susceptibility and environmental factors such as infection and trauma may initiate these conditions, that include, but are not limited to, psoriasis, rheumatoid arthritis, inflammatory bowel diseases, systemic lupus erythematosus, Sjögren syndrome, and type 1 diabetes [7,8]. Any organ system may be inflicted, and individuals may encounter a considerable reduction in quality of life, significant morbidity, and reduced lifespan [6].

Initiated and perpetuated by a dysbiotic oral microbiome, periodontitis is the most common inflammatory disease of tooth supporting tissues, with a high prevalence of up to 70% among the world's dentate adults [9,10]. The host immune and inflammatory responses disrupted by a dysbiotic microbiome are considered to be the main cause for the initiation, establishment, and progression of periodontal inflammation and tissue breakdown [11]. If left untreated, periodontitis results in progressive periodontal attachment and alveolar bone loss, which subsequently results in tooth loss. Co-existence of an IMID with another systemic inflammatory/autoimmune disease or periodontitis is not uncommon, e.g., 20–30% of patients with psoriasis will eventually develop psoriatic arthritis (PsA) [12]. Although the pathogenesis of IMIDs is not yet entirely understood and elucidated and a causative bidirectional relationship between IMIDs and periodontitis has not been proven yet, the comorbidities indicate the involvement of a dysbalanced inflammatory cytokine network in the disease processes [13–15].

As mentioned before, cytokines and antigen presentation attract and activate adaptive immune system cells. In this regard, CD4$^+$ helper T cells are pivotal players [16]. CD4$^+$ helper T cells differentiate into regulatory and effector T cell subsets i.e., Th1, Th2, Th17, follicular helper T (Tfh) cells, and regulatory T cells (Tregs), following activation. Until the discovery of other cell lineages, Th1 and Th2 were thought to be the only cells differentiating from progenitor CD4$^+$ helper T cells [17]. In this classical Th1/Th2 paradigm, Th1 cells mainly produce interleukin(IL)-2 and interferon gamma (IFN-γ) and are involved in cellular immunity [18]. Th2 cells are mainly responsible for humoral immunity via the activation of B cells, mast cells, and production of immunoglobulin E, and primarily produce IL-4, IL-5, and IL-13 [19]. The first findings that indicated the existence of a novel effector population of CD4$^+$ helper T cells were provided by an animal model of multiple sclerosis (experimental autoimmune encephalitis, EAE) [20]. According to the Th1/Th2 paradigm, it was initially hypothesized that IL-12 and, hence, Th1 cells and IFNγ were playing the central role in this inflammatory disease; however, it was demonstrated that functional Th1 pathways downregulate the onset and progression of EAE in IFNγ- and IL-12-deficient mice [21–23]. Later it was demonstrated that indeed IL-23, and not IL-12, was involved in the EAE pathogenesis [24]. This was further substantiated when the transfer of IL-17 producing T cells to healthy mice was sufficient to induce EAE [25]. In addition, IL-23-deficient animals were shown to be unable to recruit IL-17 producing T cells [26]. These and other studies led to the identification of a novel CD4$^+$ helper T cell subset named T helper 17 (Th17) cell lineage that was characterized by IL-17 production, a cytokine that Th1 and Th2 are not able to produce [17,27].

The Th1/Th2 paradigm provided a framework for understanding the pathogenesis of several conditions, such as psoriasis, rheumatoid arthritis, inflammatory bowel diseases, and periodontitis. However, the identification of Th17 cells as a distinct lineage of CD4$^+$ helper T cells has greatly expanded the understanding of autoimmunity and inflammation and filled in some of the missing gaps in host immunity that could not be fully explained by the Th1/Th2. Although there is still much to be elucidated, this review aims to provide an overview of the current knowledge about the Th17 cell lineage, the role of its key cytokine IL-17, the IL-17/IL-23 axis in health and disease, and strategies that target IL-17 related pathways. Understanding the similar mechanisms that drive the pathogenesis of these diseases will support an interdisciplinary approach between medical doctors and dentists, and thus allow proper screening, prevention, and early treatment.

2. Differentiation and Regulation of Th17 Cells

The polarization of progenitor CD4$^+$ helper T cells involves specific signal transduction mechanisms, distinct transcription factors, and local cytokine profiles for each T helper cell lineage (Figure 1). For instance, the differentiation of IFNγ producing Th1 cells is induced by IL-12 (a heterodimer consisting of a p35 and a p40 subunit) and by activation of the transcription factor STAT4 (Figure 1d) [28]. Also, IFNγ stimulates STAT1 and T-bet (a downstream transcription factor) expression in CD4$^+$ helper T cells, which in turn upregulates Th1 specific gene expression (Figure 1a) [28]. Th2 cell differentiation is, however, mainly driven by IL-4. IL-4 increases STAT6 and GATA-3 expression; thus, upregulates of Th2 differentiation (Figure 1b) [29]. The differentiation of Th1 and Th2 is mutually antagonistic, primarily due to the antagonism of IFNγ and IL-4 on molecular and cellular levels [30].

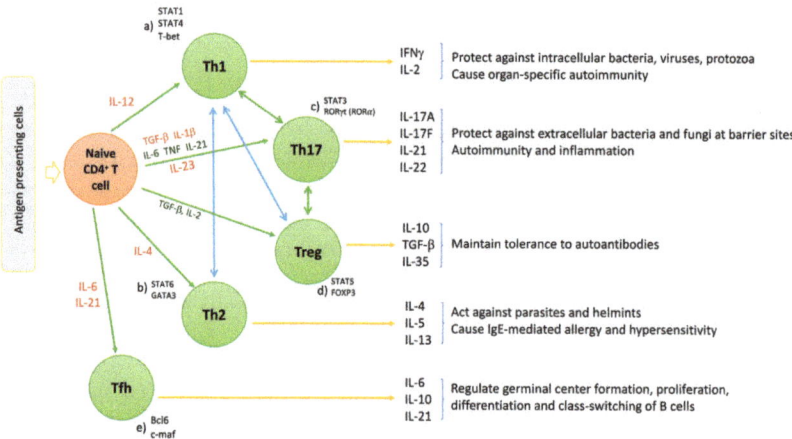

Figure 1. Differentiation of naïve CD4$^+$ cells into Th1, Th2, Th17, regulatory T cells (Treg), and follicular helper T (Tfh) cells. IL-12 leads to Th1-, IL-4 leads to Th2-, TGFβ leads to Treg-differentiation. Th17 cells differentiation is initiated by IL-1β, TGFβ, and further stimulated by TNF, IL-6, and IL-21; Th17 cells are maintained and expanded by IL-23. The transcription factors that governs Th cell subset differentiation are different, (**a**) STAT1, STAT4, and T-bet drive Th1; (**b**) STAT6 and GATA3 drive Th2; (**c**) STAT3 and RORγt (RORα, in the absence of RORγt) manage Th17 cell; (**d**) FOXP3 and STAT5 govern Treg cell differentiation; and (**e**) Bcl6 and c-maf are the regulators of Tfh cells differentiation.

Distinct from the differentiation of Th1 and Th2 cell lineages, Th17 cell differentiation is induced by STAT3 and retinoid acid related-orphan nuclear receptor γt (RORγt) that work synergistically with one another (Figure 1c) [31]. Similar to Th1/Th2 cell interaction, Tregs and Th17 cells are also maintained in an equilibrium. The transcription factor forkhead box P3 (FOXP3) is the negative regulator of RORγt and maintains the tolerance of the organism to self-antigens by inducing the differentiation of Tregs via STAT6 and downregulating differentiation of Th17 cells (Figure 1d) [32]. However, the Treg/Th17 balance is shifted in favor of Th17 in the presence of proinflammatory cytokines. In this regard, transforming growth factor beta (TGFβ) independently initiates the differentiation of Tregs from naïve CD4$^+$ helper T cells by activating FOXP3; whereas, it induces the differentiation of Th17 cells in the presence of IL-6 in mice and IL-1β in humans (Figure 1c,d) [33,34]. Exposure to TGFβ/IL-1β and IL-6 results in inhibition of FOXP3 and activation of RORγt, thus initiating the differentiation cascade of Th17 cells [35]. Furthermore, TNF and IL-1β can synergistically increase IL-6 production and contribute to further Th17 cell differentiation [36]. Following activation, RORγt promotes the expression of IL-17 and IL-23 receptor (IL-23R) [37]. In the absence of RORγt, RORα has been shown to stimulate IL-17 expression [38]. IL-23 is produced by antigen-presenting cells, such as dendritic cells and monocytes/macrophages upon activation and initiates signaling by binding to IL-23R, which in return increases the expression of RORγt and IL-17 via STAT3 (Figures 1c and 2) [39]. However, IL-23 is not able to induce Th17 cell development from naïve CD4+ helper T cells alone by itself, because IL-23R is expressed only after the differentiation of a naïve CD4$^+$ helper T cell into a Th17 cell is initiated [17]. This suggests that the role of IL-23 is rather to be seen in the maintenance, expansion, and survival of Th17 cells than in the initiation of their differentiation. IL-23 is able to maintain and expand Th17 cell populations through a positive feedback loop that upregulates IL-17, RORγt, along with TNF, IL-1β, and IL-6 [40]. In addition, IL-21 was also demonstrated to amplify Th17 cell differentiation in cooperation with TGFβ in an IL-6-independent manner through its feedback function on developing Th17 cells [31,41].

Some other general transcription factors, such as basic leucine zipper transcription factor ATF-like (BATF) and interferon regulatory factor 4 (IRF4), are also involved in the differentiation of naïve CD4+ helper T cells [42,43]. As such, IRF4 deficient mice were shown to have decreased levels of RORγt and increased levels of FOXP3 [44]. These non-nuclear transcription factors are, however, broadly expressed in both health and disease. Therefore, STAT3-induced RORγt is suggested to be the key transcriptional factor involved in Th17 differentiation. This was also supported by the finding that RORγt (*Rorc*$^{-/-}$) deficient CD4+ helper T cells failed to differentiate into Th17 [45].

Th17 cells are typically involved in vigorous proinflammatory responses, yet they also remain in the tissues, such as skin and mucosas as quiescent cells [46]. The inflammatory functions of Th17 cells depends on the different combinations of expressed cytokines in the local environment. For instance, Th17 cells were demonstrated to produce the anti-inflammatory cytokine IL-10 when stimulated with IFNα/β, thus downregulating their pathogenic functions [47]. In contrast to that, IL-23 was shown to reduce the expression levels of IL-10 in developing Th17 cells and induce pro-inflammatory Th17 cells that produce IL-17 [48]. Moreover, different subsets of TGF have also been demonstrated to induce distinct functions in Th17 cells. For instance, TGFβ1-and-IL-6-induced Th17 cells were unable to cause EAE in the absence of IL-23, whereas TGFβ3-induced Th17 cells presented highly pathogenic functions [49]. Moreover, Th-cells, especially Th17 cells, exhibit high phenotypic and functional plasticity, which means that they can transdifferentiate into other T cell subsets in different inflammatory settings [50]. As mentioned, the involvement of IL-6 during early stages of TGFβ-induced Treg differentiation can convert Treg cells into pathogenic Th17 cells [51]. Mature Th17 cells can furthermore be transformed by IL-6 into IFNγ producing Th1 cells [52]. In conclusion, differentiation and regulation of Th17 cells is mediated by a complex cytokine and transcription factor network, which may result in both pathologic and non-pathologic effector functions in inflammatory and autoimmune diseases.

3. Th17/IL-17 in Immunoprotection and Immunopathology

IL-17 is the key cytokine produced by Th17 cells and exerts versatile functions. The IL-17 receptor (IL-17R) lacks a homologous structure to other proteins; therefore, IL-17 cytokines are classified as a distinct family [53]. The IL-17 family consists of six ligands, IL-17A to IL-17F, that share similar structures and can exist as homodimers or form heterodimers, such as IL17A/F. IL-17A and IL-17F (henceforth referred to as IL-17) are produced by Th17 cells. They present 50% of structural homology and their intracellular signal transduction is dependent on the presence of the receptor heterodimer complex formed by the subunits IL-17 receptor A (IL-17RA) and IL-17 receptor C (IL-17RC) [54]. IL-17 receptor is expressed on a broad range of cells, including osteoblasts, endothelial cells, epithelial cells, fibroblast-like synoviocytes, chondrocytes, fibroblasts, keratinocytes, and macrophages (Figure 2) [40,55–57]. Although IL-17 is predominantly produced by Th17 cells, it can also be expressed by natural killer T (NKT) cells, γδ T cells, lymphoid tissue inducer cells, neutrophils, and group 3 innate lymphoid cells (ILC3s) (Figure 2) [58,59]. Moreover, Th17 cells not only produce IL-17, but also IL-21, IL-22, IFNγ, and TNF and can express CCR6, i.e., the receptor of chemokine (C-C motif) ligand 20 (CCL20) that directs IL-17 producing cells to the epithelial barrier sites [60]. IL-17-producing cells accumulate at mucosal surfaces of the oral cavity, gastrointestinal tract, lungs, vagina, and skin epithelium, and regulate protective immunity against extracellular pathogens (especially Gram-negative bacteria and fungi) by maintaining barrier integrity, promoting antimicrobial factors, and activating granulopoiesis [31,59]. Furthermore, the Th17-cytokine IL-22 was shown to contribute to IL-17-induced protective functions by enhancing the production of antimicrobial peptides and recruiting neutrophils [61]. Therefore, the disruption of IL-17 production or signaling can increase the susceptibility to bacterial and fungal infections. In this context, IL-17 receptor deficiency is associated with mortality in mice due to the inability to recruit neutrophils when being infected with *Klebsiella pneumoniae* [62]. Moreover, genetic defects in IL-17 immunity, such as in STAT3 (manifested as hyper-IgE syndrome), result in recurrent and persistent Candida spp. infections; e.g., chronic mucocutaneous candidiasis [63]. Direct IL-17 inhibition with monoclonal antibodies in patients with psoriasis or psoriatic arthritis has been shown to increase the risk of candida infections; similarly, the reactivation of latent tuberculosis infection was observed in patients treated with TNF-inhibitors [64,65]. Th17 cells are also regularly maintained in the gingival tissues, suggesting a protective role in the oral barrier; however, the mechanism that maintains these cells in the tissue is yet to be clarified [66]. Interestingly, IL-17R lacking mice are shown to be more susceptible to *Porphyromonas gingivalis (Pg)*-induced bone loss, suggesting a protective role of IL-17 in bone remodeling and homeostasis [67]. Although IL-17 may exert protective functions, several clinical human studies indicate that excessive production of IL-17 is associated with periodontitis, as well as psoriasis, rheumatoid arthritis, and other IMIDs [52,68].

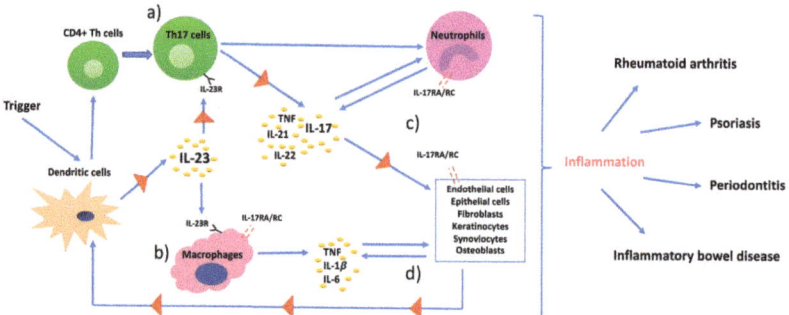

Figure 2. A pathophysiology model of immune-mediated inflammatory diseases. Dendritic cells (DCs) are triggered by a stimulus, such as environmental stress or infection, present the antigen that leads to differentiation of CD4+ helper T cells, and release IL-23. IL-23 stimulates the production of proinflammatory cytokines, such as TNF, IL-1β, and IL-17 from (**a**) Th17 cells, and IL-6 from (**b**) macrophages and DCs. (**c**) IL-17 interacts with IL-17RA/RC complex on receptor carrying cells. These cells further produce inflammatory mediators that regulate functionality of DCs and create a self-sustaining feedback loop via IL-23 (**d**).

IL-17 by itself is a weak inducer of inflammation; its potent inflammatory effects are derived from its synergistic functions with other cytokines and its ability to recruit and maintain inflammatory cells, such as neutrophils. Moreover, IL-17 eases the access of these cells to tissues through regulating the expression of chemokine (C-X-C motif) ligands (CXCL1, CXCL2, CXCL5, CXCL8), CCL20, IL-1β, MMPs, PGE2, and granulocyte- and granulocyte-macrophage colony-stimulating factors (G-CSF and GM-CSF) [51,59]. GM-CSF and G-CSF are the primary regulators of granulopoiesis and neutrophil release from the bone marrow. Its upregulation by IL-17 can lead to excessive activation and mobilization of neutrophils and production of chemokines that increase neutrophil diapedesis, which in return intensifies tissue damage. In addition to that, IL-17 works synergistically with other inflammatory cytokines, such as IL-1β, to increase CCL20 production from human gingival fibroblasts and stimulates further recruitment of Th17 cells; hence, IL-17 production [52]. Typically, neutrophils are found in inflamed periodontal tissues, but infiltration of activated Th17 cells can also be observed in inflamed sites [69,70]. This explains the upregulation of IL-17 in gingival crevicular fluid, bone, and gingiva of periodontitis patients [71–73]. In addition to the locally increased production of IL-17, the serum levels of IL-17 were also detected to be up to nine-fold higher in periodontitis patients compared to healthy controls [74]. Moreover, RORγt encoding gene (*Rorc*) expression levels were reported to be significantly higher in periodontal tissues of patients with periodontitis compared to healthy controls [75]. At last, the presence of T cell populations that can produce IL-17 in both, health and disease, demonstrates the versatile role of this cytokine.

3.1. IL-17 Dependent Processes in Psoriasis and Association with Periodontitis

Characterized by abnormal and rapid keratinocyte differentiation and thickened epidermis, psoriasis is an immune-mediated inflammatory skin disorder that affects 0.1–3% of the general population [76]. Although psoriasis is manifested in 90% of the cases in a skin plaque form called "psoriasis vulgaris", it can also manifest itself in guttate, pustular, and erythrodermic subtypes, as well as in psoriatic arthritis [77,78]. Psoriasis is also associated with other systemic conditions such as hypertension, atherosclerosis, and diabetes [79,80]. The definitive etiology of psoriatic diseases is not clear yet; however, genetic, epigenetic, and environmental factors seem to contribute to the atypical activation of the innate and adaptive immune system resulting in disease onset, progression, and comorbidities [81,82]. Streptococcal peptidoglycan was also suggested to be involved in the pathogenesis of psoriasis; however, whether the skin microbiota is significant as a primary cause or a contributing factor remains to be elucidated [83]. Psoriasis has been primarily considered a Th1-mediated disease, today it is known that the IL-23/IL-17 axis governs the accelerated progress of inflammation [84,85].

Briefly, IL-17 attracts neutrophils to the epidermis of psoriatic skin lesions through neutrophil chemoattractants and recruits additional dendritic cells via upregulation of CCL20 release from keratinocytes (Figure 3a). The dendritic cells release TNF and IL-1β and activate further differentiation of Th17 cells, and thus increased IL-17 production. IL-17 disrupts the integrity of the skin barrier through downregulation of filaggrin and adhesion molecule expression from keratinocytes, and further induces keratinocyte hyperproliferation (Figure 3a) [86]. The disease severity correlates with the numbers of IL-17 producing T cells in psoriatic lesions and their ability to increase keratinocyte proliferation and IL-17 production [87,88]. In addition, IL-22 aggravates psoriasis lesions in synergy with IL-17, although it exerts protective functions in non-psoriatic skin (Figure 3a) [89]. Also, the expression of RORγt, IL-1β, IL-6, and IL-23 was reported to be increased in psoriatic skin lesions compared to the non-psoriatic skin of patients and healthy volunteers; whereas the levels of anti-inflammatory cytokines, i.e., IL-4 and IL-10, were found to be decreased [14,86]. Besides the local changes TNF, IFNγ, IL-2, IL-17, and IL-22 levels were found to be increased in serum of psoriasis patients [14]. Increased levels of TNF, IL-1β, and IL-22 augment the inflammatory effects of IL-17 by enhancing the expression of TNF receptors, suggesting a synergistic interplay between these cytokines in psoriasis pathogenesis [90].

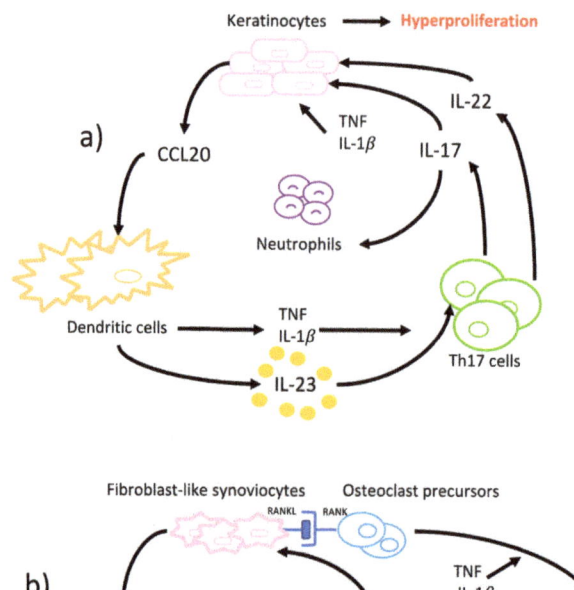
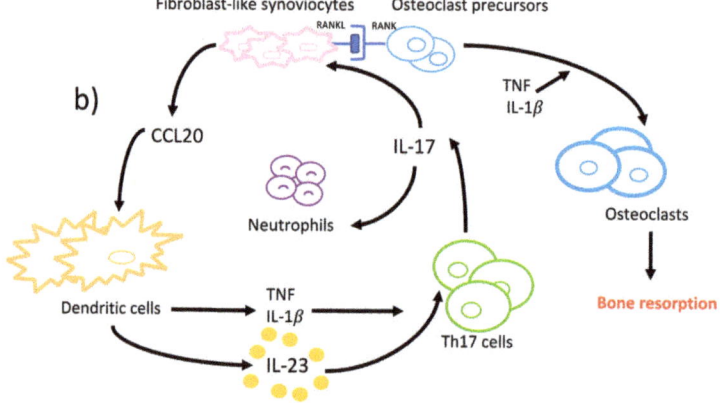

Figure 3. A simplified model of Th17 cells and the cytokines involved in the pathogenesis of (**a**) psoriasis and (**b**) rheumatoid arthritis. This figure can also be interpreted as a model of pathogenesis of gingival, periodontal, and oral mucosal inflammatory diseases, where cells such as gingival fibroblasts, keratinocytes, and epithelial cells are involved.

The role of a dysbiotic skin microbiota is controversially discussed in the pathogenesis of psoriasis. In periodontitis, however, a dysbiotic oral microbiome is known to contribute to the disease onset and progression [11]. Interestingly, it has recently been suggested that IL-17 creates a shift towards a highly pathologic bacterial environment, hence aggravating the periodontal inflammation like a vicious circle [91]. In addition, IL-23-dependent IL-17 production led to bacterial overgrowth, as demonstrated in leukocyte adhesion deficient (LAD) I periodontal phenotype mice and its inhibition reduced the bacterial overgrowth, which linked overexpression of IL-17 to microbial dysbiosis in periodontitis [92]. LAD1 is an immunodeficiency caused by a genetic mutation that results in defective neutrophil adhesion and tissue transmigration and is characterized by recurrent skin infections, oral ulcers, severe periodontal inflammation, and bone loss [93]. Although severe periodontitis in LAD1 was solely attributed to the lack of neutrophil surveillance in gingival and periodontal tissues, recent findings demonstrate that the excessive inflammatory response, mediated by IL-17, contributes to its manifestation [93,94].

Many retrospective and case-control studies have reported an association between psoriatic diseases, mainly psoriasis vulgaris and psoriatic arthritis, and periodontal disease [95–97]. A large

5-year follow-up cohort study indicated that in psoriasis patients (psoriasis subtypes not specified), chronic periodontitis showed an incidence rate of 1.88 per 1000 patient-years compared to 1.22 in the control group [98]. In accordance with these results, a longitudinal cohort study conducted in the Danish population retrospectively screened more than 5 million subjects to assess the risk for the development of periodontitis after the diagnosis of mild and severe psoriasis, and/or psoriatic arthritis [99]. Following adjustment for age, sex, co-morbidities, and smoking, the results demonstrated an increased risk for periodontitis among patients with psoriatic diseases, with the highest risk found in patients with psoriatic arthritis (risk ratio of 1.66, 2.24 and 3.48 for mild psoriasis, severe psoriasis and psoriatic arthritis, respectively). Moreover, the severity of periodontitis has been shown to be correlated with psoriasis severity [100]. Both diseases share common risk factors, i.e., smoking, obesity, and these risk factors can independently contribute to disease manifestation and severity. The risk for periodontitis was increased by six-fold in smoking psoriasis subjects compared to non-smoking psoriasis subjects [101]. Also, a significant correlation between periodontitis and psoriasis was reported after adjustment for smoking [102]. Although none of these studies could demonstrate a bidirectional causal relationship, regular periodontal screening seems to be reasonable in individuals with psoriatic diseases, since the risk for periodontitis is increased, especially in the presence of shared risk factors that negatively influence both diseases.

3.2. IL-17 Dependent Processes in Rheumatoid Arthritis and Association with Periodontitis

Rheumatoid arthritis (RA) is a chronic inflammatory and autoimmune disease of the joints, characterized by the presence of rheumatic factor and anti-citrullinated protein antibodies (ACPAs) and persistent symmetrical and erosive polyarthritis, which results in progressive articular bone and cartilage destruction [103]. The prevalence is 0.5–1% among adults, and women are affected two to three times more frequently than men [55]. The development of rheumatoid arthritis is also considered to be of genetic, epigenetic, and environmental origin [104]. HLA-DR1 and HLA-DR4-positive individuals are reported to be at significantly higher risk for manifesting ACPA-positive RA, although only about 67% of the rheumatoid arthritis patients are ACPA-positive in the early stages [105,106]. Synovitis, the inflammation of the synovial membrane in joints, causes the clinical signs and symptoms of RA. Similar to psoriasis, an interactive and complex network of immune system cells and cytokines are involved in RA pathogenesis. ACPA establishes an abnormal immune response over time that promotes inflammation, and the synovial membrane becomes highly vascularized and infiltrated with fibroblasts, macrophages, T- and B- cells, plasma cells, mast cells, dendritic cells, and neutrophils [107]. Increased TNF in the synovial fluid induces IL-1β production, T- and B-cell activation, and a cascade of inflammatory reactions that is mainly led by dendritic- and Th17-cells, that eventually leads to articular bone and cartilage destruction (Figure 3b) [57]. In the RA-affected synovium, IL-17, IL-1β, and TNF act together to induce the chemotaxis of T cells and immature dendritic cells. This results in an upregulated CCL20 production in synoviocytes and an overall increased concentration of proinflammatory cytokines in the synovial tissues [108]. The role of IL-17 in rheumatoid arthritis was clearly demonstrated when long-term intra-articular administration of IL-17 in mice resulted in rheumatoid arthritis key features like inflammation, articular bone, and cartilage destruction [109]. Furthermore, several animal models of rheumatoid arthritis reported a reduced incidence, severity, and even resistance to disease upon the induction of IL-17 deficiency [110–112].

In addition to the inflammatory effects of IL-17, the osteoclastogenic character of IL-17 puts it in the focus of interest in bone-destructing diseases. The information regarding the effects of IL-17 on bone metabolism mainly originates from studies conducted on rheumatoid arthritis; however, several studies also report its effects on periodontal bone destruction. As mentioned before, dendritic cells that are present in the synovial fluid increase the release of TNF, IL-1β, IL-6, and IL-23 and stimulate Th17-cell differentiation, and thus IL-17 production in rheumatoid arthritis joints [55]. IL-17 disturbs the bone homeostasis by inducing osteoclastogenesis, which results in extensive and rapid bone destruction [113]. This is initiated by the increase of the receptor activator of nuclear factor kappa-B ligand (RANKL) expression on fibroblasts and osteoblasts by IL-17. RANKL interacts with the receptor activator of nuclear factor kappa-B (RANK) on dendritic cells and osteoclasts and activates synovial macrophages to secrete IL-1β and TNF—both are known to induce osteoclastogenesis [114]. Similarly to the mechanism in RA, IL-17 induces RANKL expression by stimulating MMP-1, MMP-3, IL-6, and IL-8 secretion from human gingival fibroblasts and TNF release from macrophages in periodontal tissues [115]. IL-17 levels are shown to be positively correlated to RANKL expression levels in periodontal ligament cells [116,117]. Furthermore, upregulated TNF and IL-17 can synergistically lead to further stimulation of the fibroblasts and epithelial cells to secrete IL-6, IL-8, PGE2, and the neutrophil chemoattractants; thus, intensifying the inflammation [35]. Independently from IL-17, IL-22 was also demonstrated to increase synovial inflammation in rheumatoid arthritis joints and clinical attachment loss in periodontitis patients, similarly to its proinflammatory function in psoriasis [118–120].

The fact that periodontitis is reported to be twice as frequent and severe in rheumatoid arthritis patients compared to healthy controls indicates the correlated inflammatory processes in rheumatoid arthritis and periodontitis [121]. Accordingly, IL-17 levels were found to be increased in the gingival crevicular fluid of rheumatoid arthritis patients, further contributing to the inflammatory response in the gingival sulcus and the severity of periodontal inflammation [121,122]. Several links between rheumatoid arthritis and periodontitis have been suggested. One of the most striking ones is the citrullinated peptides production induced by *P. gingivalis*. Citrullinated peptides are considered to break tolerance and induce ACPA production in RA [123]. *P. gingivalis* is currently the only bacteria that is known to produce peptidyl arginine deiminase (PAD), an enzyme that leads to citrullination of the human and bacterial proteins [124]. In addition, the antibody titer against *P. gingivalis* was significantly increased in RA-patients, further supporting the role of this periodontal pathogen not only in periodontitis, but also in RA pathogenesis [125].

3.3. IL-17 Dependent Processes in Inflammatory Bowel Diseases and Association with Periodontitis

Inflammatory bowel diseases (IBD) are chronic inflammatory conditions of the gastrointestinal system and consist of ulcerative colitis (UC) and Crohn's disease (CD). Ulcerative colitis is characterized by the chronic mucosal inflammation of the colon that manifests itself with abdominal pain, haematochezia, and diarrhoea [126,127]. In Crohn's disease, however, any part of the gastrointestinal tract can be afflicted. This disease can typically be associated with extra-gastrointestinal symptoms such as anaemia, arthritis, skin rashes, oral lesions, and eye inflammations [128,129]. Although the etiology of IBDs remains largely unclear, a dysbiotic intestinal microbiome and risk factors, such as smoking and diet, were suggested to contribute to the disease onset via activation of inflammatory pathways that results in the disruption of the epithelial barrier integrity in genetically susceptible individuals [130]. The involvement of IL-23 and IL-17 in IBD is well documented; however, the different functions of IL-17 in IBD are still controversially discussed in the literature [131,132]. On the one hand, IL-17 deficient or anti-IL-17 treated mice exhibited severe epithelial damage in the colon, indicating a protective function of IL-17 [133]. This is further substantiated when inactivation of IL-17 resulted in a milder course of disease in an animal model of UC [134]. On the other hand, high IL-23 receptor and IL-17 mRNA expression levels were detected in intestinal mucosa samples of patients with active UC and CD [135,136]. Furthermore, many other studies reported increased levels of IL-17 in the intestinal mucosa and serum of active UC and CD patients [137,138].

Oral manifestations and implications of inflammatory bowel diseases are reported in a varying range from 0,5% to 37% among diseased individuals; they may appear as the first signs of the disease, especially in children, and include edema, mucogingivitis, oral ulcers, and hyperplastic lesions among others [139–141]. Involvement of upper regions of gastrointestinal tract and extra-gastrointestinal symptoms predict a more severe phenotype of the disease and may present with comorbidities due to the increased risk of systemic involvement [142]. Caries and periodontitis prevalence are reported to be often higher in individuals with CD and UC [143]. In a large nationwide cohort study, the prevalence of periodontitis was reported to be higher in patients with CD, with a hazard ratio of 1.36 (95% CI

= 1.25–1.48) compared to the control group [144]. Similarly, a meta-analysis of cross-sectional studies, including a total of 1297 subjects, reported a significantly higher prevalence of periodontitis as well as a worse decayed-missing-filled-teeth index in patients with CD and UC compared to non-IBD individuals [145]. Interestingly, worse clinical periodontal parameters were observed among smokers with UC compared to smokers with CD [143]. Unfortunately, studies regarding the effect of periodontal inflammation on CD or UC currently remain deficient [146].

3.4. IL-17 Dependent Processes in Other Immune-Mediated Inflammatory Diseases and Association with Periodontitis

IL-17 also plays an important role in the pathogenesis of other IMIDs, such as Sjögren syndrome, systemic lupus erythematosus, and type 1 diabetes, among others. Sjögren syndrome is an autoimmune disease characterized by diffuse lymphocyte infiltration into exocrine glands that results primarily in xerostomia and ocular dryness, known as "sicca symptoms" [147]. Extra-glandular tissues and organs, such as skin, lungs, nervous system, kidneys, and the gastrointestinal tract are also affected by Sjögren syndrome in at least 30% of patients, classifying it as a systemic disease [148]. Sjögren syndrome can appear independently of other conditions as a primary disease (primary Sjögren syndrome) or manifest itself secondarily as a late complication with sicca symptoms (secondary Sjögren syndrome) in the presence of other systemic conditions, such as rheumatoid arthritis, systemic lupus erythematosus, or scleroderma [149,150]. In Sjögren syndrome affected tissues, several subsets of B and T cells can be identified, predominantly consisting of CD4+ T helper cell subtypes, such as Th1, Th17, and Tfh cells [151]. The interaction between epithelial cells, dendritic cells, and B and T cells results in an increased production of Tfh and Th17 cells, which intensifies the inflammation and increases autoantibody production [152]. Tfh cells govern the ectopic germinal center formation in salivary glands and potentiate the production of autoantibodies from B cells, whereas Th17 cells secrete IL-17 and IL-22 and stimulate inflammation [153,154]. Increased levels of IL-17 in plasma of patients with primary Sjögren syndrome, as well as an abundant presence of IL-1β, TGF-β, IL-6, and IL-23 in tissues affected by the disease, demonstrate the significance of Th17 cells and IL-17 in the disease pathogenesis [155–157]. Non-surgical periodontal therapy was demonstrated to improve the salivary flow rate and decrease the subjective disease activity index in primary Sjögren syndrome patients with periodontitis [158]. However, despite this finding and common IL-17-dependent pathways in periodontitis and Sjögren syndrome, a significant association between both diseases remains to be confirmed [159,160].

Systemic lupus erythematosus (SLE) is a connective-tissue disorder characterized by T cell abnormalities and production of a wide array of autoantibodies directed against double-stranded (ds) DNA. It affects multiple tissues and organs, often causing glomerulonephritis, arthritis, and blood cell abnormalities [161]. The interaction of Th17 cells, Tfh cells, extrafollicular T helper cells (eTfh, a Tfh cell analogue $CD4^+$ subpopulation), Tregs, $CD8^+$ cells, B cell subsets, and innate immune system cells results in a reduced IL-2- and an increased IL-17-production, as well as increased antibody-production from B cells [161–163]. Since IL-17, IL-6, and IL-33 were found to be significantly elevated in the saliva of SLE/periodontitis subjects compared to periodontitis-only subjects, this systemic imbalance of cytokines may have an impact on periodontal tissues [164]. However, the long-term corticosteroid therapy may also have resulted in the observed periodontal damage [164]. In a nation-wide retrospective population-based study, the history of periodontitis was associated with an increased risk of SLE; however, the common risk factors, such as smoking status, were not adjusted [165]. Conversely, periodontal treatment in SLE/periodontitis subjects was reported to significantly improve the responsiveness of SLE patients to the immunosuppressive therapy compared to the control group [166].

The autoimmune destruction of insulin-producing β cells in the Langerhans islets of pancreas results in type 1 diabetes, which is characterized by an insufficient insulin production leading to persistent or recurrent hyperglycemia [167]. Often diagnosed in childhood, type 1 diabetes causes lifelong dependence on insulin, as well as an increased risk of cardiovascular disease, neuropathy, nephropathy, and other autoimmune and inflammatory conditions such as rheumatoid arthritis [168]. CD4$^+$ cells, especially Tregs, and CD8+ cells, autoantibody-producing B cells, and innate immune cells are involved in the disease pathogenesis [167]. IFNγ, produced by the infiltrated T cells, is a major cytokine involved in the destruction of the β cell islets; however, IL-17 was also demonstrated to play a role, when its neutralization prevented further disease development in 10-week old non-obese diabetic mice by reducing peri-islet T cell infiltration [169]. Also, increased secretion and expression of IL-17 and IL-22 were demonstrated to contribute to the disease development in type 1 diabetic children [170]. Impaired IL-2 functions that affect Treg functions lead to increased production of IL-17 and contributes to disease development in an animal model of type 1 diabetes [171]. Uncontrolled diabetes has been proven to be a predisposing risk factor for the onset and progression of periodontitis [172]. Conversely, the presence of periodontitis is suggested to affect the insulin metabolism by increasing the circulatory levels of proinflammatory cytokines [173]. Eventually, the treatment of periodontal disease has been shown to improve glycemic control, further substantiating the existing bidirectional relationship between diabetes and periodontal disease [174].

It is noteworthy to mention that the role of IL-17 has also been demonstrated in other IMIDs, such as ankylosing spondylitis, multiple sclerosis, Behcet disease, or scleroderma, in which aberrant immune and inflammatory responses also result in disease manifestation via similar mechanisms [175–178]. Unfortunately, conflicting data exists on the association of periodontitis and multiple sclerosis. In this regard, a large case control study found that no association between periodontitis and multiple sclerosis was seen between the groups after adjustment of covariates [179]. On the other hand, previous diagnosis of periodontitis was reported to be higher among female multiple sclerosis patients after adjustment of risk factors (odds ratio = 2.08; 95% CI, 1.49–2.95) [180]. In patients with scleroderma and periodontitis, a higher number of missing teeth and more clinical attachment loss were reported compared to patients with periodontitis only [181]. An association between Behcet disease severity and worse periodontal disease parameters (clinical attachment loss, bleeding on probing, and pocket probing depth) was also demonstrated in a cross-sectional study [182].

Based on the multiple interactions between genetic and environmental factors and aberrant immunological responses, multiple associations may exist between immune mediated inflammatory diseases and periodontitis. However, whether these association are causative and mutual needs to be further investigated. The findings of this research will expand the knowledge about the pathogenesis of IMIDs and periodontitis, and may help to improve the prevention, diagnosis, and the treatment of their systemic and oral complications.

4. Th17/IL-17 as Targets in the Management of IMIDs and Its Implications on Periodontal Inflammation

The treatment of immune-mediated inflammatory diseases is traditionally based on the use of glucocorticoids, non-steroidal anti-inflammatory drugs (NSAIDs), and disease-modifying antirheumatic drugs (DMARDs), such as methotrexate (MTX). They are proven to be effective against clinical signs and symptoms and are prescribed as the first-line therapy. However, intolerance, ineffectiveness, and severe adverse effects created the need for developing alternative therapies. Hence, in the early 1990s, monoclonal antibodies (mAbs) and fusion proteins, referred to as biologics or biological agents, were introduced. Biologics are a group of immunosuppressive drugs and are produced from a single clone of plasma B cells by modifying the Fc domain structures of its immunoglobulins. Initially, mAbs were only of murine origin and exhibited a reduced affinity due to the variability of the interaction of murine Fc with human Fc receptors, as well as caused the development of human anti-mouse antibodies [183–185]. To overcome these drawbacks, mAbs are nowadays bioengineered via recombinant techniques to produce chimeric, humanized, and fully human mAbs [186].

Biologics revolutionized the treatment of a wide range of immune-mediated inflammatory diseases, including but not limited to psoriasis, rheumatoid and psoriatic arthritis, ankylosing spondylitis, and inflammatory bowel diseases (Table 1). The first biologics that were introduced in the market were the TNF antagonists (Table 1). TNF antagonists act by inhibiting the binding of TNF to its receptor [186]. There are currently five TNF antagonists available, i.e., etanercept, infliximab, adalimumab, certolizumab, and golimumab. Besides others, TNF antagonists reduce IL-17 controlled inflammatory pathways (Figure 3a,b), and thus, slow down joint destruction in rheumatoid arthritis, reduce psoriatic lesions, as well as resolve chronic intestinal inflammation and ulcerations in IBD [183,187,188]. Etanercept, a TNF receptor-2 and IgG1-Fc fusion protein, reduces infiltration of polymorphonuclear cells into gingival tissues and improves periodontitis parameters in a murine model of experimental periodontitis [189]. In contrast to these anti-inflammatory functions, TNF antagonists interestingly can also cause the appearance of psoriasis-like lesions in 5–10% of treated patients, named as 'paradoxical psoriasis' [129,190]. Paradoxical psoriasis is suggested to be a side effect of all TNF antagonists, irrespective of the type and dosage, and usually disappears upon discontinuation [190,191]. In addition to paradoxical psoriasis, TNF inhibition was reported to increase susceptibility to bacterial infections [192]. The pharmacokinetic and pharmacodynamic properties differ among TNF antagonists as a result of their different molecular structures and mode of administration. Therefore, their effects show a considerable variability among individuals and diseases. Several reports indicate that in case of an ineffective response or intolerance to a specific TNF antagonist, the treatment can be continued with another TNF antagonist or replaced by a different biological drug, such as an IL-17 inhibitor [183,193]. It is noteworthy to mention that periodontitis is associated with an increased risk of etanercept discontinuation with an hazard ratio of 1.27 (95% CI, 1.01–1.60) in anti-TNF-naïve rheumatoid arthritis patients if they have been diagnosed with periodontitis within 5 years prior to or during etanercept treatment [194].

Table 1. Target cytokines involved in IL-17 pathways and approved inhibitors in the management of immune-mediated inflammatory diseases.

Targeted Cytokine	Drug	Indicated Conditions
TNF	Etanercept	Psoriasis, RA, PsA
	Infliximab	Psoriasis, RA, PsA, ankylosing spondylitis (AS), Crohn's disease (CD), ulcerative colitis
	Adalimumab	Psoriasis, RA, PsA, AS, CD, uveitis, hidradenitis suppurativa
	Certolizumab	Psoriasis, RA, PsA, AS, CD,
	Golimumab	RA, PsA, CD, ulcerative colitis, AS
IL-1	Anakinra	RA
IL-6	Tocilizumab	RA
IL-12/23	Ustenikumab	Psoriasis, PsA, CD
IL-23	Guselkumab	Psoriasis
	Tildrakizumab	Psoriasis
IL-17	Secukinumab (IL-17A)	Psoriasis, RA, PsA, CD, asthma, AS, uveitis, multiple sclerosis
	Ixekizumab (IL-17A)	Psoriasis, RA
	Brodalumab (IL-17RA)	Psoriasis, PsA, RA, Crohn's disease, asthma

Due to the synergistic effects of IL-17 and TNF in inflammation, diseases that are treated with TNF antagonists can also be managed with mAbs that target IL-17 or the IL-23/IL-17 axis [195]. Moreover, the inhibition of both TNF and IL-17 was shown to be more effective compared to TNF or IL-17 inhibition alone [196]. The first introduced anti-IL-17 drug was secukinumab, a human IgG1k monoclonal antibody, which acts by binding directly to IL-17A and inhibits its action (Figure 4b). Ixekizumab is a slightly different antibody that is developed from IgG4k, with affinity only to the IL-17A homodimer and IL-17A/F heterodimer of the IL-17 family (Figure 4c). Similarly to secukinumab, ixekizumab inhibits the IL-17 action by binding directly to this cytokine. Brodalumab, a human IgG2k mAb and the first anti-IL-17 receptor agent, inhibits the action of IL-17 by binding to the IL-17 receptor (Figure 4a) [197]. Phase II and III clinical studies proved IL-17 inhibitors as safe and efficient for the treatment of psoriasis, rheumatoid arthritis, and inflammatory bowel disease [198–201]. In psoriasis, however, the efficacy of ixekizumab was shown to be significantly superior when compared to etanercept and ustenikumab (IL-12/23 mAb) [202,203].

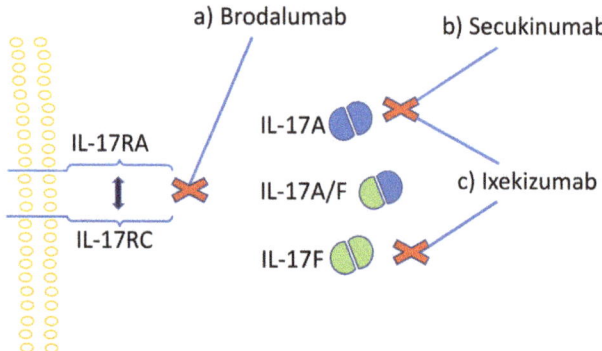

Figure 4. IL-17 cytokine inhibitors; (**a**) brodalumab, with affinity to IL-17RA/RC receptor complex, (**b**) secukinumab, with affinity to IL-17A, and (**c**) ixekizumab, with affinity to both IL-17A and IL-17F, interrupt the intracellular signaling by inhibiting the interaction between IL-17 and its receptor.

Comparative reviews on anti-IL-17 drugs reported that all three drugs were well-tolerated in patients with moderate-to-severe psoriasis; however, adverse effects, such as respiratory tract infections, were reported more frequently for ixekizumab, and it was withdrawn in some cases due to its toxicity [204,205]. A meta-analysis on efficacy of anti-IL-17 drugs on rheumatoid arthritis showed that secukinumab and ixekizumab were more effective compared to placebo; however, an increased risk of infection in the test group has also been reported [206]. Low levels of IL-17 in the synovium, heterogeneity in expression patterns of IL-17 and its receptors were shown to reduce anti-IL-17 drug effect in animal model studies, which could be the explanation to the insufficient efficacy in some patients [207].

Since the maintenance and expansion of Th17 cells are IL-23-dependent, the inhibition of IL-23 can also reduce IL-17 production and accomplish a clinical improvement. Ustekinumab is a human IgG1k monoclonal antibody that binds to the p-40 subunits of both IL-23 and IL-12 and interferes with the binding to their receptors. Long-term, multicenter, placebo-controlled phase III studies demonstrate the safety, efficacy, and superiority of ustekinumab to etanercept in patients with moderate to severe psoriasis [208–210]. However, an increased risk for neoplasia during IL-12/23 inhibitor use was reported in animal studies, which was attributed to IL-12 involvement in tumor surveillance [211,212]. Ustenikumab has also been demonstrated to reduce inflammatory responses in a patient with leukocyte adhesion deficiency type 1 (LAD1) periodontitis without serious adverse effects already after 3 weeks of treatment [213]. In addition to IL-12/IL-23 inhibitors, drugs such as guselkumab and tildrakizumab were developed to target the unique p19 subunit of IL-23 (Figure 1d,e). As expected, Th17-cell infiltration was decreased in psoriasis patients while anti-inflammatory IL-10 expression from Th1-cells was increased following the administration of IL-23 inhibitors [214,215].

As mentioned before, an increased risk of infections, especially by *Candida* spp., is often reported among patients that use these biologics over a prolonged time. Nevertheless, it is noteworthy to mention that overexpression of inflammatory cytokines may also increase infection risk, as periodontal pathogens were suggested to thrive in a highly proinflammatory cytokine environment [59].

5. Conclusions

IL-17 plays an important role in inflammatory events that lead to the manifestation of psoriasis, rheumatoid arthritis, inflammatory bowel disease, and periodontitis. Although much remains to be clarified regarding its protective and pathologic functions, the current knowledge suggests its role as a potent proinflammatory mediator and bridge between innate and adaptive immune responses. Comorbid periodontitis is often observed in patients diagnosed with an immune-mediated inflammatory disease. Although a bidirectional causal relationship is yet to be confirmed, regular screenings, preventive measures, and early treatment could reduce the burden of periodontitis in these patients, and vice versa. Many clinical randomized controlled trials prove the efficacy of cytokine inhibitors that manipulate IL-17 and related pathways in the management of psoriasis, rheumatoid arthritis, and inflammatory bowel disease. Unfortunately, reports regarding the therapeutic effects of cytokine inhibitors on gingival, periodontal, and oral mucocutaneous diseases are scant, which could be due to their restricted indication for severe systemic conditions, high costs, and adverse effects. However, further clinical research on the effects of biologics on gingival, periodontal, and oral tissues is needed to further elucidate the role of Th17-cells and the IL-23/IL-17 axis in the pathogenesis of periodontitis and its potential association with IMIDs.

Author Contributions: Conceptualization and resources, K.B. and T.B.; Investigation, K.B.; Writing—Original Draft Preparation, Review and Editing, K.B.; Writing—Review and Editing, T.B.

Acknowledgments: This research did not receive any specific grant from funding agencies in the public, commercial, or not-for-profit sectors.

Conflicts of Interest: The authors declare no conflict of interest.

References

1. Riera Romo, M.; Perez-Martinez, D.; Castillo Ferrer, C. Innate immunity in vertebrates: An overview. *Immunology* **2016**, *148*, 125–139. [CrossRef] [PubMed]
2. Rubartelli, A.; Lotze, M.T. Inside, outside, upside down: Damage-associated molecular-pattern molecules (DAMPs) and redox. *Trends Immunol.* **2007**, *28*, 429–436. [CrossRef] [PubMed]
3. Janeway, C.A., Jr. How the immune system works to protect the host from infection: A personal view. *Proc. Natl. Acad. Sci. USA* **2001**, *98*, 7461–7468. [CrossRef] [PubMed]
4. Nicholson, L.B. The immune system. *Essays Biochem.* **2016**, *60*, 275–301. [CrossRef] [PubMed]
5. Feghali, C.A.; Wright, T.M. Cytokines in acute and chronic inflammation. *Front. Biosci.* **1997**, *2*, d12–d26. [PubMed]
6. Kuek, A.; Hazleman, B.L.; Ostor, A.J. Immune-mediated inflammatory diseases (IMIDs) and biologic therapy: A medical revolution. *Postgrad. Med. J.* **2007**, *83*, 251–260. [CrossRef] [PubMed]
7. Martin, J.C.; Baeten, D.L.; Josien, R. Emerging role of IL-17 and Th17 cells in systemic lupus erythematosus. *Clin. Immunol.* **2014**, *154*, 1–12. [CrossRef]
8. McGinley, A.M.; Edwards, S.C.; Raverdeau, M.; Mills, K.H.G. Th17cells, gammadelta T cells and their interplay in EAE and multiple sclerosis. *J. Autoimmun.* **2018**, *87*, 97–108. [CrossRef]
9. Beikler, T.; Flemmig, T.F. Oral biofilm-associated diseases: Trends and implications for quality of life, systemic health and expenditures. *Periodontology* **2011**, *55*, 87–103. [CrossRef]
10. Demmer, R.T.; Papapanou, P.N. Epidemiologic patterns of chronic and aggressive periodontitis. *Periodontology* **2010**, *53*, 28–44. [CrossRef]
11. Cekici, A.; Kantarci, A.; Hasturk, H.; Van Dyke, T.E. Inflammatory and immune pathways in the pathogenesis of periodontal disease. *Periodontology* **2014**, *64*, 57–80. [CrossRef] [PubMed]
12. Krueger, J.G.; Bowcock, A. Psoriasis pathophysiology: Current concepts of pathogenesis. *Ann. Rheum. Dis.* **2005**, *64*, ii30–ii36. [CrossRef] [PubMed]
13. Wu, J.J.; Nguyen, T.U.; Poon, K.Y.; Herrinton, L.J. The association of psoriasis with autoimmune diseases. *J. Am. Acad. Derm.* **2012**, *67*, 924–930. [CrossRef] [PubMed]

14. Tan, Y.; Qi, Q.; Lu, C.; Niu, X.; Bai, Y.; Jiang, C.; Wang, Y.; Zhou, Y.; Lu, A.; Xiao, C. Cytokine Imbalance as a Common Mechanism in Both Psoriasis and Rheumatoid Arthritis. *Mediat. Inflamm.* **2017**, *2017*, 2405291. [CrossRef] [PubMed]
15. Thilagar, S.; Theyagarajan, R.; Sudhakar, U.; Suresh, S.; Saketharaman, P.; Ahamed, N. Comparison of serum tumor necrosis factor-alpha levels in rheumatoid arthritis individuals with and without chronic periodontitis: A biochemical study. *J. Indian Soc. Periodontol.* **2018**, *22*, 116–121. [CrossRef]
16. Hirahara, K.; Nakayama, T. CD4+ T-cell subsets in inflammatory diseases: Beyond the Th1/Th2 paradigm. *Int. Immunol.* **2016**, *28*, 163–171. [CrossRef]
17. Zhu, J.; Yamane, H.; Paul, W.E. Differentiation of effector CD4 T cell populations. *Annu. Rev. Immunol.* **2010**, *28*, 445–489. [CrossRef]
18. Romagnani, S. T-cell subsets (Th1 versus Th2). *Ann. Allergy Asthma Immunol.* **2000**, *85*, 9–18. [CrossRef]
19. Romagnani, S. Th1/Th2 cells. *Inflamm. Bowel Dis.* **1999**, *5*, 285–294. [CrossRef]
20. Cua, D.J.; Sherlock, J.; Chen, Y.; Murphy, C.A.; Joyce, B.; Seymour, B.; Lucian, L.; To, W.; Kwan, S.; Churakova, T.; et al. Interleukin-23 rather than interleukin-12 is the critical cytokine for autoimmune inflammation of the brain. *Nature* **2003**, *421*, 744–748. [CrossRef]
21. Chu, C.Q.; Wittmer, S.; Dalton, D.K. Failure to suppress the expansion of the activated CD4 T cell population in interferon gamma-deficient mice leads to exacerbation of experimental autoimmune encephalomyelitis. *J. Exp. Med.* **2000**, *192*, 123–128. [CrossRef] [PubMed]
22. Ferber, I.A.; Brocke, S.; Taylor-Edwards, C.; Ridgway, W.; Dinisco, C.; Steinman, L.; Dalton, D.; Fathman, C.G. Mice with a disrupted IFN-gamma gene are susceptible to the induction of experimental autoimmune encephalomyelitis (EAE). *J. Immunol.* **1996**, *156*, 5–7. [PubMed]
23. Zhang, G.X.; Gran, B.; Yu, S.; Li, J.; Siglienti, I.; Chen, X.; Kamoun, M.; Rostami, A. Induction of experimental autoimmune encephalomyelitis in IL-12 receptor-beta 2-deficient mice: IL-12 responsiveness is not required in the pathogenesis of inflammatory demyelination in the central nervous system. *J. Immunol.* **2003**, *170*, 2153–2160. [CrossRef] [PubMed]
24. Oppmann, B.; Lesley, R.; Blom, B.; Timans, J.C.; Xu, Y.; Hunte, B.; Vega, F.; Yu, N.; Wang, J.; Singh, K.; et al. Novel p19 protein engages IL-12p40 to form a cytokine, IL-23, with biological activities similar as well as distinct from IL-12. *Immunity* **2000**, *13*, 715–725. [CrossRef]
25. Langrish, C.L.; Chen, Y.; Blumenschein, W.M.; Mattson, J.; Basham, B.; Sedgwick, J.D.; McClanahan, T.; Kastelein, R.A.; Cua, D.J. IL-23 drives a pathogenic T cell population that induces autoimmune inflammation. *J. Exp. Med.* **2005**, *201*, 233–240. [CrossRef] [PubMed]
26. Murphy, C.A.; Langrish, C.L.; Chen, Y.; Blumenschein, W.; McClanahan, T.; Kastelein, R.A.; Sedgwick, J.D.; Cua, D.J. Divergent pro- and antiinflammatory roles for IL-23 and IL-12 in joint autoimmune inflammation. *J. Exp. Med.* **2003**, *198*, 1951–1957. [CrossRef] [PubMed]
27. Harrington, L.E.; Hatton, R.D.; Mangan, P.R.; Turner, H.; Murphy, T.L.; Murphy, K.M.; Weaver, C.T. Interleukin 17-producing CD4+ effector T cells develop via a lineage distinct from the T helper type 1 and 2 lineages. *Nat. Immunol.* **2005**, *6*, 1123–1132. [CrossRef]
28. Zhang, Y.; Zhang, Y.; Gu, W.; Sun, B. TH1/TH2 cell differentiation and molecular signals. *Adv. Exp. Med. Biol.* **2014**, *841*, 15–44.
29. Elo, L.L.; Jarvenpaa, H.; Tuomela, S.; Raghav, S.; Ahlfors, H.; Laurila, K.; Gupta, B.; Lund, R.J.; Tahvanainen, J.; Hawkins, R.D.; et al. Genome-wide profiling of interleukin-4 and STAT6 transcription factor regulation of human Th2 cell programming. *Immunity* **2010**, *32*, 852–862. [CrossRef]
30. Gaffen, S.L.; Hajishengallis, G. A new inflammatory cytokine on the block: Re-thinking periodontal disease and the Th1/Th2 paradigm in the context of Th17 cells and IL-17. *J. Dent. Res.* **2008**, *87*, 817–828. [CrossRef]
31. Yang, J.; Sundrud, M.S.; Skepner, J.; Yamagata, T. Targeting Th17 cells in autoimmune diseases. *Trends Pharm. Sci.* **2014**, *35*, 493–500. [CrossRef] [PubMed]
32. Fasching, P.; Stradner, M.; Graninger, W.; Dejaco, C.; Fessler, J. Therapeutic Potential of Targeting the Th17/Treg Axis in Autoimmune Disorders. *Molecules* **2017**, *22*, 134. [CrossRef] [PubMed]
33. Veldhoen, M.; Hocking, R.J.; Atkins, C.J.; Locksley, R.M.; Stockinger, B. TGFbeta in the context of an inflammatory cytokine milieu supports de novo differentiation of IL-17-producing T cells. *Immunity* **2006**, *24*, 179–189. [CrossRef] [PubMed]

34. Ichiyama, K.; Yoshida, H.; Wakabayashi, Y.; Chinen, T.; Saeki, K.; Nakaya, M.; Takaesu, G.; Hori, S.; Yoshimura, A.; Kobayashi, T. Foxp3 inhibits RORgammat-mediated IL-17A mRNA transcription through direct interaction with RORgammat. *J. Biol. Chem.* **2008**, *283*, 17003–17008. [CrossRef] [PubMed]
35. Wang, M.; Tian, T.; Yu, S.; He, N.; Ma, D. Th17 and Treg cells in bone related diseases. *Clin. Dev. Immunol.* **2013**, *2013*, 203705. [CrossRef] [PubMed]
36. Ruddy, M.J.; Wong, G.C.; Liu, X.K.; Yamamoto, H.; Kasayama, S.; Kirkwood, K.L.; Gaffen, S.L. Functional cooperation between interleukin-17 and tumor necrosis factor-alpha is mediated by CCAAT/enhancer-binding protein family members. *J. Biol. Chem.* **2004**, *279*, 2559–2567. [CrossRef] [PubMed]
37. Khan, D.; Ansar Ahmed, S. Regulation of IL-17 in autoimmune diseases by transcriptional factors and microRNAs. *Front. Genet.* **2015**, *6*, 236. [CrossRef] [PubMed]
38. Yang, X.O.; Pappu, B.P.; Nurieva, R.; Akimzhanov, A.; Kang, H.S.; Chung, Y.; Ma, L.; Shah, B.; Panopoulos, A.D.; Schluns, K.S.; et al. T helper 17 lineage differentiation is programmed by orphan nuclear receptors ROR alpha and ROR gamma. *Immunity* **2008**, *28*, 29–39. [CrossRef] [PubMed]
39. Gooderham, M.J.; Papp, K.A.; Lynde, C.W. Shifting the focus—the primary role of IL-23 in psoriasis and other inflammatory disorders. *J. Eur. Acad. Derm. Venereol.* **2018**, *32*, 1111–1119. [CrossRef]
40. Iwakura, Y.; Ishigame, H. The IL-23/IL-17 axis in inflammation. *J. Clin. Investig.* **2006**, *116*, 1218–1222. [CrossRef]
41. Korn, T.; Bettelli, E.; Gao, W.; Awasthi, A.; Jager, A.; Strom, T.B.; Oukka, M.; Kuchroo, V.K. IL-21 initiates an alternative pathway to induce proinflammatory T(H)17 cells. *Nature* **2007**, *448*, 484–487. [CrossRef] [PubMed]
42. Ciofani, M.; Madar, A.; Galan, C.; Sellars, M.; Mace, K.; Pauli, F.; Agarwal, A.; Huang, W.; Parkhurst, C.N.; Muratet, M.; et al. A validated regulatory network for Th17 cell specification. *Cell* **2012**, *151*, 289–303. [CrossRef] [PubMed]
43. Bystrom, J.; Taher, T.E.; Muhyaddin, M.S.; Clanchy, F.I.; Mangat, P.; Jawad, A.S.; Williams, R.O.; Mageed, R.A. Harnessing the Therapeutic Potential of Th17 Cells. *Mediat. Inflamm.* **2015**, *2015*, 205156. [CrossRef] [PubMed]
44. Brustle, A.; Heink, S.; Huber, M.; Rosenplanter, C.; Stadelmann, C.; Yu, P.; Arpaia, E.; Mak, T.W.; Kamradt, T.; Lohoff, M. The development of inflammatory T(H)-17 cells requires interferon-regulatory factor 4. *Nat. Immunol.* **2007**, *8*, 958–966. [CrossRef] [PubMed]
45. Ivanov, I.I.; McKenzie, B.S.; Zhou, L.; Tadokoro, C.E.; Lepelley, A.; Lafaille, J.J.; Cua, D.J.; Littman, D.R. The orphan nuclear receptor RORgammat directs the differentiation program of proinflammatory IL-17+ T helper cells. *Cell* **2006**, *126*, 1121–1133. [CrossRef] [PubMed]
46. Kryczek, I.; Zhao, E.; Liu, Y.; Wang, Y.; Vatan, L.; Szeliga, W.; Moyer, J.; Klimczak, A.; Lange, A.; Zou, W. Human TH17 cells are long-lived effector memory cells. *Sci. Transl. Med.* **2011**, *3*, 104ra100. [CrossRef]
47. Guo, B. IL-10 Modulates Th17 Pathogenicity during Autoimmune Diseases. *J. Clin. Cell. Immunol.* **2016**, 7. [CrossRef]
48. McGeachy, M.J.; Bak-Jensen, K.S.; Chen, Y.; Tato, C.M.; Blumenschein, W.; McClanahan, T.; Cua, D.J. TGF-beta and IL-6 drive the production of IL-17 and IL-10 by T cells and restrain T(H)-17 cell-mediated pathology. *Nat. Immunol.* **2007**, *8*, 1390–1397. [CrossRef]
49. Lee, Y.; Awasthi, A.; Yosef, N.; Quintana, F.J.; Xiao, S.; Peters, A.; Wu, C.; Kleinewietfeld, M.; Kunder, S.; Hafler, D.A.; et al. Induction and molecular signature of pathogenic TH17 cells. *Nat. Immunol.* **2012**, *13*, 991–999. [CrossRef]
50. Hirota, K.; Duarte, J.H.; Veldhoen, M.; Hornsby, E.; Li, Y.; Cua, D.J.; Ahlfors, H.; Wilhelm, C.; Tolaini, M.; Menzel, U.; et al. Fate mapping of IL-17-producing T cells in inflammatory responses. *Nat. Immunol.* **2011**, *12*, 255–263. [CrossRef]
51. Veldhoen, M. Interleukin 17 is a chief orchestrator of immunity. *Nat. Immunol.* **2017**, *18*, 612–621. [CrossRef] [PubMed]
52. Zenobia, C.; Hajishengallis, G. Basic biology and role of interleukin-17 in immunity and inflammation. *Periodontology* **2015**, *69*, 142–159. [CrossRef]
53. Gaffen, S.L. Life before seventeen: Cloning of the IL-17 receptor. *J. Immunol.* **2011**, *187*, 4389–4391. [CrossRef] [PubMed]
54. Pappu, R.; Ramirez-Carrozzi, V.; Sambandam, A. The interleukin-17 cytokine family: Critical players in host defence and inflammatory diseases. *Immunology* **2011**, *134*, 8–16. [CrossRef] [PubMed]

55. Sharif, K.; Sharif, A.; Jumah, F.; Oskouian, R.; Tubbs, R.S. Rheumatoid arthritis in review: Clinical, anatomical, cellular and molecular points of view. *Clin. Anat.* **2018**, *31*, 216–223. [CrossRef] [PubMed]
56. Mitra, A.; Raychaudhuri, S.K.; Raychaudhuri, S.P. IL-17 and IL-17R: An auspicious therapeutic target for psoriatic disease. *Actas Dermosifiliogr.* **2014**, *105*, 21–33. [CrossRef]
57. Ganesan, R.; Rasool, M. Fibroblast-like synoviocytes-dependent effector molecules as a critical mediator for rheumatoid arthritis: Current status and future directions. *Int. Rev. Immunol.* **2017**, *36*, 20–30. [CrossRef]
58. Matsuzaki, G.; Umemura, M. Interleukin-17 family cytokines in protective immunity against infections: Role of hematopoietic cell-derived and non-hematopoietic cell-derived interleukin-17s. *Microbiol. Immunol.* **2018**, *62*, 1–13. [CrossRef]
59. Abusleme, L.; Moutsopoulos, N.M. IL-17: Overview and role in oral immunity and microbiome. *Oral Dis.* **2017**, *23*, 854–865. [CrossRef]
60. Bedoya, S.K.; Lam, B.; Lau, K.; Larkin, J. Th17 cells in immunity and autoimmunity. *Clin. Dev. Immunol.* **2013**, *2013*, 986789. [CrossRef]
61. Valeri, M.; Raffatellu, M. Cytokines IL-17 and IL-22 in the host response to infection. *Pathog. Dis.* **2016**, *74*, ftw111. [CrossRef] [PubMed]
62. Ye, P.; Rodriguez, F.H.; Kanaly, S.; Stocking, K.L.; Schurr, J.; Schwarzenberger, P.; Oliver, P.; Huang, W.; Zhang, P.; Zhang, J.; et al. Requirement of interleukin 17 receptor signaling for lung CXC chemokine and granulocyte colony-stimulating factor expression, neutrophil recruitment, and host defense. *J. Exp. Med.* **2001**, *194*, 519–527. [CrossRef] [PubMed]
63. Ling, Y.; Puel, A. IL-17 and infections. *Actas Dermosifiliogr.* **2014**, *105*, 34–40. [CrossRef]
64. Saunte, D.M.; Mrowietz, U.; Puig, L.; Zachariae, C. Candida infections in patients with psoriasis and psoriatic arthritis treated with interleukin-17 inhibitors and their practical management. *Br. J. Derm.* **2017**, *177*, 47–62. [CrossRef] [PubMed]
65. Souto, A.; Maneiro, J.R.; Salgado, E.; Carmona, L.; Gomez-Reino, J.J. Risk of tuberculosis in patients with chronic immune-mediated inflammatory diseases treated with biologics and tofacitinib: A systematic review and meta-analysis of randomized controlled trials and long-term extension studies. *Rheumatology* **2014**, *53*, 1872–1885. [CrossRef] [PubMed]
66. Dutzan, N.; Abusleme, L.; Bridgeman, H.; Greenwell-Wild, T.; Zangerle-Murray, T.; Fife, M.E.; Bouladoux, N.; Linley, H.; Brenchley, L.; Wemyss, K.; et al. On-going Mechanical Damage from Mastication Drives Homeostatic Th17 Cell Responses at the Oral Barrier. *Immunity* **2017**, *46*, 133–147. [CrossRef] [PubMed]
67. Yu, J.J.; Ruddy, M.J.; Wong, G.C.; Sfintescu, C.; Baker, P.J.; Smith, J.B.; Evans, R.T.; Gaffen, S.L. An essential role for IL-17 in preventing pathogen-initiated bone destruction: Recruitment of neutrophils to inflamed bone requires IL-17 receptor-dependent signals. *Blood* **2007**, *109*, 3794–3802. [CrossRef]
68. Awang, R.A.; Lappin, D.F.; MacPherson, A.; Riggio, M.; Robertson, D.; Hodge, P.; Ramage, G.; Culshaw, S.; Preshaw, P.M.; Taylor, J.; et al. Clinical associations between IL-17 family cytokines and periodontitis and potential differential roles for IL-17A and IL-17E in periodontal immunity. *Inflamm. Res.* **2014**, *63*, 1001–1012. [CrossRef]
69. Ito, H.; Honda, T.; Domon, H.; Oda, T.; Okui, T.; Amanuma, R.; Nakajima, T.; Yamazaki, K. Gene expression analysis of the CD4+ T-cell clones derived from gingival tissues of periodontitis patients. *Oral Microbiol Immunol.* **2005**, *20*, 382–386. [CrossRef]
70. Cheng, W.C.; Hughes, F.J.; Taams, L.S. The presence, function and regulation of IL-17 and Th17 cells in periodontitis. *J. Clin. Periodontol.* **2014**, *41*, 541–549. [CrossRef]
71. Cardoso, C.R.; Garlet, G.P.; Crippa, G.E.; Rosa, A.L.; Junior, W.M.; Rossi, M.A.; Silva, J.S. Evidence of the presence of T helper type 17 cells in chronic lesions of human periodontal disease. *Oral Microbiol. Immunol.* **2009**, *24*, 1–6. [CrossRef] [PubMed]
72. Vernal, R.; Dutzan, N.; Chaparro, A.; Puente, J.; Antonieta Valenzuela, M.; Gamonal, J. Levels of interleukin-17 in gingival crevicular fluid and in supernatants of cellular cultures of gingival tissue from patients with chronic periodontitis. *J. Clin. Periodontol.* **2005**, *32*, 383–389. [CrossRef] [PubMed]
73. Adibrad, M.; Deyhimi, P.; Ganjalikhani Hakemi, M.; Behfarnia, P.; Shahabuei, M.; Rafiee, L. Signs of the presence of Th17 cells in chronic periodontal disease. *J. Periodontal Res.* **2012**, *47*, 525–531. [CrossRef] [PubMed]
74. Schenkein, H.A.; Koertge, T.E.; Brooks, C.N.; Sabatini, R.; Purkall, D.E.; Tew, J.G. IL-17 in sera from patients with aggressive periodontitis. *J. Dent. Res.* **2010**, *89*, 943–947. [CrossRef] [PubMed]

75. Behfarnia, P.; Birang, R.; Pishva, S.S.; Hakemi, M.G.; Khorasani, M.M. Expression levels of th-2 and th-17 characteristic genes in healthy tissue versus periodontitis. *J. Dent.* **2013**, *10*, 23–31.
76. Furue, K.; Ito, T.; Tsuji, G.; Kadono, T.; Nakahara, T.; Furue, M. Autoimmunity and autoimmune co-morbidities in psoriasis. *Immunology* **2018**, *154*, 21–27. [CrossRef]
77. Raychaudhuri, S.K.; Maverakis, E.; Raychaudhuri, S.P. Diagnosis and classification of psoriasis. *Autoimmun. Rev.* **2014**, *13*, 490–495. [CrossRef]
78. Boehncke, W.H.; Schon, M.P. Psoriasis. *Lancet* **2015**, *386*, 983–994. [CrossRef]
79. Takeshita, J.; Grewal, S.; Langan, S.M.; Mehta, N.N.; Ogdie, A.; Van Voorhees, A.S.; Gelfand, J.M. Psoriasis and comorbid diseases: Epidemiology. *J. Am. Acad. Derm.* **2017**, *76*, 377–390. [CrossRef]
80. Stuart, P.E.; Nair, R.P.; Tsoi, L.C.; Tejasvi, T.; Das, S.; Kang, H.M.; Ellinghaus, E.; Chandran, V.; Callis-Duffin, K.; Ike, R.; et al. Genome-wide association analysis of psoriatic arthritis and cutaneous psoriasis reveals differences in their genetic architecture. *Am. J. Hum. Genet.* **2015**, *97*, 816–836. [CrossRef]
81. Gudjonsson, J.E.; Krueger, G. A role for epigenetics in psoriasis: Methylated Cytosine-Guanine sites differentiate lesional from nonlesional skin and from normal skin. *J. Investig. Derm.* **2012**, *132*, 506–508. [CrossRef] [PubMed]
82. Nibali, L.; Henderson, B.; Sadiq, S.T.; Donos, N. Genetic dysbiosis: The role of microbial insults in chronic inflammatory diseases. *J. Oral Microbiol.* **2014**, *6*, 22962. [CrossRef]
83. Fry, L.; Baker, B.S.; Powles, A.V.; Engstrand, L. Psoriasis is not an autoimmune disease? *Exp. Derm.* **2015**, *24*, 241–244. [CrossRef] [PubMed]
84. Mease, P.J. Inhibition of interleukin-17, interleukin-23 and the TH17 cell pathway in the treatment of psoriatic arthritis and psoriasis. *Curr. Opin. Rheumatol.* **2015**, *27*, 127–133. [CrossRef] [PubMed]
85. Chhabra, S.; Narang, T.; Joshi, N.; Goel, S.; Sawatkar, G.; Saikia, B.; Dogra, S.; Bansal, F.; Minz, R. Circulating T-helper 17 cells and associated cytokines in psoriasis. *Clin. Exp. Derm.* **2016**, *41*, 806–810. [CrossRef] [PubMed]
86. Raychaudhuri, S.K.; Saxena, A.; Raychaudhuri, S.P. Role of IL-17 in the pathogenesis of psoriatic arthritis and axial spondyloarthritis. *Clin. Rheumatol.* **2015**, *34*, 1019–1023. [CrossRef] [PubMed]
87. Di Cesare, A.; Di Meglio, P.; Nestle, F.O. The IL-23/Th17 axis in the immunopathogenesis of psoriasis. *J. Investig. Derm.* **2009**, *129*, 1339–1350. [CrossRef] [PubMed]
88. Grine, L.; Dejager, L.; Libert, C.; Vandenbroucke, R.E. An inflammatory triangle in psoriasis: TNF, type I IFNs and IL-17. *Cytokine Growth Factor Rev.* **2015**, *26*, 25–33. [CrossRef]
89. Ekman, A.K.; Bivik Eding, C.; Rundquist, I.; Enerback, C. IL-17 and IL-22 promote keratinocyte stemness in the germinative compartment in psoriasis. *J. Investig. Derm.* **2019**, *139*, 1564–1573. [CrossRef]
90. Chabaud, M.; Fossiez, F.; Taupin, J.L.; Miossec, P. Enhancing effect of IL-17 on IL-1-induced IL-6 and leukemia inhibitory factor production by rheumatoid arthritis synoviocytes and its regulation by Th2 cytokines. *J. Immunol.* **1998**, *161*, 409–414.
91. Graves, D.T.; Correa, J.D.; Silva, T.A. The Oral Microbiota Is Modified by Systemic Diseases. *J. Dent. Res.* **2019**, *98*, 148–156. [CrossRef] [PubMed]
92. Hajishengallis, G.; Moutsopoulos, N.M. Role of bacteria in leukocyte adhesion deficiency-associated periodontitis. *Microb. Pathog.* **2016**, *94*, 21–26. [CrossRef] [PubMed]
93. Moutsopoulos, N.M.; Konkel, J.; Sarmadi, M.; Eskan, M.A.; Wild, T.; Dutzan, N.; Abusleme, L.; Zenobia, C.; Hosur, K.B.; Abe, T.; et al. Defective neutrophil recruitment in leukocyte adhesion deficiency type I disease causes local IL-17-driven inflammatory bone loss. *Sci. Transl. Med.* **2014**, *6*, 229ra40. [CrossRef] [PubMed]
94. Hajishengallis, G.; Moutsopoulos, N.M. Etiology of leukocyte adhesion deficiency-associated periodontitis revisited: Not a raging infection but a raging inflammatory response. *Expert Rev. Clin. Immunol.* **2014**, *10*, 973–975. [CrossRef] [PubMed]
95. Su, N.Y.; Huang, J.Y.; Hu, C.J.; Yu, H.C.; Chang, Y.C. Increased risk of periodontitis in patients with psoriatic disease: A nationwide population-based retrospective cohort study. *PeerJ* **2017**, *5*, e4064.
96. Mendes, V.S.; Cota, L.O.M.; Costa, A.A.; Oliveira, A.; Costa, F.O. Periodontitis as another comorbidity associated with psoriasis: A case-control study. *J. Periodontol.* **2018**, *90*, 358–366. [CrossRef] [PubMed]
97. Lazaridou, E.; Tsikrikoni, A.; Fotiadou, C.; Kyrmanidou, E.; Vakirlis, E.; Giannopoulou, C.; Apalla, Z.; Ioannides, D. Association of chronic plaque psoriasis and severe periodontitis: A hospital based case-control study. *J. Eur. Acad. Derm. Venereol.* **2013**, *27*, 967–972. [CrossRef]

98. Keller, J.J.; Lin, H.C. The effects of chronic periodontitis and its treatment on the subsequent risk of psoriasis. *Br. J. Derm.* **2012**, *167*, 1338–1344. [CrossRef]
99. Egeberg, A.; Mallbris, L.; Gislason, G.; Hansen, P.R.; Mrowietz, U. Risk of periodontitis in patients with psoriasis and psoriatic arthritis. *J. Eur. Acad. Derm. Venereol.* **2017**, *31*, 288–293. [CrossRef]
100. Sharma, A.; Raman, A.; Pradeep, A.R. Association of chronic periodontitis and psoriasis: Periodontal status with severity of psoriasis. *Oral Dis.* **2015**, *21*, 314–319. [CrossRef]
101. Gheorghita, D.; Antal, M.A.; Nagy, K.; Kertesz, A.; Braunitzer, G. Smoking and Psoriasis as Synergistic Risk Factors in Periodontal disease. *Fogorv. Szle.* **2016**, *109*, 119–124.
102. Antal, M.; Braunitzer, G.; Mattheos, N.; Gyulai, R.; Nagy, K. Smoking as a permissive factor of periodontal disease in psoriasis. *PloS ONE* **2014**, *9*, e92333. [CrossRef] [PubMed]
103. Hueber, W.; Tomooka, B.H.; Zhao, X.; Kidd, B.A.; Drijfhout, J.W.; Fries, J.F.; van Venrooij, W.J.; Metzger, A.L.; Genovese, M.C.; Robinson, W.H. Proteomic analysis of secreted proteins in early rheumatoid arthritis: Anti-citrulline autoreactivity is associated with up regulation of proinflammatory cytokines. *Ann. Rheum. Dis.* **2007**, *66*, 712–719. [CrossRef] [PubMed]
104. Viatte, S.; Plant, D.; Raychaudhuri, S. Genetics and epigenetics of rheumatoid arthritis. *Nat. Rev. Rheumatol.* **2013**, *9*, 141–153. [CrossRef] [PubMed]
105. Guo, Q.; Wang, Y.; Xu, D.; Nossent, J.; Pavlos, N.J.; Xu, J. Rheumatoid arthritis: Pathological mechanisms and modern pharmacologic therapies. *Bone Res.* **2018**, *6*, 15. [CrossRef] [PubMed]
106. Veale, D.J.; Orr, C.; Fearon, U. Cellular and molecular perspectives in rheumatoid arthritis. *Semin. Immunopathol.* **2017**, *39*, 343–354. [CrossRef] [PubMed]
107. Firestein, G.S.; McInnes, I.B. Immunopathogenesis of Rheumatoid Arthritis. *Immunity* **2017**, *46*, 183–196. [CrossRef]
108. Hirota, K.; Yoshitomi, H.; Hashimoto, M.; Maeda, S.; Teradaira, S.; Sugimoto, N.; Yamaguchi, T.; Nomura, T.; Ito, H.; Nakamura, T.; et al. Preferential recruitment of CCR6-expressing Th17 cells to inflamed joints via CCL20 in rheumatoid arthritis and its animal model. *J. Exp. Med.* **2007**, *204*, 2803–2812. [CrossRef]
109. Lubberts, E.; Joosten, L.A.; van de Loo, F.A.; Schwarzenberger, P.; Kolls, J.; van den Berg, W.B. Overexpression of IL-17 in the knee joint of collagen type II immunized mice promotes collagen arthritis and aggravates joint destruction. *Inflamm. Res.* **2002**, *51*, 102–104. [CrossRef]
110. Nakae, S.; Nambu, A.; Sudo, K.; Iwakura, Y. Suppression of immune induction of collagen-induced arthritis in IL-17-deficient mice. *J. Immunol.* **2003**, *171*, 6173–6177. [CrossRef]
111. Hirota, K.; Hashimoto, M.; Yoshitomi, H.; Tanaka, S.; Nomura, T.; Yamaguchi, T.; Iwakura, Y.; Sakaguchi, N.; Sakaguchi, S. T cell self-reactivity forms a cytokine milieu for spontaneous development of IL-17+ Th cells that cause autoimmune arthritis. *J. Exp. Med.* **2007**, *204*, 41–47. [CrossRef] [PubMed]
112. Jaller Char, J.J.; Jaller, J.A.; Waibel, J.S.; Bhanusali, D.G.; Bhanusali, N. The Role of IL-17 in the Human Immune System and Its Blockage as a Treatment of Rheumatoid Arthritis, Ankylosing Spondylitis, and Psoriatic Arthritis. *J. Drugs Derm.* **2018**, *17*, 539–542.
113. Sato, K.; Suematsu, A.; Okamoto, K.; Yamaguchi, A.; Morishita, Y.; Kadono, Y.; Tanaka, S.; Kodama, T.; Akira, S.; Iwakura, Y.; et al. Th17 functions as an osteoclastogenic helper T cell subset that links T cell activation and bone destruction. *J. Exp. Med.* **2006**, *203*, 2673–2682. [CrossRef] [PubMed]
114. Kurebayashi, Y.; Nagai, S.; Ikejiri, A.; Koyasu, S. Recent advances in understanding the molecular mechanisms of the development and function of Th17 cells. *Genes Cells* **2013**, *18*, 247–265. [CrossRef] [PubMed]
115. Beklen, A.; Ainola, M.; Hukkanen, M.; Gurgan, C.; Sorsa, T.; Konttinen, Y.T. MMPs, IL-1, and TNF are regulated by IL-17 in periodontitis. *J. Dent. Res.* **2007**, *86*, 347–351. [CrossRef] [PubMed]
116. Dutzan, N.; Gamonal, J.; Silva, A.; Sanz, M.; Vernal, R. Over-expression of forkhead box P3 and its association with receptor activator of nuclear factor-kappa B ligand, interleukin (IL)-17, IL-10 and transforming growth factor-beta during the progression of chronic periodontitis. *J. Clin. Periodontol.* **2009**, *36*, 396–403. [CrossRef] [PubMed]
117. Lin, D.; Li, L.; Sun, Y.; Wang, W.; Wang, X.; Ye, Y.; Chen, X.; Xu, Y. IL-17 regulates the expressions of RANKL and OPG in human periodontal ligament cells via TRAF6/TBK1-JNK/NF-kappaB pathways. *Immunology* **2014**, *3*, 472–485.
118. Van Hamburg, J.P.; Corneth, O.B.; Paulissen, S.M.; Davelaar, N.; Asmawidjaja, P.S.; Mus, A.M.; Lubberts, E. IL-17/Th17 mediated synovial inflammation is IL-22 independent. *Ann. Rheum. Dis.* **2013**, *72*, 1700–1707. [CrossRef]

119. Miyazaki, Y.; Nakayamada, S.; Kubo, S.; Nakano, K.; Iwata, S.; Miyagawa, I.; Ma, X.; Trimova, G.; Sakata, K.; Tanaka, Y. Th22 Cells Promote Osteoclast Differentiation via Production of IL-22 in Rheumatoid Arthritis. *Front. Immunol.* **2018**, *9*, 2901. [CrossRef]
120. Diaz-Zuniga, J.; Melgar-Rodriguez, S.; Rojas, L.; Alvarez, C.; Monasterio, G.; Carvajal, P.; Vernal, R. Increased levels of the T-helper 22-associated cytokine (interleukin-22) and transcription factor (aryl hydrocarbon receptor) in patients with periodontitis are associated with osteoclast resorptive activity and severity of the disease. *J. Periodontal Res.* **2017**, *52*, 893–902.
121. De Pablo, P.; Dietrich, T.; McAlindon, T.E. Association of periodontal disease and tooth loss with rheumatoid arthritis in the US population. *J. Rheumatol.* **2008**, *35*, 70–76. [PubMed]
122. Gumus, P.; Buduneli, E.; Biyikoglu, B.; Aksu, K.; Sarac, F.; Nile, C.; Lappin, D.; Buduneli, N. Gingival crevicular fluid, serum levels of receptor activator of nuclear factor-kappaB ligand, osteoprotegerin, and interleukin-17 in patients with rheumatoid arthritis and osteoporosis and with periodontal disease. *J. Periodontol.* **2013**, *84*, 1627–1637. [PubMed]
123. Correa, M.G.; Sacchetti, S.B.; Ribeiro, F.V.; Pimentel, S.P.; Casarin, R.C.; Cirano, F.R.; Casati, M.Z. Periodontitis increases rheumatic factor serum levels and citrullinated proteins in gingival tissues and alter cytokine balance in arthritic rats. *PLoS ONE* **2017**, *12*, e0174442. [CrossRef] [PubMed]
124. Arunachalam, L.T. Autoimmune correlation of rheumatoid arthritis and periodontitis. *J. Indian Soc. Periodontol.* **2014**, *18*, 666–669. [CrossRef] [PubMed]
125. Mikuls, T.R.; Payne, J.B.; Reinhardt, R.A.; Thiele, G.M.; Maziarz, E.; Cannella, A.C.; Holers, V.M.; Kuhn, K.A.; O'Dell, J.R. Antibody responses to Porphyromonas gingivalis (P. gingivalis) in subjects with rheumatoid arthritis and periodontitis. *Int. Immunopharmacol.* **2009**, *9*, 38–42. [CrossRef] [PubMed]
126. Ordas, I.; Eckmann, L.; Talamini, M.; Baumgart, D.C.; Sandborn, W.J. Ulcerative colitis. *Lancet* **2012**, *380*, 1606–1619. [CrossRef]
127. Adams, S.M.; Bornemann, P.H. Ulcerative colitis. *Am. Fam. Physician* **2013**, *87*, 699–705.
128. Baumgart, D.C.; Sandborn, W.J. Crohn's disease. *Lancet* **2012**, *380*, 1590–1605. [CrossRef]
129. Iida, T.; Hida, T.; Matsuura, M.; Uhara, H.; Nakase, H. Current clinical issue of skin lesions in patients with inflammatory bowel disease. *Clin. J. Gastroenterol.* **2019**, *5*, 1–10. [CrossRef]
130. Zhang, Y.Z.; Li, Y.Y. Inflammatory bowel disease: Pathogenesis. *World J. Gastroenterol.* **2014**, *20*, 91–99. [CrossRef]
131. Siakavellas, S.I.; Bamias, G. Role of the IL-23/IL-17 axis in Crohn's disease. *Discov. Med.* **2012**, *14*, 253–262. [PubMed]
132. Kobayashi, T.; Okamoto, S.; Hisamatsu, T.; Kamada, N.; Chinen, H.; Saito, R.; Kitazume, M.T.; Nakazawa, A.; Sugita, A.; Koganei, K.; et al. IL23 differentially regulates the Th1/Th17 balance in ulcerative colitis and Crohn's disease. *Gut* **2008**, *57*, 1682–1689. [CrossRef]
133. Ogawa, A.; Andoh, A.; Araki, Y.; Bamba, T.; Fujiyama, Y. Neutralization of interleukin-17 aggravates dextran sulfate sodium-induced colitis in mice. *Clin. Immunol.* **2004**, *110*, 55–62. [CrossRef] [PubMed]
134. Ito, R.; Kita, M.; Shin-Ya, M.; Kishida, T.; Urano, A.; Takada, R.; Sakagami, J.; Imanishi, J.; Iwakura, Y.; Okanoue, T.; et al. Involvement of IL-17A in the pathogenesis of DSS-induced colitis in mice. *Biochem. Biophys. Res. Commun.* **2008**, *377*, 12–16. [CrossRef] [PubMed]
135. Sugihara, T.; Kobori, A.; Imaeda, H.; Tsujikawa, T.; Amagase, K.; Takeuchi, K.; Fujiyama, Y.; Andoh, A. The increased mucosal mRNA expressions of complement C3 and interleukin-17 in inflammatory bowel disease. *Clin. Exp. Immunol.* **2010**, *160*, 386–393. [CrossRef] [PubMed]
136. Song, L.; Zhou, R.; Huang, S.; Zhou, F.; Xu, S.; Wang, W.; Yi, F.; Wang, X.; Xia, B. High intestinal and systemic levels of interleukin-23/T-helper 17 pathway in Chinese patients with inflammatory bowel disease. *Mediat. Inflamm.* **2013**, *2013*, 425915. [CrossRef] [PubMed]
137. Fujino, S.; Andoh, A.; Bamba, S.; Ogawa, A.; Hata, K.; Araki, Y.; Bamba, T.; Fujiyama, Y. Increased expression of interleukin 17 in inflammatory bowel disease. *Gut* **2003**, *52*, 65–70. [CrossRef] [PubMed]
138. Seiderer, J.; Elben, I.; Diegelmann, J.; Glas, J.; Stallhofer, J.; Tillack, C.; Pfennig, S.; Jurgens, M.; Schmechel, S.; Konrad, A.; et al. Role of the novel Th17 cytokine IL-17F in inflammatory bowel disease (IBD): Upregulated colonic IL-17F expression in active Crohn's disease and analysis of the IL17F p.His161Arg polymorphism in IBD. *Inflamm. Bowel Dis.* **2008**, *14*, 437–445. [CrossRef]
139. Chi, A.C.; Neville, B.W.; Krayer, J.W.; Gonsalves, W.C. Oral manifestations of systemic disease. *Am. Fam. Physician* **2010**, *82*, 1381–1388.

140. Eckel, A.; Lee, D.; Deutsch, G.; Maxin, A.; Oda, D. Oral manifestations as the first presenting sign of Crohn's disease in a pediatric patient. *J. Clin. Exp. Dent.* **2017**, *9*, e934–e938. [CrossRef]
141. Tan, C.X.; Brand, H.S.; de Boer, N.K.; Forouzanfar, T. Gastrointestinal diseases and their oro-dental manifestations: Part 1: Crohn's disease. *Br. Dent. J.* **2016**, *221*, 794–799. [CrossRef] [PubMed]
142. Feuerstein, J.D.; Cheifetz, A.S. Crohn Disease: epidemiology, diagnosis, and management. *Mayo Clin. Proc.* **2017**, *92*, 1088–1103. [CrossRef] [PubMed]
143. Brito, F.; de Barros, F.C.; Zaltman, C.; Carvalho, A.T.; Carneiro, A.J.; Fischer, R.G.; Gustafsson, A.; Figueredo, C.M. Prevalence of periodontitis and DMFT index in patients with Crohn's disease and ulcerative colitis. *J. Clin. Periodontol.* **2008**, *35*, 555–560. [CrossRef] [PubMed]
144. Chi, Y.C.; Chen, J.L.; Wang, L.H.; Chang, K.; Wu, C.L.; Lin, S.Y.; Keller, J.J.; Bai, C.H. Increased risk of periodontitis among patients with Crohn's disease: A population-based matched-cohort study. *Int. J. Colorectal Dis.* **2018**, *33*, 1437–1444. [CrossRef] [PubMed]
145. Papageorgiou, S.N.; Hagner, M.; Nogueira, A.V.; Franke, A.; Jager, A.; Deschner, J. Inflammatory bowel disease and oral health: Systematic review and a meta-analysis. *J. Clin. Periodontol.* **2017**, *44*, 382–393. [CrossRef] [PubMed]
146. Lira-Junior, R.; Figueredo, C.M. Periodontal and inflammatory bowel diseases: Is there evidence of complex pathogenic interactions? *World J. Gastroenterol.* **2016**, *22*, 7963–7972. [CrossRef] [PubMed]
147. Fox, R.I. Sjogren's syndrome. *Lancet* **2005**, *366*, 321–331. [CrossRef]
148. Brito-Zeron, P.; Ramos-Casals, M. Advances in the understanding and treatment of systemic complications in Sjogren's syndrome. *Curr. Opin. Rheumatol.* **2014**, *26*, 520–527. [CrossRef] [PubMed]
149. Carsons, S.E.; Patel, B.C. Sjogren Syndrome. In *StatPearls*; StatPearls Publishing LLC.: Treasure Island, FL, USA, 2019.
150. Bowman, S.J. Primary Sjogren's syndrome. *Lupus* **2018**, *27*, 32–35. [CrossRef] [PubMed]
151. Saito, M.; Otsuka, K.; Ushio, A.; Yamada, A.; Arakaki, R.; Kudo, Y.; Ishimaru, N. Unique Phenotypes and Functions of Follicular Helper T Cells and Regulatory T Cells in Sjogren's Syndrome. *Curr. Rheumatol. Rev.* **2018**, *14*, 239–245. [CrossRef] [PubMed]
152. Hillen, M.R.; Ververs, F.A.; Kruize, A.A.; Van Roon, J.A. Dendritic cells, T-cells and epithelial cells: A crucial interplay in immunopathology of primary Sjogren's syndrome. *Expert Rev. Clin. Immunol.* **2014**, *10*, 521–531. [CrossRef] [PubMed]
153. Matsui, K.; Sano, H. T Helper 17 Cells in Primary Sjogren's Syndrome. *J. Clin. Med.* **2017**, *65*. [CrossRef] [PubMed]
154. Weinstein, J.S.; Herman, E.I.; Lainez, B.; Licona-Limon, P.; Esplugues, E.; Flavell, R.; Craft, J. TFH cells progressively differentiate to regulate the germinal center response. *Nat. Immunol.* **2016**, *17*, 1197–1205. [CrossRef] [PubMed]
155. Katsifis, G.E.; Rekka, S.; Moutsopoulos, N.M.; Pillemer, S.; Wahl, S.M. Systemic and local interleukin-17 and linked cytokines associated with Sjogren's syndrome immunopathogenesis. *Am. J. Pathol.* **2009**, *175*, 1167–1177. [CrossRef] [PubMed]
156. Kwok, S.K.; Cho, M.L.; Her, Y.M.; Oh, H.J.; Park, M.K.; Lee, S.Y.; Woo, Y.J.; Ju, J.H.; Park, K.S.; Kim, H.Y.; et al. TLR2 ligation induces the production of IL-23/IL-17 via IL-6, STAT3 and NF-kB pathway in patients with primary Sjogren's syndrome. *Arthritis Res.* **2012**, *14*, R64. [CrossRef] [PubMed]
157. Pollard, R.P.; Abdulahad, W.H.; Bootsma, H.; Meiners, P.M.; Spijkervet, F.K.; Huitema, M.G.; Burgerhof, J.G.; Vissink, A.; Kroese, F.G. Predominantly proinflammatory cytokines decrease after B cell depletion therapy in patients with primary Sjogren's syndrome. *Ann. Rheum. Dis.* **2013**, *72*, 2048–2050. [CrossRef] [PubMed]
158. Ambrosio, L.M.; Rovai, E.S.; Franca, B.N.; Balzarini, D.A.; Abreu, I.S.; Lopes, S.B.; Nunes, T.B.; Lourenco, S.V.; Pasoto, S.G.; Saraiva, L.; et al. Effects of periodontal treatment on primary sjogren's syndrome symptoms. *Braz. Oral Res.* **2017**, *31*, e8. [CrossRef]
159. Lugonja, B.; Yeo, L.; Milward, M.R.; Smith, D.; Dietrich, T.; Chapple, I.L.; Rauz, S.; Williams, G.P.; Barone, F.; de Pablo, P.; et al. Periodontitis prevalence and serum antibody reactivity to periodontal bacteria in primary Sjogren's syndrome: A pilot study. *J. Clin. Periodontol.* **2016**, *43*, 26–33. [CrossRef]
160. De Goes Soares, L.; Rocha, R.L.; Bagordakis, E.; Galvao, E.L.; Douglas-de-Oliveira, D.W.; Falci, S.G.M. Relationship between sjogren syndrome and periodontal status: A systematic review. *Oral Surg. Oral Med. Oral Pathol. Oral Radiol.* **2018**, *125*, 223–231. [CrossRef]

161. Koga, T.; Ichinose, K.; Tsokos, G.C. T cells and IL-17 in lupus nephritis. *Clin. Immunol.* **2017**, *185*, 95–99. [CrossRef]
162. Kluger, M.A.; Nosko, A.; Ramcke, T.; Goerke, B.; Meyer, M.C.; Wegscheid, C.; Luig, M.; Tiegs, G.; Stahl, R.A.; Steinmetz, O.M. RORgammat expression in Tregs promotes systemic lupus erythematosus via IL-17 secretion, alteration of Treg phenotype and suppression of Th2 responses. *Clin. Exp. Immunol.* **2017**, *188*, 63–78. [CrossRef] [PubMed]
163. Moulton, V.R.; Suarez-Fueyo, A.; Meidan, E.; Li, H.; Mizui, M.; Tsokos, G.C. Pathogenesis of Human Systemic Lupus Erythematosus: A Cellular Perspective. *Trends Mol. Med.* **2017**, *23*, 615–635. [CrossRef] [PubMed]
164. Mendonca, S.M.S.; Correa, J.D.; Souza, A.F.; Travassos, D.V.; Calderaro, D.C.; Rocha, N.P.; Vieira, E.L.M.; Teixeira, A.L.; Ferreira, G.A.; Silva, T.A. Immunological signatures in saliva of systemic lupus erythematosus patients: Influence of periodontal condition. *Clin. Exp. Rheumatol.* **2019**, *37*, 208–214. [PubMed]
165. Wu, Y.D.; Lin, C.H.; Chao, W.C.; Liao, T.L.; Chen, D.Y.; Chen, H.H. Association between a history of periodontitis and the risk of systemic lupus erythematosus in Taiwan: A nationwide, population-based, case-control study. *PLoS ONE* **2017**, *12*, e0187075. [CrossRef] [PubMed]
166. Fabbri, C.; Fuller, R.; Bonfa, E.; Guedes, L.K.; D'Alleva, P.S.; Borba, E.F. Periodontitis treatment improves systemic lupus erythematosus response to immunosuppressive therapy. *Clin. Rheumatol.* **2014**, *33*, 505–509. [CrossRef] [PubMed]
167. Bluestone, J.A.; Herold, K.; Eisenbarth, G. Genetics, pathogenesis and clinical interventions in type 1 diabetes. *Nature* **2010**, *464*, 1293–1300. [CrossRef]
168. Wu, Y.L.; Ding, Y.P.; Gao, J.; Tanaka, Y.; Zhang, W. Risk factors and primary prevention trials for type 1 diabetes. *Int. J. Biol. Sci.* **2013**, *9*, 666–679. [CrossRef]
169. Emamaullee, J.A.; Davis, J.; Merani, S.; Toso, C.; Elliott, J.F.; Thiesen, A.; Shapiro, A.M. Inhibition of Th17 cells regulates autoimmune diabetes in NOD mice. *Diabetes* **2009**, *58*, 1302–1311. [CrossRef]
170. Honkanen, J.; Nieminen, J.K.; Gao, R.; Luopajarvi, K.; Salo, H.M.; Ilonen, J.; Knip, M.; Otonkoski, T.; Vaarala, O. IL-17 immunity in human type 1 diabetes. *J. Immunol.* **2010**, *185*, 1959–1967. [CrossRef]
171. Marwaha, A.K.; Panagiotopoulos, C.; Biggs, C.M.; Staiger, S.; Del Bel, K.L.; Hirschfeld, A.F.; Priatel, J.J.; Turvey, S.E.; Tan, R. Pre-diagnostic genotyping identifies T1D subjects with impaired Treg IL-2 signaling and an elevated proportion of FOXP3(+)IL-17(+) cells. *Genes Immun.* **2017**, *18*, 15–21. [CrossRef]
172. Novotna, M.; Podzimek, S.; Broukal, Z.; Lencova, E.; Duskova, J. Periodontal Diseases and Dental Caries in Children with Type 1 Diabetes Mellitus. *Mediat. Inflamm.* **2015**, *2015*, 379626. [CrossRef] [PubMed]
173. Preshaw, P.M.; Alba, A.L.; Herrera, D.; Jepsen, S.; Konstantinidis, A.; Makrilakis, K.; Taylor, R. Periodontitis and diabetes: A two-way relationship. *Diabetologia* **2012**, *55*, 21–31. [CrossRef] [PubMed]
174. Simpson, T.C.; Weldon, J.C.; Worthington, H.V.; Needleman, I.; Wild, S.H.; Moles, D.R.; Stevenson, B.; Furness, S.; Iheozor-Ejiofor, Z. Treatment of periodontal disease for glycaemic control in people with diabetes mellitus. *Cochrane Database Syst. Rev.* **2015**, *11*, Cd004714. [CrossRef] [PubMed]
175. Emmi, G.; Silvestri, E.; Bella, C.D.; Grassi, A.; Benagiano, M.; Cianchi, F.; Squatrito, D.; Cantarini, L.; Emmi, L.; Selmi, C.; et al. Cytotoxic Th1 and Th17 cells infiltrate the intestinal mucosa of Behcet patients and exhibit high levels of TNF-alpha in early phases of the disease. *Medicine* **2016**, *95*, e5516. [CrossRef] [PubMed]
176. Lei, L.; Zhao, C.; Qin, F.; He, Z.Y.; Wang, X.; Zhong, X.N. Th17 cells and IL-17 promote the skin and lung inflammation and fibrosis process in a bleomycin-induced murine model of systemic sclerosis. *Clin. Exp. Rheumatol.* **2016**, *34*, 14–22. [PubMed]
177. Jethwa, H.; Bowness, P. The interleukin (IL)-23/IL-17 axis in ankylosing spondylitis: New advances and potentials for treatment. *Clin. Exp. Immunol.* **2016**, *183*, 30–36. [CrossRef] [PubMed]
178. Li, Y.F.; Zhang, S.X.; Ma, X.W.; Xue, Y.L.; Gao, C.; Li, X.Y. Levels of peripheral Th17 cells and serum Th17-related cytokines in patients with multiple sclerosis: A meta-analysis. *Mult. Scler. Relat. Disord.* **2017**, *18*, 20–25. [CrossRef]
179. Gustavsen, M.W.; Celius, E.G.; Moen, S.M.; Bjolgerud, A.; Berg-Hansen, P.; Nygaard, G.O.; Sandvik, L.; Lie, B.A.; Harbo, H.F. No association between multiple sclerosis and periodontitis after adjusting for smoking habits. *Eur. J. Neurol.* **2015**, *22*, 588–590. [CrossRef]
180. Sheu, J.J.; Lin, H.C. Association between multiple sclerosis and chronic periodontitis: A population-based pilot study. *Eur. J. Neurol.* **2013**, *20*, 1053–1059. [CrossRef]

181. Isola, G.; Williams, R.C.; Lo Gullo, A.; Ramaglia, L.; Matarese, M.; Iorio-Siciliano, V.; Cosio, C.; Matarese, G. Risk association between scleroderma disease characteristics, periodontitis, and tooth loss. *Clin. Rheumatol.* **2017**, *36*, 2733–2741. [CrossRef]
182. Habibagahi, Z.; Khorshidi, H.; Hekmati, S. Periodontal health status among patients with Behcet's Disease. *Scientifica* **2016**, *2016*, 7506041. [CrossRef] [PubMed]
183. Ma, X.; Xu, S. TNF inhibitor therapy for rheumatoid arthritis. *Biomed. Rep.* **2013**, *1*, 177–184. [CrossRef] [PubMed]
184. Kalden, J.R.; Schulze-Koops, H. Immunogenicity and loss of response to TNF inhibitors: Implications for rheumatoid arthritis treatment. *Nat. Rev. Rheumatol.* **2017**, *13*, 707–718. [CrossRef] [PubMed]
185. Nissim, A.; Chernajovsky, Y. Historical development of monoclonal antibody therapeutics. *Handb. Exp. Pharmacol.* **2008**, *181*, 3–18.
186. Breedveld, F.C. Therapeutic monoclonal antibodies. *Lancet* **2000**, *355*, 735–740. [CrossRef]
187. Levin, A.D.; Wildenberg, M.E.; van den Brink, G.R. Mechanism of Action of Anti-TNF Therapy in Inflammatory Bowel Disease. *J. Crohn's Colitis* **2016**, *10*, 989–997. [CrossRef] [PubMed]
188. Yost, J.; Gudjonsson, J.E. The role of TNF inhibitors in psoriasis therapy: New implications for associated comorbidities. *F1000 Med. Rep.* **2009**, *1*. [CrossRef]
189. Di Paola, R.; Mazzon, E.; Muia, C.; Crisafulli, C.; Terrana, D.; Greco, S.; Britti, D.; Santori, D.; Oteri, G.; Cordasco, G.; et al. Effects of etanercept, a tumour necrosis factor-alpha antagonist, in an experimental model of periodontitis in rats. *Br. J. Pharmacol.* **2007**, *150*, 286–297. [CrossRef]
190. Mylonas, A.; Conrad, C. Psoriasis: Classical vs. Paradoxical. The Yin-Yang of TNF and Type I Interferon. *Front. Immunol.* **2018**, *9*, 2746. [CrossRef]
191. Brown, G.; Wang, E.; Leon, A.; Huynh, M.; Wehner, M.; Matro, R.; Linos, E.; Liao, W.; Haemel, A. Tumor necrosis factor-alpha inhibitor-induced psoriasis: Systematic review of clinical features, histopathological findings, and management experience. *J. Am. Acad. Derm.* **2017**, *76*, 334–341. [CrossRef]
192. Segaert, S.; Hermans, C. Clinical Signs, Pathophysiology and Management of Cutaneous Side Effects of Anti-Tumor Necrosis Factor Agents. *Am. J. Clin. Dermatol.* **2017**, *18*, 771–787. [CrossRef] [PubMed]
193. Blanco, F.J.; Moricke, R.; Dokoupilova, E.; Codding, C.; Neal, J.; Andersson, M.; Rohrer, S.; Richards, H. Secukinumab in Active Rheumatoid Arthritis: A Phase III Randomized, Double-Blind, Active Comparator- and Placebo-Controlled Study. *Arthritis Rheumatol.* **2017**, *69*, 1144–1153. [CrossRef] [PubMed]
194. Chen, H.H.; Chen, D.Y.; Lai, K.L.; Chen, Y.M.; Chou, Y.J.; Chou, P.; Lin, C.H.; Huang, N. Periodontitis and etanercept discontinuation risk in anti-tumor necrosis factor-naive rheumatoid arthritis patients: A nationwide population-based cohort study. *J. Clin. Rheumatol.* **2013**, *19*, 432–438. [CrossRef] [PubMed]
195. Miossec, P. Diseases that may benefit from manipulating the Th17 pathway. *Eur. J. Immunol.* **2009**, *39*, 667–669. [CrossRef] [PubMed]
196. Alzabin, S.; Abraham, S.M.; Taher, T.E.; Palfreeman, A.; Hull, D.; McNamee, K.; Jawad, A.; Pathan, E.; Kinderlerer, A.; Taylor, P.C.; et al. Incomplete response of inflammatory arthritis to TNFalpha blockade is associated with the Th17 pathway. *Ann. Rheum. Dis.* **2012**, *71*, 1741–1748. [CrossRef]
197. Beck, K.M.; Koo, J. Brodalumab for the treatment of plaque psoriasis: Up-to-date. *Expert Opin. Biol. Ther.* **2019**, *19*, 287–292. [CrossRef]
198. Genovese, M.C.; Durez, P.; Richards, H.B.; Supronik, J.; Dokoupilova, E.; Mazurov, V.; Aelion, J.A.; Lee, S.H.; Codding, C.E.; Kellner, H.; et al. Efficacy and safety of secukinumab in patients with rheumatoid arthritis: A phase II, dose-finding, double-blind, randomised, placebo controlled study. *Ann. Rheum. Dis.* **2013**, *72*, 863–869. [CrossRef]
199. Genovese, M.C.; Braun, D.K.; Erickson, J.S.; Berclaz, P.Y.; Banerjee, S.; Heffernan, M.P.; Carlier, H. Safety and Efficacy of Open-label Subcutaneous Ixekizumab Treatment for 48 Weeks in a Phase II Study in Biologic-naive and TNF-IR Patients with Rheumatoid Arthritis. *J. Rheumatol.* **2016**, *43*, 289–297. [CrossRef]
200. Leonardi, C.; Matheson, R.; Zachariae, C.; Cameron, G.; Li, L.; Edson-Heredia, E.; Braun, D.; Banerjee, S. Anti-interleukin-17 monoclonal antibody ixekizumab in chronic plaque psoriasis. *N. Engl. J. Med.* **2012**, *366*, 1190–1199. [CrossRef]
201. Hueber, W.; Patel, D.D.; Dryja, T.; Wright, A.M.; Koroleva, I.; Bruin, G.; Antoni, C.; Draelos, Z.; Gold, M.H.; Durez, P.; et al. Effects of AIN457, a fully human antibody to interleukin-17A, on psoriasis, rheumatoid arthritis, and uveitis. *Sci. Transl. Med.* **2010**, *2*, 52ra72. [CrossRef]

202. Shelton, S.K.; Bai, S.R.; Jordan, J.K.; Sheehan, A.H. Ixekizumab: A Review of Its Use for the Management of Moderate to Severe Plaque Psoriasis. *Ann. Pharmacother.* **2019**, *53*, 276–284. [CrossRef] [PubMed]
203. Blauvelt, A.; Lomaga, M.; Burge, R.; Zhu, B.; Shen, W.; Shrom, D.; Dossenbach, M.; Pinter, A. Greater Cumulative Benefits from Ixekizumab versus Ustekinumab Treatment over 52 Weeks for Patients with Moderate-to-Severe Psoriasis in a Randomized, Double-Blinded Phase 3b Clinical Trial. *J. Dermatol. Treat.* **2019**, 1–21. [CrossRef] [PubMed]
204. Amin, M.; Darji, K.; No, D.J.; Bhutani, T.; Wu, J.J. Review of IL-17 inhibitors for psoriasis. *J. Dermatol. Treat.* **2017**, 1–6. [CrossRef] [PubMed]
205. Bilal, J.; Berlinberg, A.; Bhattacharjee, S.; Trost, J.; Riaz, I.B.; Kurtzman, D.J.B. A systematic review and meta-analysis of the efficacy and safety of the interleukin (IL)-12/23 and IL-17 inhibitors ustekinumab, secukinumab, ixekizumab, brodalumab, guselkumab and tildrakizumab for the treatment of moderate to severe plaque psoriasis. *J. Dermatol. Treat.* **2018**, *29*, 569–578. [CrossRef] [PubMed]
206. Kunwar, S.; Dahal, K.; Sharma, S. Anti-IL-17 therapy in treatment of rheumatoid arthritis: A systematic literature review and meta-analysis of randomized controlled trials. *Rheumatol. Int.* **2016**, *36*, 1065–1075. [CrossRef] [PubMed]
207. Van Baarsen, L.G.; Lebre, M.C.; van der Coelen, D.; Aarrass, S.; Tang, M.W.; Ramwadhdoebe, T.H.; Gerlag, D.M.; Tak, P.P. Heterogeneous expression pattern of interleukin 17A (IL-17A), IL-17F and their receptors in synovium of rheumatoid arthritis, psoriatic arthritis and osteoarthritis: Possible explanation for nonresponse to anti-IL-17 therapy? *Arthritis Res. Ther.* **2014**, *16*, 426. [CrossRef] [PubMed]
208. Griffiths, C.E.; Strober, B.E.; van de Kerkhof, P.; Ho, V.; Fidelus-Gort, R.; Yeilding, N.; Guzzo, C.; Xia, Y.; Zhou, B.; Li, S.; et al. Comparison of ustekinumab and etanercept for moderate-to-severe psoriasis. *N. Engl. J. Med.* **2010**, *362*, 118–128. [CrossRef] [PubMed]
209. Leonardi, C.L.; Kimball, A.B.; Papp, K.A.; Yeilding, N.; Guzzo, C.; Wang, Y.; Li, S.; Dooley, L.T.; Gordon, K.B. Efficacy and safety of ustekinumab, a human interleukin-12/23 monoclonal antibody, in patients with psoriasis: 76-week results from a randomised, double-blind, placebo-controlled trial (PHOENIX 1). *Lancet* **2008**, *371*, 1665–1674. [CrossRef]
210. Papp, K.A.; Langley, R.G.; Lebwohl, M.; Krueger, G.G.; Szapary, P.; Yeilding, N.; Guzzo, C.; Hsu, M.C.; Wang, Y.; Li, S.; et al. Efficacy and safety of ustekinumab, a human interleukin-12/23 monoclonal antibody, in patients with psoriasis: 52-week results from a randomised, double-blind, placebo-controlled trial (PHOENIX 2). *Lancet* **2008**, *371*, 1675–1684. [CrossRef]
211. Ghosh, S.; Gensler, L.S.; Yang, Z.; Gasink, C.; Chakravarty, S.D.; Farahi, K.; Ramachandran, P.; Ott, E.; Strober, B.E. Ustekinumab Safety in Psoriasis, Psoriatic Arthritis, and Crohn's Disease: An Integrated Analysis of Phase II/III Clinical Development Programs. *Drug Saf.* **2019**, *42*, 751–768. [CrossRef]
212. Ustekinumab: New drug. Suspicion of carcinogenicity: Too great a risk for psoriasis patients. *Prescrire Int.* **2009**, *18*, 202–204.
213. Moutsopoulos, N.M.; Zerbe, C.S.; Wild, T.; Dutzan, N.; Brenchley, L.; DiPasquale, G.; Uzel, G.; Axelrod, K.C.; Lisco, A.; Notarangelo, L.D.; et al. Interleukin-12 and Interleukin-23 Blockade in Leukocyte Adhesion Deficiency Type 1. *N. Engl. J. Med.* **2017**, *376*, 1141–1146. [CrossRef] [PubMed]
214. Machado, A.; Torres, T. Guselkumab for the Treatment of Psoriasis. *Biodrugs Clin. Immunother. Biopharm. Gene Ther.* **2018**, *32*, 119–128. [CrossRef] [PubMed]
215. Kolli, S.S.; Gabros, S.D.; Pona, A.; Cline, A.; Feldman, S.R. Tildrakizumab: A Review of Phase II and III Clinical Trials. *Ann. Pharmacother.* **2019**, *53*, 413–418. [CrossRef] [PubMed]

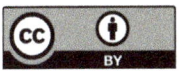

© 2019 by the authors. Licensee MDPI, Basel, Switzerland. This article is an open access article distributed under the terms and conditions of the Creative Commons Attribution (CC BY) license (http://creativecommons.org/licenses/by/4.0/).

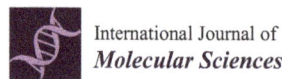

Review

The Association of Periodontitis and Peripheral Arterial Occlusive Disease—A Systematic Review

Mark Kaschwich [1,2,*], Christian-Alexander Behrendt [1], Guido Heydecke [3], Andreas Bayer [2], Eike Sebastian Debus [1], Udo Seedorf [3] and Ghazal Aarabi [3]

1   Department of Vascular Medicine, University Heart Center Hamburg, University Medical Center Hamburg-Eppendorf, 20251 Hamburg, Germany; ch.behrendt@uke.de (C.-A.B.); s.debus@uke.de (E.S.D.)
2   Department of Surgery, University Medical Centre Schleswig-Holstein, Campus Luebeck, Ratzeburger Allee 160, 23538 Luebeck, Germany; andreas.bayer@uksh.de
3   Department of Prosthetic Dentistry, Center for Dental and Oral Medicine, University Medical Center Hamburg-Eppendorf, 20246 Hamburg, Germany; g.heydecke@uke.de (G.H.); u.seedorf@uke.de (U.S.); g.aarabi@uke.de (G.A.)
*   Correspondence: mark.kaschwich@uksh.de; Tel.: +49 451-500-50874; Fax: +49 451-500-40924

Received: 6 May 2019; Accepted: 12 June 2019; Published: 15 June 2019

Abstract: Background: Observational studies support an association between periodontitis (PD) and atherosclerotic vascular disease, but little is known specifically about peripheral arterial occlusive disease (PAOD). Objectives: To systematically review the evidence for an association between PD and PAOD. Data Sources: Medline via PubMed. Review Methods: We searched the Pubmed database for original studies, case reports, case series, meta-analyses and systematic reviews that assessed whether there is an association between PD (all degrees of severity) and PAOD (all degrees of severity). The reporting of this systematic review was in accordance with the Preferred Reporting Items for Systematic Reviews and Meta-Analyses (PRISMA) statement following the Population, Intervention, Control, and Outcome (PICO) format. Results: 17 out of 755 detected studies were included in the qualitative synthesis. Nine studies demonstrated associations between PD and PAOD, and two studies reported associations between tooth loss and PAOD. Six studies addressed the pathomechanism regarding PD as a possible trigger for PAOD. No study that dismissed an association could be detected. Odds ratios or hazard ratios ranged from 1.3 to 3.9 in four large cohort studies after adjusting for established cardiovascular risk factors. Conclusions: The presented evidence supports a link between PD and PAOD. Further studies which address the temporality of PD and PAOD and randomized controlled intervention trials examining the causal impact of PD on PAOD are needed. Although our results cannot confirm a causal role of PD in the development of PAOD, it is likely that PD is associated with PAOD and plays a contributing role.

Keywords: oral disease; periodontitis; PD; peripheral arterial occlusive disease; PAOD; systematic review

1. Introduction

As a consequence of demographic changes and the proliferation of the western lifestyle, peripheral arterial occlusive disease (PAOD) has developed into a widespread disease with globally over 200 million persons affected [1–3]. PAOD preferably effects the peripheral limb vessels of the lower extremity. It limits a person's ability to walk, may require revascularization, or worse yet, can result in the loss of a limb. But it is not simply a disease of the legs. PAOD is one of multiple clinical manifestations of atherosclerotic vascular disease. It is a clinical manifestation of a systemic disease, that is frequently associated with ischemic heart disease, stroke, abdominal aortic aneurysms, and other serious health issues [4]. In addition to its clinical aspects that limit the patient's quality of life, it has a profound cost impact on the healthcare system [5].

Despite the benefit of modern medicine, to date, there is no curative treatment available, and all non-invasive or invasive approaches aim to address the symptoms or disease progression. Hence, screening and prevention programs have gained more attention to identify new PAOD risk factors. It is well known that PAOD is associated with tobacco use, diabetes, high cholesterol, and higher age [3]. With respect to prevention of PAOD, the identification of additional risk factors is of high clinical importance.

Nowadays, there is scientific consensus that the development of PAOD is also associated with chronic subclinical inflammation [6–8]. The inflammatory genesis has been demonstrated to be multifactorial, and there is evidence that local inflammatory processes can spread systemically and trigger inflammation of the vessel wall [9]. One inflammatory focus in humans is the oral cavity, and it was proposed that chronic oral inflammations, e.g., periodontitis (PD) and caries, lead to degradation of the tooth-supporting structures [8] and may, in concert with other established risk factors, be able to trigger PAOD. PD is caused by the outgrowth of oral microorganisms, which induce a destructive host inflammatory response that contributes to progressive periodontal tissue destruction and loss of the alveolar bone around the teeth, resulting in gingival pocket formation and clinical attachment loss and, if untreated, tooth loss [10]. Tailored options are available for periodontitis treatment at various stages [11]. Approximately 47% of adults aged ≥30 years in the United States have chronic periodontitis (CP), with 30% having moderate and 8.5% severe PD [12]. PD is a complex inflammatory disease, with genetic and epigenetic factors having a role along with lifestyle and environmental factors, such as smoking, oral hygiene, nutrition, and stress, as well as other widespread systemic diseases, such as diabetes. Hereditary factors, age-dependent mutagenesis, and epigenetic changes have also been involved in the development of certain head and neck cancers, such as squamous cell carcinomas [13]. Chronic PD and obesity have been shown to be associated with pro-atherogenic lipid profiles, which are also risk factors for PAOD [14].

PD has been shown to be associated with atherosclerotic vascular disease. At least four basic pathogenic mechanisms are currently hypothesized that may explain how PD may promote atherosclerosis [15]: (1) Oral bacteria enter the blood stream and invade the arterial wall by chronic low level bacteremia; (2) inflammatory mediators released from the sites of the oral inflammation into the blood stream cause an acute phase reaction, which is pro-atherogenic; (3) specific components of oral pathogens trigger a host immune response, thereby promoting autoimmunity; (4) specific bacterial toxins that are produced by oral pathogenic bacteria have pro-atherogenic effects. A connection between PD as a trigger for the development of PAOD has been controversially discussed for years.

Therefore, the goals of this systematic review were: (1) to collect evidence for an association between PD or tooth loss and PAOD from the published literature and (2) to look for clinical studies that investigated the pathomechanism that might be involved in a potential cause-effect relationship between PD and PAOD.

2. Results

Seven hundred and fifty-one studies were detected by the search formula (shown in the method section), and four additional studies were identified through other sources and added in December 2018. Seven hundred and two studies were excluded following the screening algorithm (see Methods section). Full-text articles were assessed for eligibility. Thirty-six studies were excluded because no full-text article was available, the paper did not match the eligibility criteria, or it had limitations regarding the definition of PAOD or PD. Following application of the eligibility criteria, 17 studies out of the detected 755 studies were included in the qualitative synthesis. Nine studies demonstrated associations between PD and PAOD and two studies associations between tooth loss and PAOD. Six studies addressed the pathomechanism regarding PD as a trigger for PAOD and were included in the discussion. No study that dismissed an association was detected. Figure 1 summarizes the search-results using the Preferred Reporting Items for Systematic Reviews and Meta-Analyses (PRISMA) flow diagram.

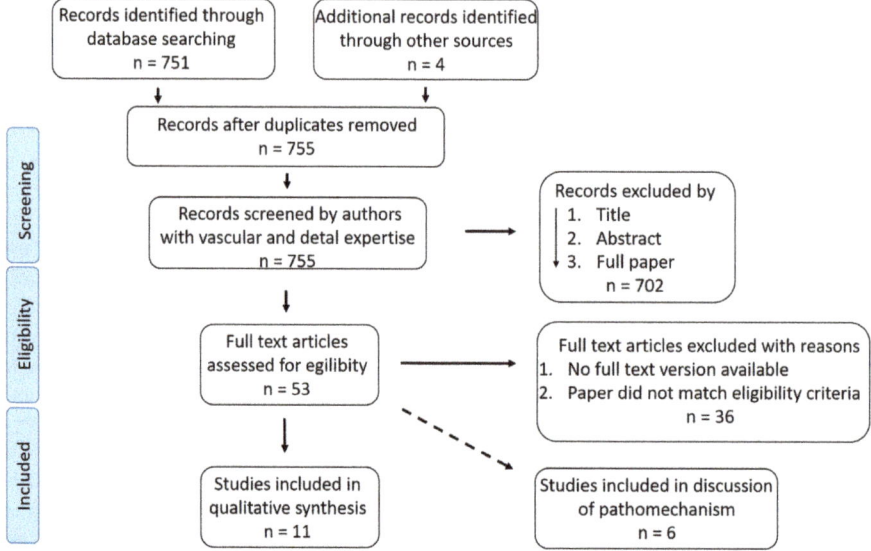

Figure 1. Preferred Reporting Items for Systematic Reviews and Meta-Analyses (PRISMA) flow diagram, the detected studies regarding the pathomechanism were also inserted into the PRISMA diagram (represented by a dashed line).

2.1. Association between PD or Tooth Loss and PAOD

The first study to demonstrate an association between PD and PAOD was a longitudinal study published by Mendez et al. in 1998 [16]. One thousand, one hundred and ten men were followed for up to 30 years, and a 2.27-fold increased incidence rate (95% CI: 1.32–3.9, $p = 0.003$) of developing PAOD was observed in men with clinically significant PD at baseline compared to men with no or only mild PD at baseline. Subsequently, an evaluation of the prospective Health Professionals Follow-up Study [17], which was based on 45,136 male health professionals free of cardiovascular diseases at baseline and 342 incidences of PAOD that had occurred during 12 years of follow-up, showed that incident tooth loss caused by PD was significantly associated with elevated risk of PAOD (relative risk (RR) for history of PD: 1.41, RR for any tooth loss during follow-up: 1.39, after controlling for traditional risk factors of cardiovascular disease) [17].

In a cross-sectional evaluation of data from the National Health and Nutrition Examination Survey (NHANES), 172 of 3585 participants were diagnosed to have PAOD. PD was significantly associated with PAOD with an odds ratio (OR) of over two in men and women [18]. Moreover, systemic markers of inflammation, such as C-reactive protein (CRP), white blood cell count, and fibrinogen, were also associated with PAOD and PD.

Munoz-Torres et al. [19] assessed the association between baseline number of teeth and recent tooth loss and the risk of PAOD in over 70,000 women participating in the Nurses' Health Study. During 16 years of follow-up, a significant association between incident tooth loss and the hazard of PAOD (hazard ratio (HR) = 1.31 95% CI: 1.00–1.71) could be demonstrated.

A recently reported meta-analysis that included a total of 4,307 participants from seven independent studies, confirmed these findings. The study showed a significantly increased risk of PD in PAOD patients compared with non-PAOD patients (RR = 1.70, 95% CI = 1.25–2.29, $p = 0.01$). PAOD patients also had more missing teeth than non-PAOD participants (weighted mean difference, WMD = 3.75,

95% CI = 1.31–6.19, p = 0.003), while no significant difference was found with respect to the clinical attachment loss between PAOD patients and non-PAOD participants (WMD = −0.05, 95% CI = −0.03–0.19, p = 0.686) [20].

Association between PD and PAOD was not only detected in cross-sectional and longitudinal studies, but also in several case-control studies. A strong association was observed by Soto-Barreras et al. [21] based on a small case-control study that included 30 patients with PAOD and 30 healthy controls. Patients with ≥30% of the teeth with an attachment loss ≥4 mm had a six-fold increased risk of PAOD compared to controls (OR = 8.18, 95% CI = 1.21 to 35.23, p = 0.031). The results also indicated that PAOD patients had higher CRP levels (p = 0.0413) and a higher mean decayed missing filled teeth (DMFT) index value (p = 0.0002) along with an elevated number of missing teeth (p = 0.0459) compared to the control group. The study also addressed the potential mechanism of the association. The CRP level was significantly higher (p = 0.0413), and there was also a difference in the decayed-missing-filled-teeth (DMFT) index (p = 0.0002), with a higher number of missing teeth (p = 0.0459) in the PAOD group compared to the control group. However, there were no significant differences regarding the frequency of bacteria in serum and subgingival plaque samples.

A strong association between PAOD and PD was also reported by Calapkorur et al. [22] who found an OR of 5.8 after adjusting for confounders (age, gender, diabetes, hypertension, and body mass index (BMI)) based on a case-control study including 40 patients with PAOD and 20 healthy controls. In a multicenter, population-based, case-control study that included 212 young women with PAOD and 475 healthy women from the Netherlands, PD was associated with PAOD with an OR of 3.0 (95% CI: 1.4–6.3) [23].

In a case-control, retrospective study based on chart reviews, Molloy et al. [24] evaluated self-reported systemic conditions and smoking history of 2006 selected patients attending the University of Minnesota dental clinics. In addition, the number of missing teeth and the degree of alveolar bone loss were recorded. After adjustments for age, sex, diabetes, and smoking, vascular disease and vascular surgery were significantly associated with alveolar bone loss and the number of missing teeth. The association could be demonstrated not only in people of mostly European descent but also in Asians. Ahn et al. observed an OR of 2.03 (95% CI: 1.05–3.93) for the association between severe PD and PAOD in a Korean community cohort of adults aged over 40 years (N = 1343) [25].

Chen et al. [26], observed that PD was significantly associated with PAOD (OR: 5.45, 95% CI: 1.57–18.89 after adjusting for age, gender, diabetes, and smoking) in a Japanese case-control sample of 25 patients with aorto-iliac and/or femoro-popliteal occlusive disease and 32 generally healthy patients who were employed as controls. Table 1 summarizes the results presented above.

Table 1. Summary of the strength of the association between PD or tooth loss and PAOD. RR = risk ratio; OR = odds ratio; HR = hazard ratio; WMD = weighted mean difference. * PAOD patients had more missing teeth than non-PAOD participants. ** conditions that were significantly related to bone loss or number of missing teeth.

Ref	Study Design	Strength of the Association between PD or Tooth Lost and PAOD	Participants	Limitations
[20]	systematic review and meta-analysis	RR = 1.70 (95% CI: 1.3–2.3; p = 0.01) * WMD = 3.75 (95% CI: 1.3–6.2; p = 0.003)	4.307	
[22]	cross-sectional study	OR = 5.8 (95% CI: 1.5–21.9; p = 0.009)	60	
[19]	cohort study	HR = 1.3 (95% CI: 1.0–1.7)	79.663	no adjustment for smoking only women
[25]	cross-sectional study	OR = 2.0 (95% CI: 1.0–3.9; p = 0.036)	1.343	
[21]	case-control study	OR = 8.2 (95% CI: 1.2–35.2; p = 0.031)	60	
[26]	case-control study	OR = 5.5 (95% CI: 1.6–18.9; p = 0.007)	57	
[18]	cross-sectional study	OR = 2.3 (95% CI: 1.2–4.2; p = 0.004)	3.585	
[24]	case-control study	**vascular disease p-value 0.014; **vascular surgery p-value 0.001	2.006	
[17]	cohort study	RR = 1.41 (95% CI: 1.1–1.8)	45.136	only men
[23]	case-control study	OR = 3.0 (95% CI: 1.4–6.3)	687	only women
[16]	cohort study	OR = 2.27 (95% CI: 1.3–3.9; p = 0.003)	1.110	only men

2.2. Pathomechanism

For this systematic review, six studies were found that addressed the potential pathomechanism that may be involved in the association and may explain how PD could induce or aggravate PAOD (see supplementary Table S1 for details). These studies suggest at least three basic mechanisms (Figure 2): (1) Periodontal pathogenic bacteria were demonstrated to enter the bloodstream and to invade atherosclerotic lesions at damaged sites of the arterial wall [27,28]; (2) experimental data showed that inflammatory mediators, such as serum amyloid A and anti-inflammatory mediators, are released from the oral sites affected by PD into the bloodstream, thereby modulating systemic inflammation [29,30]; (3) it was demonstrated in patients with PD that autoimmunity to the host protein heat shock protein 60 (HSP60) resulted from the host immune response to the bacterial HSP60 homolog GroEL produced by *Phorphyromonas gingivalis* (the main oral pathogens involved in PD) [31].

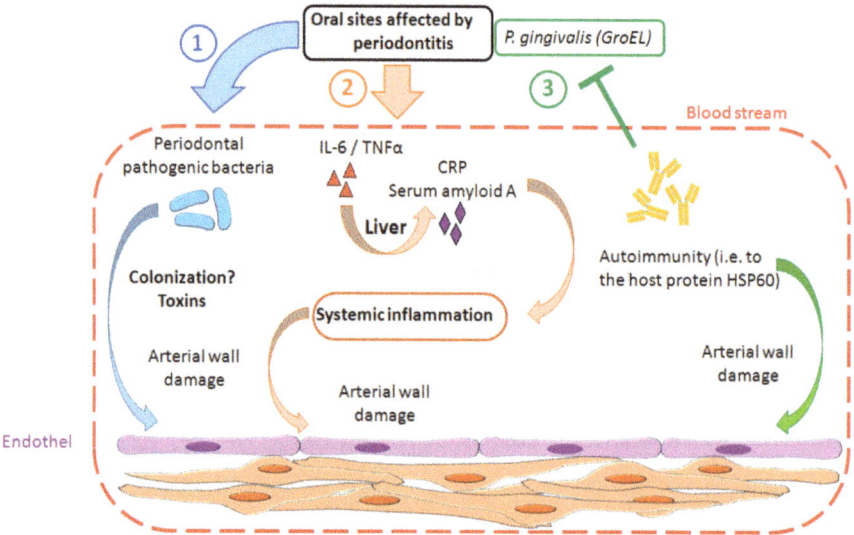

Figure 2. Potential pathomechanism that may be involved in the association of PD and PAOD; (1) periodontal pathogenic bacteria enter the bloodstream, invade and damage the arterial wall; (2) release of inflammatory mediators into the bloodstream, such as serum amyloid A, interleukin-6 (IL-6), tumor necrosis factor α (TNFα), and C-reactive protein (CRP) causing a systemic inflammation that also damages the arterial wall; (3) autoimmunity to host proteins (i.e., heat shock protein 60, HSP60) resulting from the host immuno response to the bacterial proteins, such as the HSP60 homolog GroEL.

In a blinded randomized controlled trial, Li et al. [32] could show that treatment of PD lowered the number of circulating CD34+ cells relative to untreated controls. The reduction of circulating CD34+ cells correlated with the treatment-induced decrease in sites showing bleeding on probing and the number of periodontal pockets with a depth of ≥4 mm, suggesting that treatment of PD reduced the level of systemic inflammation. On the other hand, treatment of PD did not improve endothelial function in this study.

3. Discussion

This systematic review supports that PD is associated with PAOD, which may lead to the hypothesis that PD may be a risk factor for PAOD. To date, many studies describe associations between periodontitis or oral disease and atherosclerosis in general. Therefore, we wanted to specifically focus on studies that concern peripheral vascular disease (PAOD) as a potential consequence of periodontitis in this systematic review. However, it has to be stated that the published literature is not absolutely certain about the term PAOD for "peripheral artery occlusive disease". In publications, it is frequently used for lower extremity artery disease (LEAD). Indeed, other peripheral localizations, including the carotid and vertebral, upper extremities, mesenteric and renal arteries, are also frequently affected, mainly by atherosclerosis, and complete the family of peripheral arterial diseases [6]. In addition, there is sometimes no differentiation between extracranial and cerebral atherosclerotic pathologies. Hence, for this systematic review, we excluded studies that were linked to carotid/cerebral sclerosis, coronary sclerosis as well as vascular sclerosis in general. We also excluded animal studies as we wanted to focus on clinical evidence for an association between the two pathologies.

All studies that were included in this systematic review could detect an association between PD or tooth loss and PAOD irrespective of study design, outcome measure, and study population.

This supports that the consistency of the association is high. It must be noted, however, that there is inherent bias, since risk factors for PAOD also can cause PD. Standardized effect sizes, which provide a measure of the strength of the association, have mostly been determined by logistic regression analyses and reported as ORs together with 95% CIs. After making adjustments for age, gender, and other cardio vascular disease (CVD) risk factors, the reported ORs ranged from somewhat over two in NHANES [18] to over eight in the small case-control study published by Soto-Barreras et al. [21]. In general, the smaller case-control studies yielded higher ORs than the larger cohort studies. Measures of hazard ratios or relative risk estimates are available from only a few studies. Data from the Nurses' Health Study demonstrated a significant association between incident tooth loss and PAOD and reported a hazard ratio of 1.3 for PAOD in women with PD vs. women without PD. The meta-analysis published by Yang et al. 2018 [20] reported a statistically significant relative risk of 1.7 for PAOD in people with PD vs. those without PD.

Taken together, these results suggest that severe PD increases the risk for PAOD to a similar extent as PD increases the risk for cardiovascular events, which with respect to the latter was shown to be ≈1.20-fold in adjusted models from meta-analyses of prospective cohort studies [33,34]. Smoking, a profound risk factor for PAOD, is associated with PAOD with odds ratios ranging between 1.7 and 7.4 [3]. With respect to diabetes, a twofold increased rate of macroalbuminuria and a threefold increased rate of end-stage renal disease were found in diabetics who also had severe periodontitis compared to diabetics without severe periodontitis [35]. Moreover, cardiorenal mortality resulting from ischaemic heart disease and diabetic nephropathy was three times higher in diabetics with severe PD compared to periodontally healthy diabetics [36]. The risk of PD for preterm delivery ranged between 4.45 and 7.07, depending on the gestational age [37]. Severe maternal PD was also shown to be associated with preterm low birth weight with an odds ratio of 7.5 [38]. All referenced studies considered a wide range of suspected confounders and included corresponding adjustments. Thus, PD may be a risk factor for multiple, widespread diseases. On the other hand, the possibility that some of the weak associations may be due to residual confounding by unrecognized confounders should not be neglected.

If PD is a causal or, at the least, an important contributor involved in the pathogenesis of PAOD, one would expect that PD precedes the onset of PAOD. However, only very limited information exists with respect to the temporality of both diseases. According to results from the prospective Health Professionals Follow-up Study, tooth loss seemed to precede PAOD, since the incidence of PAOD was most strongly associated with tooth loss in a period of 2 to 6 years prior to the occurrence of PAOD [17]. The fact that tooth loss in the previous 2 to 6 years was more strongly associated with PAOD than tooth loss in the previous 2 years or 6 to 8 years suggests that 6 years may be too distant and 2 years may be too recent for tooth loss to have an impact on PAOD. However, these reported time-dependent differences in the strength of the association were based on only the disparity of only a few PAOD incidences and may, thus, have been chance findings.

The plausibility of a causal or, at least, an important involvement of PD in the development of PAOD mostly relates to experimental data showing that inflammation is involved in the pathophysiology of atherosclerosis, which in turn is involved in the development of PAOD. This inflammation could be caused by a direct involvement of periodontal pathogenic bacteria, which enter the vascular wall via the bloodstream. The study by Figuero et al. used nested polymerase chain reaction (PCR) to detect three periodontal pathogens in subgingival, vascular, and blood samples. Although positive test results were obtained in high fractions of the subgingival samples (>70%) and the vascular and blood samples (7 to 11.4%), patients with and without PD did not differ with respect to the levels of the targeted bacteria. Therefore, a direct involvement of the bacteria seems inconclusive at this stage.

The studies by Nishida et al. 2016 [30] and Armingohar et al. 2015 [29] support that inflammatory mediators, such as serum amyloid A and anti-inflammatory mediators, such as interleukin-10, which are released from the oral sites affected by PD into the bloodstream, thereby modulating systemic inflammation may be involved in the pathomechanism of PD-induced PAOD. In addition, autoimmunity induced by PD via the immune response of the host to the bacterial HSP60 homolog GroEL produced by *P. gingivalis* (the main oral pathogen involved in PD) could play a role [31]. Support for this mechanism comes from the study by Choi et al., who successfully established *P. gingivalis*–specific T-cell lines from atheroma lesions isolated from PD patients. However, the study included only two patients, and the origin of the lesions remained unclear.

It is evident from the results section that our search-strategy yielded only a few publications that dealt with the pathomechanism of the association between PD and PAOD. A large fraction of the published mechanistic studies concerned animal, in vitro and ex vivo studies describing the link between PD and vascular sclerosis in general rather than that between PD and PAOD specifically. These studies were, however, not eligible for this review based on the pre-defined exclusion criteria shown in Figure 3. Roles of oral infections in the pathomechanism of atherosclerosis, in general, were discussed in great detail in a recent review published by Aarabi et al. [15]. Briefly, there is a wealth of support for at least four plausible pathogenic mechanisms: (1) low-level bacteremia by which oral bacteria enter the bloodstream and invade and damage the arterial wall; (2) systemic inflammation induced by inflammatory mediators, which are released from the sites of the oral inflammation into the bloodstream; (3) autoimmunity to host proteins which results from the host immune response to specific components of oral pathogens; (4) pro-atherogenic effects resulting from specific bacterial toxins that are produced by oral pathogenic bacteria. In addition, recent genome-wide association studies supported that PD and PAOD share at least one important predisposing genetic risk haplotype that is located at chromosome 9p21.3 in a locus known as *ANRIL/CDKN2B-AS1* [39,40]. The risk haplotype affects the structure and expression of ANRIL, which is a long non-coding RNA (lncRNA) that, such as other lncRNAs, regulates genome methylation, thereby affecting the expression of multiple genes by *cis* and *trans* mechanisms. How precisely ANRIL contributes to the risk of PD and PAOD on the molecular level is currently unclear.

So far, many, but not all, studies demonstrated the presence of bacterial DNA in a large number of atheromas, but only very few could demonstrate the successful isolation of viable bacteria from an atherosclerotic plaque. In fact, to the best of our knowledge, there is not a single study available that could demonstrate isolation and cultivation of viable *P. gingivalis* from atherosclerotic tissue. In addition, it should be noted that long-term treatment with antibiotics, such as roxithromycin and rifalazil, showed no benefit in patients with an established diagnosis of PAOD [41,42]. Nevertheless, it seems prudent at this stage to recommend that patients with PAOD should be routinely referred to a dentist, and periodontitis should be appropriately treated if present.

4. Methods

4.1. Literature Search

This systematic review considered all studies listed in PubMed until 30 September 2018. For additional studies, we double-checked in EMBASE and supplemented with additional hits obtained from Google Scholar. Grey literature was not part of the review process. It was reported in accordance with the Preferred Reporting Items for Systematic Reviews and Meta-Analyses statement

(PRISMA) [43]. For the PRISMA checklist, see http://www.prisma-statement.org. We employed the Population, Intervention, Control, and Outcome (PICO) format to answer the following PICO questions:

Is PD associated with the occurrence of PAOD?

Population = All patients with PD (all degrees of severity) who were detected in the selected literature

Intervention = None

Comparison = Patients with and without PD

Outcome = PAOD of the lower extremity

We first determined a list of synonyms and MeSH-terms (Medical Subject Headings) for PAOD and PD. Using these lists, we defined the following search-formula.

(peripheral arterial disease OR peripheral artery disease OR PAD OR occlusive vascular disease OR IC OR intermittent claudication OR CLI OR peripheral arterial occlusive disease OR peripheral artery occlusive disease OR PAOD OR lower limb ischemia OR DFS OR vascular surgery)

AND (periodontitis OR gum disease OR pyorrhea OR periodontal disease OR periodontal infection OR periodontal conditions OR chronic periodontitis OR periodontal health OR tooth loss OR attachment loss OR probing pocket depth)

4.2. Study Selection and Data Extraction

All studies were reviewed by two independent authors, one with vascular expertise (MK) and one with oral health expertise (US). Reviewers were blinded to each other results. Both reviewers screened all papers selected by the search formula to identify inclusion criteria. Any disagreements between reviewers at each stage of selection were resolved by consensus. Cohen's kappa coefficient (κ) demonstrated good agreement between the two reviewers (κ = 0.9) (Appendix A Figure A1). The studies were processed according to the PRISMA flow diagram shown in Figure 1. To sort the studies, we developed a screening-algorithm (Figure 3).

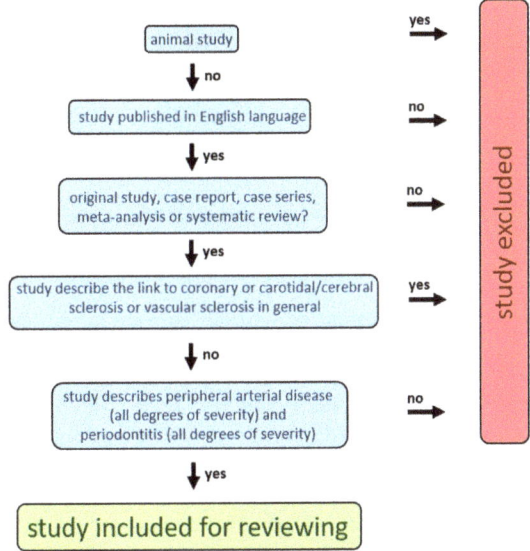

Figure 3. Screening algorithm.

Following this algorithm, we decided whether the eligibility criteria were met; first by title, and if the title led to an uncertainty regarding the eligibility criteria, additionally by the abstract. If there was still uncertainty, the whole paper was read. Animal studies, studies that were published in non-English, studies that did not correspond to original papers, case reports, case series, meta-analyses, or systemic reviews were excluded. In addition, studies on coronary or carotidal/cerebral sclerosis or vascular sclerosis were excluded in general because the aim of this systematic review was to focus on PAOD. Studies describing an association between PD (all degrees of severity) and PAOD (all degrees of severity) were included and further processed according to the PRISMA flow diagram (Figure 1). Studies that were identified by additional manual searches were also added. No duplicates were identified. Citations were managed throughout the different stages of preparing the review with the Mendeley reference management software.

4.3. Quality Assessment

The risk of bias was assessed by using the Newcastle–Ottawa Scale [44] for case-control studies and cohort studies. For the quality assessment of cross-sectional studies, we used a modified version of the Newcastle–Ottawa Scale [45]. The results of the quality assessment are shown in Figure 4.

author	study design	Quality score	Selection	Comparability	Outcome/Exposure/Outcome
Munoz-Torres FJ et al. 2017	cohort study	4	*	*	**
Hsin-Chia Hung et al. 2003	cohort study	5	*	*	***
Mendez M et al. 1998	cohort study	7	**	**	***
Soto-Barreras U et al. 2013	case-control study	4	*	**	*
Chen Y.-W. et al. 2008	case-control study	7	***	**	**
Molloy J et al. 2004	case-control study	3	*	*	*
Bloemenkamp D et al. 2002	case-control study	7	***	**	**
Lu B et al. 2008	cross-sectional study	9	****	**	***
M. Unlu Calapkorur et al. 2017	cross-sectional study	9	****	**	***
Ahn Y-B et al. 2016	cross-sectional study	9	****	**	***

Thresholds for converting the Newcastle-Ottawa scales to AHRQ standards (good, fair, and poor):
Good quality: 3 or 4 stars in selection domain AND 1 or 2 stars in comparability domain AND 2 or 3 stars in outcome/exposure domain
Fair quality: 2 stars in selection domain AND 1 or 2 stars in comparability domain AND 2 or 3 stars in outcome/exposure domain
Poor quality: 0 or 1 star in selection domain OR 0 stars in comparability domain OR 0 or 1 stars in outcome/exposure domain

Figure 4. Results of the quality assessment.

5. Conclusions

In conclusion, the present evidence supports a link between PD and PAOD. Further studies which address the temporality of PD and PAOD are warranted. Thus, a causal, or at least, an important contributing role of PD in the development of PAOD can currently not be confirmed but may be suspected. Clearly, the ultimate proof of causality would depend on data from randomized controlled invention trials to show that treatment of PD can diminish or even prevent PAOD. Such data does, to the best of our knowledge, currently not exist.

Supplementary Materials: Supplementary Materials can be found at http://www.mdpi.com/1422-0067/20/12/2936/s1.

Funding: This work was supported by the Innovation Fund of the Joint Federal Committee, Berlin, Germany [grant number 01VSF16008] and the Else Kröner-Fresenius-Foundation, Bad Homburg, Germany [grant number 2016_A166].

Conflicts of Interest: The authors declare no conflict of interest.

Appendix A

Cohens Kappa coefficient

κ= 0,90

p_0= 0,99

p_e= 0,88

		Reviewer II (US)		sum
		included	excluded	
Reviewer I (MK)	included	45	1	46
	excluded	8	701	709
	sum	53	702	755

Figure A1. Cohens Kappa coefficient calculation.

References

1. Vos, T.; Flaxman, A.D.; Naghavi, M.; Lozano, R.; Michaud, C.; Ezzati, M.; Shibuya, K.; Salomon, J.A.; Abdalla, S.; Aboyans, V.; et al. Years lived with disability (YLDs) for 1160 sequelae of 289 diseases and injuries 1990–2010: A systematic analysis for the Global Burden of Disease Study 2010. *Lancet* **2012**, *380*, 2163–2196. [CrossRef]
2. Sampson, U.K.A.; Fowkes, F.G.R.; McDermott, M.M.; Criqui, M.H.; Aboyans, V.; Norman, P.E.; Forouzanfar, M.H.; Naghavi, M.; Song, Y.; Harrell, F.E., Jr.; et al. Global and Regional Burden of Death and Disability from Peripheral Artery Disease: 21 World Regions, 1990 to 2010. *Glob. Heart* **2014**, *9*, 145–158. [CrossRef]
3. Fowkes, F.G.R.; Rudan, D.; Rudan, I.; Aboyans, V.; Denenberg, J.O.; McDermott, M.M.; Norman, P.E.; Sampson, U.K.; Williams, L.J.; Mensah, G.A.; et al. Comparison of global estimates of prevalence and risk factors for peripheral artery disease in 2000 and 2010: A systematic review and analysis. *Lancet* **2013**, *382*, 1329–1340. [CrossRef]
4. Creager, M.A. The Crisis of Vascular Disease and the Journey to Vascular Health. *Circulation* **2016**, *133*, 2593–2598. [CrossRef] [PubMed]
5. Malyar, N.; Fürstenberg, T.; Wellmann, J.; Meyborg, M.; Lüders, F.; Gebauer, K.; Bunzemeier, H.; Roeder, N.; Reinecke, H. Recent trends in morbidity and in-hospital outcomes of in-patients with peripheral arterial disease: A nationwide population-based analysis. *Eur. Heart J.* **2013**, *34*, 2706–2714. [CrossRef] [PubMed]
6. Aboyans, V.; Ricco, J.B.; Bartelink, M.E.L.; Björck, M.; Brodmann, M.; Cohnert, T.; Collet, J.P.; Czerny, M.; De Carlo, M.; Debus, S.; et al. 2017 ESC Guidelines on the Diagnosis and Treatment of Peripheral Arterial Diseases, in collaboration with the European Society for Vascular Surgery (ESVS). *Eur. Heart J.* **2018**, *39*, 763–816. [CrossRef] [PubMed]
7. Hamburg, N.M.; Creager, M.A. Pathophysiology of Intermittent Claudication in Peripheral Artery Disease. *Circ. J.* **2017**, *81*, 281–289. [CrossRef]
8. Taleb, S. Inflammation in atherosclerosis. *Arch. Cardiovasc. Dis.* **2016**, *109*, 708–715. [CrossRef]
9. Miao, C.-Y.; Li, Z.-Y. The role of perivascular adipose tissue in vascular smooth muscle cell growth. *Br. J. Pharmacol.* **2012**, *165*, 643–658. [CrossRef]
10. Armitage, G.C. Periodontal diagnoses and classification of periodontal diseases. *Periodontol. 2000* **2004**, *34*, 9–21. [CrossRef]

11. Matarese, G.; Ramaglia, L.; Fiorillo, L.; Cervino, G.; Lauritano, F.; Isola, G. Implantology and Periodontal Disease: The Panacea to Problem Solving? *Open Dent. J.* **2017**, *11*, 460–465. [CrossRef] [PubMed]
12. Thornton-Evans, G.; Eke, P.; Wei, L.; Palmer, A.; Moeti, R.; Hutchins, S.; Borrell, L.N. Periodontitis among adults aged ≥30 years—United States, 2009–2010. *MMWR Suppl.* **2013**, *62*, 129–135. [PubMed]
13. Ferlazzo, N.; Currò, M.; Zinellu, A.; Caccamo, D.; Isola, G.; Ventura, V.; Carru, C.; Matarese, G.; Ientile, R. Influence of MTHFR Genetic Background on p16 and MGMT Methylation in Oral Squamous Cell Cancer. *Int. J. Mol. Sci.* **2017**, *18*, 724. [CrossRef] [PubMed]
14. Cury, E.Z.; Santos, V.R.; da Silva Maciel, S.; Gonçalves, T.E.D.; Zimmermann, G.S.; Mota, R.M.S.; Figueiredo, L.C.; Duarte, P.M. Lipid parameters in obese and normal weight patients with or without chronic periodontitis. *Clin. Oral Investig.* **2018**, *22*, 161–167. [CrossRef] [PubMed]
15. Aarabi, G.; Heydecke, G.; Seedorf, U. Roles of Oral Infections in the Pathomechanism of Atherosclerosis. *Int. J. Mol. Sci.* **2018**, *19*, 1978. [CrossRef] [PubMed]
16. Mendez, M.V.; Scott, T.; LaMorte, W.; Vokonas, P.; Menzoian, J.O.; Garcia, R. An Association between Periodontal Disease and Peripheral Vascular Disease. *Am. J. Surg.* **1998**, *176*, 153–157. [CrossRef]
17. Hung, H.-C.; Willett, W.; Merchant, A.; Rosner, B.A.; Ascherio, A.; Joshipura, K.J. Oral Health and Peripheral Arterial Disease. *Circulation* **2003**, *107*, 1152–1157. [CrossRef]
18. Lu, B.; Parker, D.; Eaton, C.B. Relationship of periodontal attachment loss to peripheral vascular disease: An analysis of NHANES 1999–2002 data. *Atherosclerosis* **2008**, *200*, 199–205. [CrossRef]
19. Muñoz-Torres, F.J.; Mukamal, K.J.; Pai, J.K.; Willett, W.; Joshipura, K.J. Relationship between Tooth Loss and Peripheral Arterial Disease among Women. *J. Clin. Periodontol.* **2017**, *44*, 989–995. [CrossRef]
20. Yang, S.; Zhao, L.S.; Cai, C.; Shi, Q.; Wen, N.; Xu, J. Association between periodontitis and peripheral artery disease: A systematic review and meta-analysis. *BMC Cardiovasc. Disord.* **2018**, *18*, 141. [CrossRef]
21. Soto-Barreras, U.; Olvera-Rubio, J.O.; Loyola-Rodríguez, J.P.; Reyes-Macías, J.F.; Martinez-Martinez, R.E.; Patiño-Marin, N.; Martinez-Castanon, G.-A.; Aradillas-García, C.; Little, J.W. Peripheral Arterial Disease Associated with Caries and Periodontal Disease. *J. Periodontol.* **2013**, *84*, 486–494. [CrossRef] [PubMed]
22. Çalapkorur, M.U.; Alkan, B.A.; Tasdemir, Z.; Akcali, Y.; Saatci, E. Association of peripheral arterial disease with periodontal disease: Analysis of inflammatory cytokines and an acute phase protein in gingival crevicular fluid and serum. *J. Periodontal Res.* **2017**, *52*, 532–539. [CrossRef] [PubMed]
23. Bloemenkamp, D.G.; van den Bosch, M.A.; Mali, W.P.; Tanis, B.C.; Rosendaal, F.R.; Kemmeren, J.M.; Algra, A.; Visseren, F.L.; Van Der Graaf, Y. Novel risk factors for peripheral arterial disease in young women. *Am. J. Med.* **2002**, *113*, 462–467. [CrossRef]
24. Molloy, J.; Wolff, L.F.; Lopez-Guzman, A.; Hodges, J.S. The association of periodontal disease parameters with systemic medical conditions and tobacco use. *J. Clin. Periodontol.* **2004**, *31*, 625–632. [CrossRef] [PubMed]
25. Ahn, Y.-B.; Shin, M.-S.; Han, D.-H.; Sukhbaatar, M.; Kim, M.-S.; Shin, H.-S.; Kim, H.-D. Periodontitis is associated with the risk of subclinical atherosclerosis and peripheral arterial disease in Korean adults. *Atherosclerosis* **2016**, *251*, 311–318. [CrossRef] [PubMed]
26. Chen, Y.-W.; Umeda, M.; Nagasawa, T.; Takeuchi, Y.; Huang, Y.; Inoue, Y.; Iwai, T.; Izumi, Y.; Ishikawa, I. Periodontitis May Increase the Risk of Peripheral Arterial Disease. *Eur. J. Vasc. Endovasc. Surg.* **2008**, *35*, 153–158. [CrossRef]
27. Armingohar, Z.; Jørgensen, J.J.; Kristoffersen, A.K.; Abesha-Belay, E.; Olsen, I. Bacteria and bacterial DNA in atherosclerotic plaque and aneurysmal wall biopsies from patients with and without periodontitis. *J. Oral Microbiol.* **2014**, *6*, 23408. [CrossRef]
28. Figuero, E.; Lindahl, C.; Marín, M.J.; Renvert, S.; Herrera, D.; Ohlsson, O.; Wetterling, T.; Sanz, M. Quantification of Periodontal Pathogens in Vascular, Blood, and Subgingival Samples from Patients with Peripheral Arterial Disease or Abdominal Aortic Aneurysms. *J. Periodontol.* **2014**, *85*, 1182–1193. [CrossRef]
29. Armingohar, Z.; Jørgensen, J.J.; Kristoffersen, A.K.; Schenck, K.; Dembic, Z. Polymorphisms in the interleukin-10 gene and chronic periodontitis in patients with atherosclerotic and aortic aneurysmal vascular diseases. *J. Oral Microbiol.* **2015**, *7*, 26051. [CrossRef]
30. Nishida, E.; Aino, M.; Kobayashi, S.-I.; Okada, K.; Ohno, T.; Kikuchi, T.; Hayashi, J.-I.; Yamamoto, G.; Hasegawa, Y.; Mitani, A. Serum Amyloid A Promotes E-Selectin Expression via Toll-Like Receptor 2 in Human Aortic Endothelial Cells. *Mediat. Inflamm.* **2016**, *2016*, 7150509. [CrossRef]

31. Choi, J.-I.; Chung, S.-W.; Kang, H.-S.; Rhim, B.Y.; Kim, S.-J.; Kim, S.-J. Establishment of *Porphyromonas gingivalis* Heat-shock-protein-specific T-cell Lines from Atherosclerosis Patients. *J. Dent. Res.* **2002**, *81*, 344–348. [CrossRef] [PubMed]
32. Li, X.; Tse, H.F.; Yiu, K.H.; Li, L.S.W.; Jin, L. Effect of periodontal treatment on circulating CD34+ cells and peripheral vascular endothelial function: A randomized controlled trial. *J. Clin. Periodontol.* **2011**, *38*, 148–156. [CrossRef] [PubMed]
33. Leng, W.-D.; Zeng, X.-T.; Kwong, J.S.; Hua, X.-P. Periodontal disease and risk of coronary heart disease: An updated meta-analysis of prospective cohort studies. *Int. J. Cardiol.* **2015**, *201*, 469–472. [CrossRef] [PubMed]
34. Humphrey, L.L.; Fu, R.; Buckley, D.I.; Freeman, M.; Helfand, M. Periodontal Disease and Coronary Heart Disease Incidence: A Systematic Review and Meta-analysis. *J. Gen. Intern. Med.* **2008**, *23*, 2079–2086. [CrossRef] [PubMed]
35. Shultis, W.A.; Weil, E.J.; Looker, H.C.; Curtis, J.M.; Shlossman, M.; Genco, R.J.; Knowler, W.C.; Nelson, R.G. Effect of Periodontitis on Overt Nephropathy and End-Stage Renal Disease in Type 2 Diabetes. *Diabetes Care* **2007**, *30*, 306–311. [CrossRef] [PubMed]
36. Saremi, A.; Nelson, R.G.; Tulloch-Reid, M.; Hanson, R.L.; Sievers, M.L.; Taylor, G.W.; Shlossman, M.; Bennett, P.H.; Genco, R.; Knowler, W.C. Periodontal disease and mortality in type 2 diabetes. *Diabetes Care* **2005**, *28*, 27–32. [CrossRef]
37. Jeffcoat, M.K.; Geurs, N.C.; Reddy, M.S.; Cliver, S.P.; Goldenberg, R.L.; Hauth, J.C. Periodontal infection and preterm birth: Results of a prospective study. *J. Am. Dent. Assoc.* **2001**, *132*, 875–880. [CrossRef]
38. Offenbacher, S.; Katz, V.; Fertik, G.; Collins, J.; Boyd, D.; Maynor, G.; McKaig, R.; Beck, J. Periodontal Infection as a Possible Risk Factor for Preterm Low Birth Weight. *J. Periodontol.* **1996**, *67*, 1103–1113. [CrossRef]
39. Belkin, N.; Damrauer, S.M. Peripheral Arterial Disease Genetics: Progress to Date and Challenges Ahead. *Curr. Cardiol. Rep.* **2017**, *19*, 131. [CrossRef]
40. Aarabi, G.; Zeller, T.; Heydecke, G.; Munz, M.; Schäfer, A.; Seedorf, U. Roles of the Chr.9p21.3 ANRIL Locus in Regulating Inflammation and Implications for Anti-Inflammatory Drug Target Identification. *Front. Cardiovasc. Med.* **2018**, *5*, 47. [CrossRef]
41. Jaff, M.R.; Dale, R.A.; Creager, M.A.; Lipicky, R.J.; Constant, J.; Campbell, L.A.; Hiatt, W.R. Anti-Chlamydial Antibiotic Therapy for Symptom Improvement in Peripheral Artery Disease. Prospective Evaluation of Rifalazil Effect on Vascular Symptoms of Intermittent Claudication and Other Endpoints in *Chlamydia pneumoniae* Seropositive Patients (PROVIDENCE-1). *Circulation* **2009**, *119*, 452–458. [CrossRef] [PubMed]
42. Joensen, J.B.; Juul, S.; Henneberg, E.; Thomsen, G.; Ostergaard, L.; Lindholt, J.S. Can long-term antibiotic treatment prevent progression of peripheral arterial occlusive disease? A large, randomized, double-blinded, placebo-controlled trial. *Atherosclerosis* **2008**, *196*, 937–942. [CrossRef] [PubMed]
43. Moher, D.; Shamseer, L.; Clarke, M.; Ghersi, D.; Liberati, A.; Petticrew, M.; Shekelle, P.; Stewart, L.A. Preferred reporting items for systematic review and meta-analysis protocols (PRISMA-P) 2015 statement. *Syst. Rev.* **2015**, *4*, 1. [CrossRef] [PubMed]
44. Wells, G.A.; Shea, B.; O'Connell, D.; Peterson, J.; Welch, V.; Losos, M.; Tugwell, P. The Newcastle-Ottawa Scale (NOS) for Assessing the Quality of Nonrandomised Studies in Meta-Analyses. Ottawa Hospital Research Institute. Available online: http://www.ohri.ca/programs/clinical_epidemiology/oxford.asp (accessed on 23 July 2015).
45. Herzog, R.; Álvarez-Pasquin, M.J.; Díaz, C.; Del Barrio, J.L.; Estrada, J.M.; Gil, A. Are healthcare workers' intentions to vaccinate related to their knowledge, beliefs and attitudes? A systematic review. *BMC Public Health* **2013**, *13*, 154. [CrossRef] [PubMed]

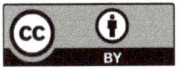

© 2019 by the authors. Licensee MDPI, Basel, Switzerland. This article is an open access article distributed under the terms and conditions of the Creative Commons Attribution (CC BY) license (http://creativecommons.org/licenses/by/4.0/).

MDPI
St. Alban-Anlage 66
4052 Basel
Switzerland
Tel. +41 61 683 77 34
Fax +41 61 302 89 18
www.mdpi.com

International Journal of Molecular Sciences Editorial Office
E-mail: ijms@mdpi.com
www.mdpi.com/journal/ijms

www.ingramcontent.com/pod-product-compliance
Lightning Source LLC
LaVergne TN
LVHW070632100526
838202LV00012B/790